Themes in Modern European History 1890–1945

The Europe of 1945 bore only the most superficial resemblance to that of 1890; its position in world affairs was utterly different. Europeans at the turn of the century were the assured masters of the globe: only a generation later Europe was a political and economic wreck. The collapse of the Eurocentric system opened the way for the Cold War and fixed relationships for almost half a century.

This collection of essays traces the important issues during this period and sets them in the context of what had hitherto been seen as the norms of political, economic and social life. The book deals with continuity – or lack of it – with the past and the rapid breaking of the threads which normally bind the lives of one generation to its predecessors and successors. Emphasis is on cultural change; the shifting balance of European, and world, power which led to the Cold War and post-Cold War period is closely examined. Linking together developments in society, the economy, politics and culture, this volume elucidates the very different paths followed by the major European states.

This book offers an up-to-date thematic account of developments, focusing on cultural and societal issues as well as politics. It will be of great value to university and sixth-form students who need to gain a fuller appreciation of the context behind the world reordering events of this period.

THEMES IN MODERN EUROPEAN HISTORY
General editor: Michael Biddiss, University of Reading

Already published

Themes in Modern European History 1830–90
Edited by Bruce Waller

Themes in Modern European History 1890–1945

Edited by Paul Hayes

First published 1992
by Routledge
11 New Fetter Lane, London EC4P 4EE

Simultaneously published in the USA and Canada
by Routledge
29 West 35th Street, New York, NY 10001

Reprinted 1994

The collection as a whole © 1992 Paul Hayes; individual chapters
© 1992 the respective contributors

Photoset in 10 on 12 point Times by
Redwood Press Limited, Melksham, Wiltshire
Printed in Great Britain by
Redwood Press Limited

British Library Cataloguing in Publication Data
A catalogue record for this book is available from the British Library.

Library of Congress Cataloguing in Publication Data
Hayes, Paul
    Themes in European history, 1890–1945 / Paul Hayes.
        p.   cm.
    Includes bibliographical references and index.
    1. Europe – History – 1871–1918.   2. Europe – History – 1918–1945.
I. Title.
D395.H29   1992
940.2'8 – dc20   91-46074

ISBN 0–415–07904–7
        0–415–07905–5 (pbk)

Contents

List of contributors

Edward Acton is Professor of Modern History at the University of East Anglia. Publications include *Alexander Herzen and the Role of the Intellectual Revolutionary* (1979), *Russia: the Present and the Past* (1986), and *Rethinking the Russian Revolution* (1990).

Nicholas Atkin is Lecturer in History at the University of Reading. Publications include *Church and Schools in Vichy France, 1940–44* (1991) and several articles on France during the Nazi occupation. He is currently preparing a biography of Marshal Pétain.

Philip Bell is Reader in History at the University of Liverpool. Publications include *A Certain Eventuality. Britain and the Fall of France* (1974) and *The Origins of the Second World War in Europe* (1986).

Michael Biddiss is Professor of History at the University of Reading. Publications include *The Father of Racist Ideology: The Social and Political Thought of Count Gobineau* (1970) *The Age of the Masses: Ideas and Society in Europe since 1870* (1977). He is General Editor of the series.

Paul Hayes (editor) is Fellow and Tutor in Modern History and Politics, Keble College, Oxford. Publications include *Quisling* (1971), *Fascism* (1973), *British Foreign Policy in the Nineteenth Century, 1814–80* (1975) and *British Foreign Policy in the Twentieth Century, 1880–1939* (1978). He is joint editor and contributor to *War Strategy, and International Politics: Essays in Honour of Sir Michael Howard* (1992).

1 Introduction

Paul Hayes

In May 1945 European power and influence stood at its lowest point for centuries. The collapse of the Third Reich ushered in the Cold War, thus promoting the division of Europe into two armed camps dominated by the USA and USSR. Neither of these powers was truly European. While the USA had a strong ethnic and cultural base primarily of European origin, neither its leaders nor its people saw issues with European eyes. It was fortunate for much of Europe that what was in its interests so often coincided with American interests in the course of the next forty years or so. The USSR in the post-1945 era, as Russia had been before 1914, was involved in European affairs, had European interests, and, occasionally, looked at questions in a European way. But its interests stretched beyond Europe, and the USSR possessed a cultural and ethnic base which was far from being European in character; the USSR, then, even at the height of the Cold War did not always give priority to Europe. Furthermore, the nature of Stalinism – ostensibly derived from a European ideology – struck most Europeans as barbarous and alien. Europeans in 1945, and for long after, were forcibly reminded of their continent's decline; the most powerful symbol of the change in status was the division of Berlin and, from 1961 onwards, the wall which physically separated West from East.

If Europeans found in concrete and barbed wire the clearest possible evidence of decline and division, in fact there was an abundance of equally significant clues. There were changes in the boundaries of states, loss of colonies, a decline in economic influence, widespread social changes, the rise of political extremism, rapid scientific advance and technological development (in which Europeans did not usually play the leading part, unlike in the nineteenth century), and the retreat of cultural influence; all these were characteristic of Europe's decline between 1890 and 1945. If the war of 1914–18 weakened European dominance, that of 1939–45 marked its end. As A. J. P. Taylor observed in mid-century,

> Europe has ceased to be the centre of the world. Though it is always unsafe to guess how the present will appear to the eyes of the future, this is a generalization which is likely to stand the test of time; it is the greatest shift in the world balance since the upheavals of the fifteenth century.[1]

It is to a general examination of this shift that it is now necessary to turn.

The most obvious and striking fact of the political map of 1945 is how different it looked from that of 1890. Boundary changes were the result of a number of different factors; most commonly the result of wars, sometimes the consequence of deals struck between major powers, and, very occasionally, the product of evolution. In these circumstances, therefore, there was no consistency in the changes. Russia lost large areas of territory in 1918 but regained most of these in 1945, together with some areas not controlled in 1914. Germany ruled over much of eastern Europe during both the war of 1914–18 and that of 1939–45, but suffered serious reductions in territory in 1919 and again in 1945. As a result of the Cold War Germany then remained divided until 1989. Is it possible then to ascertain any thematic development during this period of war, revolution and political upheaval?

The answer is a cautious affirmative. Taking the period as a whole it is possible to discern an evolution away from the large multinational states which so characterized nineteenth-century Europe towards smaller entities. This was, however, neither entirely consistent, nor always uninterrupted. The revival of Russian power in 1944–5 led not only to a reassertion of control over the three small Baltic states, but also to the annexation of areas which were predominantly German, Polish, Ruthene and Romanian in character (part of east Prussia, eastern Poland, eastern Czechoslovakia, and parts of Bukovina, Moldavia and all of Bessarabia, respectively). It is at the very least arguable that in 1945 the USSR was just as much a multinational empire as Russia had been in 1890. Yet, in fact, this was an exception, albeit politically a very significant one, to the general development of states.

In 1918–19 the states with large and diverse ethnic groups all underwent substantial transformation. Germany lost large numbers of French and Poles, and a smaller number of Danes. The USSR was obliged to concede independence to the new states of Finland, Latvia, Lithuania and Estonia, as well as territory to a revived Poland and an enlarged Romania. Austria-Hungary disintegrated; some territory was transferred to existing states such as Italy and Romania, some went to newly-created entities such as Czechoslovakia and Yugoslavia, some went to Poland. The Austrians and the Hungarians perforce set up their own states. The war of 1914–18 in effect completed the process of Turkish withdrawal from Europe, although the main blows to Turkish domination were felt in the Levant rather than in south-eastern Europe. Even if some of the new boundaries posed their own problems – such as those of Italy with Austria and Yugoslavia, or those of Romania with Hungary and the USSR – no attempt was made by the victors in 1919 to create their own grand multinational states in Europe. Of course, if Russia had been numbered among the victors in 1919 then it is fair to assume that matters might have been rather different. Where diverse ethnic groups were placed together in new forms of association, as in Czechoslovakia and Yugoslavia, this was not so much the product of deliberate engineering by the victorious powers, but rather a combination of weariness and lack of interest and knowledge on their part, together with the assertion of political muscle by the dominant Czechs and Serbs in those two states. In neither case was the amalgamation of different groups to prove a substantial success before or after 1945.

Thus, a number of new, or revived, states emerged out of these collapsed or reduced states. The results were far from perfect. Commentators have frequently pointed to the large number of Europeans who continued to be ruled, often badly, by those not of their own ethnic group. The fact remains that, large though the number was, it was smaller than in 1914. While individual mistakes might have been corrected, particularly in less frantic and more dispassionate circumstances than existed in 1919, it is hard to see how a more generally acceptable settlement could have been reached given the political realities of the time. Europe might have been subdivided to a greater extent, but would that necessarily have enhanced economic and political stability? Perhaps major movements of peoples would have helped (as occurred forcibly towards the end of the period and after 1945), though the experiences of the post-1945 period scarcely bear out the value of such a policy. The only other answer would have been the enforced integration of small groups, with the ultimate sanction of genocide if they refused to be integrated. Where such policies were pursued, both before and after 1945, they have rightly been regarded as repellent.

The evolution towards smaller entities, especially in eastern Europe, was thus effectively limited both by the requirements of international politics and trade and the large number of potentially autonomous ethnic groups. In any event, in most of Europe success or failure in establishing independence largely depended on the outcome of conflicts between powerful nations rather than the merits or defects of particular cases. There were, however, some exceptions to this pattern. Finland secured its independence from Russia in the aftermath of the revolutions of 1917 and, despite a series of misjudgements in the war of 1939–45, was not forcibly reincorporated into the USSR. The price paid was a dismal subservience to the USSR which lasted some forty years. Norway secured its independence from Sweden in 1905, essentially because the Swedish government came to realize that an unwanted union could not be forced on a genuine Norwegian nationalist movement. Finally, although the process was not properly completed until 1949, from the early 1920s onwards the southern parts of Ireland in effect constituted a separate state from the rest of the British Isles. Irish nationalism was too strong to be contained within the United Kingdom, and after years of futile negotiation and still more futile conflict this was formally recognized in 1921.

There was, then, a limited advance towards the concept of the nation-state during this period, though the process was much interrupted by the acquisitive propensities of Mussolini, Stalin and Hitler. Changing boundaries created enormous problems for both governments and governed, especially when those ruled were not members of the majority or most important ethnic group. As might be expected, it was with rare exceptions the smallest, the least educated, and the least economically powerful groups which tended to suffer most from changes in sovereignty. Typical examples may be found in the treatment of Albanians in Yugoslavia, of Ruthenes in Czechoslovakia, or of Macedonians in Greece. The two groups which suffered enormously and which were large in size, economically significant, and generally exceptionally well-educated, were the German and Jewish minorities to be found in many European states. The fate of the German minorities, or *Volksdeutsche*, was not viewed with great sympathy by most Europeans – for understandable, if not very creditable, reasons. In areas in which Germans had ruled before 1914 their treatment of minorities had often been heavy-handed and clumsy. Their economic and cultural ascendancy in eastern Europe was by no means destroyed during 1914–18, and post-1918 Germany remained a powerful state. After the rise of Hitler to power anti-German sentiment was often held in check by an only too accurate assessment that there would be an unpleasant price to be paid later for any self-indulgence. The treatment received by German minorities was thus very mixed. Generally the authorities in Denmark, Belgium, France, Hungary, Romania, and the Baltic states behaved well, and their conduct was met with an appropriate response from their German-speaking citizens. The Germans in Czechoslovakia were also well treated, but there their response was much less accommodating, as the career of Henlein showed. The Italians, rather surprisingly, pursued an active policy of Italianization in the South Tirol with almost entirely undesirable results; however, the evolution of a close relationship between Hitler and Mussolini relegated this question to the bottom of the political agenda. Only Poland and the USSR treated their German minorities really badly, and this treatment proved an important element in fanning anti-Slav feelings in Germany, and in the promotion of severe anti-Polish and anti-Russian measures during German occupation in the course of the war of 1939–45. After the end of the war the Germans suffered in their turn. Many Germans fled westwards, many were forced out, some were sent into internal exile in the USSR, largely German-speaking areas were transferred to Poland and the USSR, and Germany was divided into what became two separate states. Sympathy for German misfortunes was, unsurprisingly, in short supply.

The Europeans who suffered most from the political convulsions of the era were, of course, the Jews. Anti-Semitism was a potent force in many states during the nineteenth century. The results could be seen in mass emigration, especially to the USA. But, if anything, anti-Semitism increased rather than diminished; the rise of nation-states was not infrequently accompanied by the search for scapegoats for the failures of their governments. Conveniently for others, the Jews had no powerful state to protect them; their energy, education, culture, and enterprise marked them out and promoted envy and jealousy. The results of government-inspired hostility were horrific. Mass emigration was followed by forced exile and, finally, genocide. The exact figures will never be known, but the general consensus is that between five and six million Jews perished during the Holocaust; the Germans found many willing accomplices among their neighbours, so the guilt was not theirs alone. To this figure should be added an unknown, but substantial, number who perished at the hands of Stalin's government. To put this in context, it is as if the total population of the Baltic states had suddenly disappeared. Because the death of so many Jews had no impact upon European political boundaries it is all too easy to underestimate the enormous political, cultural and economic consequences of the virtual elimination of a people which had for centuries played an important role in so many states.

The fate of the Jews illustrates the point that it is futile to think that the most important political changes are always those involving frontiers. What mattered at least as much was what political choices, if any, people had, how they were governed, how their institutions worked, and what ideas or beliefs were dominant. This was a period of violent political convulsions during which the pattern of life was often dramatically altered. If pluralism, political participation and democracy advanced in some areas, there was also a retreat in others. Often the process of change was so fast, as in Russia in 1917, that the ordinary citizen had little idea either of what was happening or the implications of these events.

During these years the democratic process was enhanced in the British Isles, Scandinavia, Switzerland, the Low Countries, and France – though in the case of many of these countries democracy was suspended as a result of events in 1940. More unhappily, many of the supposed democracies set up in central and eastern Europe during 1918–19 either never were proper democracies or succumbed to internal *coups d'état* long before the advance of German power destroyed what democracy had survived. Russia lurched from one autocracy to another during 1917, an exchange which proved very much for the worse as the tsarist system had at least possessed the redeeming feature of gross inefficiency. Democratic development was halted in Italy (1922), Portugal (1926), Germany (1933), Greece (1935), and Spain (1936), while Czechoslovakia was abandoned in 1938–9. The advances of the Red Army after 1944 merely replaced one form of undemocratic rule with another.

The advance of democracy, whether temporary or permanent, could best be seen in the extension of voting rights. This, however, should not be confused with the surrender of power by existing élites, which often found institutional practices an effective safeguard against radical change.[2] But there was some progress, and to the reactionary or the politically unsophisticated the changes seemed almost revolutionary. In 1914 universal adult suffrage existed in none of the four most populous states of western Europe. Many voters did not vote; sometimes obstacles were put in their way, sometimes there were no contests in the areas in which they lived, sometimes their vote would obviously be wasted because of out-of-date constituency boundaries, and many did not vote because they could see no point in it. In Italy the franchise was significantly extended by the legislation of 1911–12, but it was not until 1946 that women obtained the vote. Similarly, French women had to wait until the Liberation before they were enfranchised. In Germany, in reaction to the Wilhelmine era, the 1919 Weimar

Constitution introduced 'the universal, equal, direct and secret suffrage of all men and women of the German Reich, upon the principles of proportional representation'.[3] This lasted until 1933; in passing it should be noted that in 1949 the Bundesrepublik adopted a less radical form of proportional representation. Although in Britain universal male adult suffrage truly existed after 1918, it was not until 1928 that women were able to vote on equal terms. In Britain, France and Italy there was pressure for proportional representation well before 1914, but this never seemed likely to be accepted by their parliaments.

The effects of extension of voting rights were mixed. The existence of large numbers of new voters, often without previous political attachments, gave opportunities for the development of new parties and ideas. It also opened the way for the emergence of charismatic leaders. When parties were responsive to legitimate concerns and grievances they aided the development of democracy. This was particularly important as, for a variety of reasons, the pre-1914 political systems had often been quite inadequate. Old parties that could not adapt to the needs of a mass electorate were reduced in importance, or even swept away. By 1920 the political landscapes in Britain, Germany, and Italy looked quite different from a decade earlier. Parties clearly of the Left had advanced in all three countries, both in terms of votes and seats. In Britain the Conservatives' fortunes had also improved, and in Italy the Popolari had emerged as a significant force. In Germany the ultra-conservative groups had sustained a severe reverse from which they were never to recover fully. These changes were swift and dramatic; they were not, of course, viewed with enthusiasm by all, but they represented the popular will, and the parties which profited were firmly democratic in character. The experience of a shift to the Left or Centre-Left in the major states was, to a large extent, shared by the smaller democracies of the region. By the early 1930s the largest party in all three Scandinavian states was to be found on the Left, a situation which has endured to the present day. In Norway, for example, the Arbeiderparti held 18 seats in parliament in 1918 (out of 125), and by 1933 70 seats (out of 150).

Changing electorates and changing parties put pressure on existing institutions, élites, interests, hierarchies and pressure groups. In some cases the collapse of established interests was spectacular – for example, the end of the monarchy in Germany or Spain. In countries where the monarch had been less obviously involved in politically contentious ways, however, even the advent of apparently radical governments of the Left did not lead to significant pressure to establish a republic. Constitutional monarchies survived in much of western

Europe, and the fact that the role to be played by the head of state did not become a genuine political issue proved an important element in the preservation of political consensus during the difficult inter-war years.

In many democratic states, however, the creation of a mass electorate did little to check or control established interests. The existence of unstable governments, or the ephemeral nature of electoral support actually strengthened the powers of the establishment in several states. It is hard to argue that the radical, democratic constitutions of 1911 in Portugal, and of 1919 in Germany in any significant way weakened the largely conservative forces to be found in the Church and the army, or among civil servants and judges. Parliamentary control of such bodies, where it existed at all, tended to be occasional and tenuous. Even in those states where entry to the armed forces or the civil service was made more open, it is fairly clear that the changes made little difference to the type of person recruited or, presumably, to the values held. Those who, in the aftermath of war in 1918, believed that not only would a new and better world be established, but that the newly-enfranchised masses would have a share in the shaping of it, were for the most part in error. It was not at all unusual for those with power and influence to think that by conceding the right to vote they would not merely avoid revolution, but would gain time to strengthen their position against any subsequent assault. Nor were they always wrong. Many of those who had gained the vote had little interest in anything more than mild reform or the rectification of specific grievances. Few in western Europe were enthusiastic for revolution – whether social, economic or political – and, deprived of revolutionary opportunities, even fewer were willing to try the strategy of the long march through the institutions.

In much of Europe, however, mass participation in politics co-incided with the achievement of independence. Governments in newly-created states tend to be sensitive on questions involving either external or internal sovereignty, and the inter-war period proved no exception to this general rule. As a result, minority interests were commonly ignored, and not infrequently deliberately suppressed. States were reluctant to recognize the legitimacy of basic rights when these apparently conflicted with the utility of infringing them.[4] Given the ethnic, social and economic tensions prevalent in eastern and central Europe it was not long before popular democracy was almost everywhere replaced with dictatorships or oligarchic rule. Powerful interest groups were usually able to ensure continuing influence while institutions were used to promote tighter state control. Dissidents were harshly treated and elections, when they took place, were largely meaningless. The regimes of Dollfuss in Austria and of Horthy in Hungary provide two good examples of the destruction of democracy in states with well-educated and sophisticated populations. In states such as Romania and Bulgaria, afflicted by mass illiteracy, the collapse of democracy can perhaps be more easily understood.

The most serious challenges to the peaceful and gradual growth of Western-style democracy came not from the instability generated by the collapsed systems in eastern Europe, nor from the obstructionism of vested interests in western Europe, but from the social and economic frustrations so characteristic of the inter-war years. Because of the damage done to the European economies during the war of 1914–18 it proved very difficult to make much, let alone rapid, progress towards that degree of well-being which so many people had hoped for, and had been promised, in 1918. Impatient for improvement, and armed with the right to vote, the masses offered a tempting target to unscrupulous politicians and demagogues. The apparent failure of ostensibly democratic systems to deliver an increased standard of living to many in employment, the lack of provision for the unemployed, and the failure to maintain the value of pensions for the old or those disabled in war, created an ever-growing army of the enfranchised and the disenchanted. It ought to be remembered too that these failures followed not only the demands for great sacrifices during the war – many of which seemed futile even by 1919 – but also that before 1914 Western societies had been 'rent by deep divisions ... partly ... an outcome of the rise in food prices, which held down the workers' standard of living'.[5] The disappointments of the immediate post-war period led to the overthrow of democracy in several states in eastern Europe and to the rise of Mussolini. The post-1929 collapse led to further reverses for democracy in eastern Europe, and to Hitler's ascendancy in Germany. Even in those states where democracy survived there were great shifts in electoral fortune, sometimes accompanied by demands for strong leadership. It was a measure of the established strength of the democratic process in much of western Europe that the appeal of the Fascists proved so limited. But while the cautious conservatism of so many voters and leaders in western Europe was an invaluable asset in the fight against domestic extremism and the inroads of demagogy, it was a serious handicap in the task of coordinating resistance against the dictators.

Political developments in Russia further complicated the picture. Few in the West lamented the fall of the tsarist system; the general reaction among the Allies was that it relieved them of the embarrassment of claiming to fight for democracy and self-determination while associated with a state whose government clearly believed in neither. It was also supposed that 'the new constitutional administration would put out all its strength into a real effort to win the war'.[6] Instead, the Provisional Government was overwhelmed with problems and gave way, by means of a *coup d'état*, to the Bolsheviks in the autumn of 1917. The result of Lenin's bold stroke was the establishment of 'another centralized tyranny'[7] – bizarrely enough in the name of international, proletarian revolution. After Lenin's death Stalin continued, and extended the process of repression. The democratic states soon discovered that the existence of this regime seriously complicated their attempts to promote international stability; this problem was not resolved in 1939, and was a primary cause of the outbreak of war. A second unpleasant consequence was that most states were faced with communist parties which, once the possibility of immediate revolution had been abandoned, set themselves to work to try to destroy democratic institutions and movements, becoming in the process agents of the foreign policy of the USSR, rather than the catalysts of genuine reform. The communist parties, especially those which were well supported, as in France and Germany, took advantage of ambiguity in the position of socialists and progressives and helped to weaken and divide the Left. The KPD played a central part in the destruction of democracy in Germany, especially during 1929–33, and the PCF played the key role in paralysing the Popular Front in France. The revolutionary rhetoric to which these parties adhered also played an important part in strengthening the determination of anti-democratic forces on the Right to resist change, and, by alarming those who had something to lose, encouraged many citizens who were not reactionaries to seek refuge in the arms of leaders such as Mussolini and Hitler.

The introduction or development of democracy brought to the fore the problem of how democrats, of whatever political hue, were to cope with the emergence of anti-democratic parties and movements. The existence of a mass franchise did not necessarily mean that votes would be cast more wisely than in the past. The gradual increases in freedom, especially of the press, did not ensure that that freedom was not abused. Hitler and Stalin were as one in their contempt for, and hostility to, democratic institutions and values. They saw the processes of debate and compromise as evidence of weakness and uncertainty. The economic and social conditions of the inter-war years enabled those who were ready to act ruthlessly, and who claimed to know where they were going, to profit at the expense of those whose claims were more modest. It is not surprising, then, that democratic development was patchy and liable to sudden reversals.

It has already been asserted that social and economic pressures were essential in determining the pace and nature of political change within states. In some states, such as the USSR, it is also evident that political survival dictated social and economic change. Lenin's attitude towards the New Economic Policy, or Stalin's towards the purges, are fairly clear examples of the pre-eminence of political considerations of a tactical kind. Yet, with rare exceptions, as in the past, political developments tended to follow – sometimes tardily – social and economic changes. In this period these changes were so substantial that it is scarcely possible to do more than mention the main outlines of developments in societies and economies. First, however, it is important to mention two causes of the rapidity with which change took place: the influence of war, and the influence of scientific and technological advance.

It has often been argued that conflict, particularly if prolonged, has been a seed-bed for change. The war of 1914–18 provides substantial support for this assertion, having been fought on a scale inconceivable half a century earlier. There were bitter battles between the European powers well outside the European theatre, especially at sea and in East Africa,[8] but it was in Europe that efforts were concentrated. Much of the continent became a battleground, and behind the lines became an arsenal and a granary. Millions of men were conscripted into the armed forces, disrupting economic life and shattering relationships among families and society in the larger sense. Special attention is often paid to Britain, traditionally a country with a small army, because the strain upon her manpower was largely unexpected. During the war over five million men served in the British army, nearly half of whom did so as volunteers.[9] The tragic impact of the resultant loss of life was well captured in an aside by Flora Thompson:

> And all the time boys were being born or growing up in the parish, expecting to follow the plough all their lives, or, at most, to do a little mild soldiering or to go to work in a town. Gallipoli? Kut? Vimy Ridge? Ypres? What did they know of such places? But they were to know them and when the time came they did not flinch. Eleven of that tiny community never came back again.[10]

The destruction of communities was not confined to the villages, either. The losses sustained by units based on particular cities, especially among the Pals Battalions, were on the same scale and had equally strong effects.

The true social and political consequences of mass conscription are hard to estimate, not least because they cannot easily be separated from the effects of other actions by governments during wartime. However, it is at least arguable that the influences on British life were particularly marked. Alone of the major powers Britain possessed, despite its imperial acquisitiveness, a strong anti-militarist tradition. Conscription had been accepted as part of the way of life in much of continental Europe for decades before 1914, so the social and economic effects of conscription, though substantially increased during wartime, were not entirely compressed within a short period of time. In fact, in peacetime military service had provided opportunities for conscripts to improve their education and skills. One historian has argued that in France 'the army turned out to be an agency for emigration, acculturation, and in the final analysis, civilization, an agency as potent in its way as the schools, about which we tend to talk a great deal more'.[11] During war, as previously in peacetime, the issue of conscription produced heated political debate in Britain, and, in the end, damaging political convulsions. The nature of pre-1914 Britain, especially the emphasis upon minimal government and a *laissez-faire* economic system, made the notion of government intervention much more controversial; the dispute over conscription, though important, was in one sense merely representative of an established economic, social, and political system struggling to come to terms with new conditions, imperatives and ideas.

If other countries' governments were more accustomed to intervention than those in Britain, the scale and speed of the adjustment required was still vast. This was particularly evident in the exercise of governmental control over the economy. Banks, industrial enterprises, and trading houses found that their independence was curtailed or even extinguished. Taxation was hugely increased, and governments printed money at a rate which was highly inflationary, as well as borrowing large sums. The direction of labour became a crucial element in attempts to put states on a war footing. Key workers in certain industries, such as mines, chemicals, railways, and engineering, found that even the right to volunteer to fight was denied them. The munitions industry took over factories producing other goods, and a whole system of priority allocation of resources was established. The role of women in industrial and agricultural production was considerably enhanced, and governments proved ready to shift labour from one occupation to another, and from one place to another. Rationing was introduced and the production of non-essential goods was largely eliminated. The service industries found that not only were their activities reduced by war but also that conscription fell particularly heavily upon their employees. In short, the economic patterns which had evolved during European industrialization were almost completely changed. Many jobs were destroyed for ever, and the level of indebtedness incurred by governments changed the public perception of economic prospects, now viewed much more gloomily than at any point since the industrial revolution had begun.

There were other aspects of government intervention which also left a mark upon society. Perhaps the most significant of these was the extension of propaganda, coupled with the development of censorship. The truth was hard to get at during wartime, even for parliamentary representatives. The maintenance of the war effort, and hence morale, habitually took precedence over the admission of failure or incompetence. Initially, of course, the reckoning was more immediately painful for those governments which lost the war, namely Russia, Austria-Hungary, and Germany. In the long term, however, disillusionment concerning the gap between what had been expected and promised, and what could be achieved, was no less prevalent among the victor states. The extension of governmental powers during wartime also helped change the attitude of people towards their governments. After 1918 governments were expected to do more; there was a shift from the notion of individual to collective responsibility – a process which was particularly evident in Britain.

Yet, at the same time, there was a greater tendency to question established authority. The experiences of many soldiers caused them to doubt the capacity (and sometimes the sanity) of those who governed and commanded them. This attitude was reinforced by knowledge of the privation endured by the families of many servicemen. The failure to satisfy the expectations of those who had fought and lived, and, equally, of those whose menfolk had died, was a regular cause of political unrest and volatility in the inter-war period, even in those countries where democracy survived. These frustrations were intensified by continuing disappointment in the 1920s and 1930s, culminating in the outbreak of war in 1939. The renewal of demands by states for sacrifices to be made produced a widespread desire to modify the international system held responsible for the wars. It also increased already strong pressure for real social and economic change in individual states, as was clearly shown in the immediate aftermath of war in 1945.

The preoccupation of governments and peoples with organizing for victory largely blinded them to the global significance of the changes which occurred. It was during the war of 1914–18 that European domination of the world economy was destroyed. Those countries which had controlled the bulk of international trade through their capital resources, their financial skills, their technological and scientific supremacy, and their occupation of territories with vast quantities of raw materials, found in 1919 that the situation had changed dramatically. The accumulated savings of generations had been expended on war, and the savings of future generations were committed to the repayment of debts or reparations. The financial services in which the most advanced nations had specialized suffered from the lack of trade during the war, from insurance losses, and from lack of capital. While technological and scientific efforts had been directed towards the waging of war – and had made the European nations highly proficient at that – ordinary commercial developments, as well as pure research, had suffered. Even the territorial ascendancy of the Europeans was under threat, as the rise of nationalism in the Middle East and parts of Asia showed.

After 1918 the USA possessed the most important economy in the world. Curiously, this was a fact of life that was sometimes acknowledged, and sometimes not, on both sides of the Atlantic. There was in Europe a reluctance, both politically and culturally, to recognize this fundamental shift in resources and power. Equally, there were those in the USA who did not wish to take on the responsibilities which were tied to economic primacy. This unhappy state of affairs led not only to many misunderstandings, but also contributed to disastrous economic and political decisions during the 1920s and 1930s. Failure to recognize that economic and political capacities were closely linked helped pave the way to war in 1939. However, after 1941, among leading American politicians there was a clear recognition of the need to integrate policies. This then led them towards proposals, such as those made at Bretton Woods and Dumbarton Oaks, which attempted to design policies on a global scale.

The war of 1939–45 was less dramatic in its economic effects, though it was perhaps more important in inspiring demands for specific changes, such as for the maintenance of full employment. What the war did do was to confirm and reinforce the developments of 1914–18. Not only were precious resources, especially of skilled manpower, squandered, but the trading positions of the European nations were still further weakened. After 1945 the dead hand of Stalinism then effectively precluded any chance of recovery in eastern Europe. Scientific and technological supremacy had already passed to the USA, but European shortages of skills – even in uninvaded Britain – were dramatically exposed during the conflict.[12] Furthermore, the nature of the German occupation of much of Europe from 1940 to 1944, and the destruction which accompanied the German retreat, damaged the industrial base of Europe far more than the largely static conflicts of 1914–18. Finally, the dramatic collapses of European imperial authority in Asia made it clear to all but the wishful thinking that the old order was gone forever.

It should thus be of no surprise that the effect of the two wars upon class relationships was shattering. Old money was largely lost, and the social distinctions attached to its possession seemed increasingly irrelevant and irritating. The catastrophic events of 1914–18 greatly reduced public confidence in the notion of paternalistic government, and economic mismanagement in the inter-war years gnawed away at what faith remained. The ruling classes and élites also lost a good deal of their self-confidence, and their pessimism led them to act in ways which could only end in disaster. The enthusiasm of Italian and German élites for Mussolini and Hitler is a case in point. The heavy toll in the trenches, in which an unusually high proportion of middle- and upper-class soldiers were killed, severely reduced the numbers, though not the pretensions, of the élite. Occupation and destruction of land and property, combined with high taxation, further changed the picture. The evolution of new parties, the development of different ideologies, the establishment of organizations representing very different interests – such as the trade unions – all contributed to the collapse of the old certainties. While deference continued to be an important element in social and political life, it and the hierarchies sustained by it were declining forces, ruined by wars and revolutions.

If war was a powerful agent for change, so too was science and technology. The railway, long established in western Europe, exerted a strong influence on economic development and social change in eastern Europe and Russia by 1914. The late nineteenth century witnessed a further revolution in transport when first trams, and then underground trains, were introduced in many of Europe's leading cities. At more or less the same time appeared the motor car, and a little later buses. In a period of only a quarter-century to 1914 the lives of ordinary people were revolutionized. The availability of cheap, rapid forms of transport promoted the growth of cities and suburbs. The effects on trade, industry, housing, utilities and schools were immeasurable. The invention of the telephone vastly improved communications, and the development of oil-fired engines changed the shipping industry. Later, air transport became possible, though it was not until the jet engine was invented that remote parts of the world became swiftly accessible.

If ordinary lives were much altered by these developments, still more important discoveries were in train. Electrical and chemical engineers began the process of revolutionizing all manner of industrial processes – the manufacture of steel, photography, printing, dyes, machine-tools and glassware. The development of the dynamo, the diesel engine, the gas turbine, hydroelectric power, and the petrochemical industry, all have their origins in the late nineteenth century. The modern study of genetics was revived at the turn of the century, given a stimulus by the discovery of Mendel's long-forgotten work. This was an age of great discovery in physics; the work of Kelvin was coming to an end, but Rutherford, Thomson, Boltzmann and Planck were producing seminal research. Einstein published his famous paper 'The Electrodynamics of Moving Bodies' in 1905, and a decade later his *General Theory of Relativity*. The earlier work of the great chemist, Mendeleev, took on new meaning after the publication of Thomson's work on electrons. Röntgen and Marie Curie pursued their work on radioactive compounds with great consequences for both physics and medicine. After the war, and mainly because of it, research into many areas with commercial applicability became concentrated in the USA. Even so, there was much important work done in Europe, including the development of television, computers, penicillin, and sulphur drugs. In the fields of nuclear physics, mathematics and chemistry much of the best research was by Europeans – Bohr, von Neumann, Fermi, von Laue, Born, Heisenberg, Schrödinger, Szilard – even if many of them, usually under the pressure of political events, ended in the USA. The advance of knowledge affected the peoples of Europe increasingly in the 1920s and 1930s. At great pace they were being rushed into the age of high technology, computation, plastics, pharmaceuticals, atomic energy, radiography, cancer research, genetic engineering and immunology.

Those who lived through this period were well aware of the pace of change, but were often confused, understandably enough, as to where such developments would lead. There were those, usually socialists or Marxists, who professed great confidence in the application of 'scientific' principles to politics, economics, and society. Indeed it was not uncommon to believe 'in the power of science to solve all problems, and, more particularly, all political problems which confront men in the modern age'.[13] Socialism was depicted as a more scientific form of political belief than other ideologies, though this was usually the product of prejudice, rather than the result of examination of evidence. In fact this was a period of careful analysis of the structure of societies, the operation of economics, and the basis of human belief.

The work of distinguished sociologists, economists and psychologists – such as Weber, Freud, Jung, Adler, Mannheim, Schumpeter, Pareto and Durkheim – showed how diverse were structures, choices, reasoning, and behaviour. It was unfortunate that the savants so often came to such different conclusions when a widespread desire, in an age of change, was for the clarity of certainty. The scientific revolution when extended into the social sciences helped demolish old beliefs but put little that was agreed in their place. Quite inadvertently this aided those whose beliefs were immune from uncertainty, and who offered simple answers to problems.

Given all these changes and uncertainties, this was inevitably an era of rapid cultural development. An important element in this was the advance of literacy, though there was still mass illiteracy, or very limited literacy, in some areas of Europe. This advance opened the way for a few to higher education. More significantly, the mass circulation of newspapers presented an opportunity for contact with a different world, and, in providing such an opportunity, helped change the world still more rapidly. Improvements in printing and photography, and a better transport system, aided the dissemination of information. But without increased education the process would have been slower and more limited. Market forces determined that mass circulation newspapers were cheap and written in a readily comprehensible way. From the turn of the century onwards, at least in western Europe, newspapers were read avidly by the poor and the disadvantaged in society. This enabled newspapers to represent and to mould the opinions of those who in an earlier period would have had either no views or precious little chance of expressing them. Once a mass franchise had come into existence, demands for which were certainly increased by improved knowledge of social, political and economic life, the political potential of the press became immense.

The twentieth century thus witnessed the development of popular culture in a way which was quite different from the past. What the newspapers began was continued with the development of radio and cinema. Once sound and vision were united in the cinema an exceptionally potent influence was established, unrivalled until the spread of television after 1945. The rise of the press, radio and cinema produced a certain familiarity with the famous figures of the day; familiarity in some cases bred contempt. Politicians were certainly less revered than in the nineteenth century; it is difficult to argue that in general they were worse, but what is more likely is that they were better-known and thus usually regarded as less than godlike figures. It is highly significant that dictators were exceptionally sensitive to what was written about their regimes, and how ready they were to suppress domestic comment and, when possible, even foreign comment. But at another level, non-political figures, such as entertainers or sportsmen, were elevated to positions of fame, or notoriety. The activities of criminals, a matter of great interest in the previous century, came into the public eye in a different way. There was a market in exposing the peccadilloes of those regarded as pillars of society which had been largely untapped in the past. Scandal-mongering and sensationalism sold newspapers, but also helped to chip away at already crumbling institutions and values. The shrewd and unscrupulous were able to take advantage of this craving for the novel, or for the titillating, or the absurd.

Popular culture was also enhanced by the press, radio and cinema. There was much good discussion of serious issues. Political and economic debates were not always trivialized. There were many informative articles and programmes on a whole range of topics which helped educate the general public about art, music, literature, history, geography and science. The sophistication of news presentation increased and a better-informed public was not backward in expressing its own views, though these were not necessarily always helpful. Selective presentation of news to reflect the views of the proprietor or the government, or to appeal to the prejudices of the reader or listener, was characteristic of every country. The reluctance to face up to the nastiness of Hitler's regime during the appeasement period was paralleled by the gushing praise of 'Uncle Joe' after 1941. In both cases not only was the public deceived, but it was made more difficult for necessary policy changes to be made.[14]

It was not only newspapers which were read. There was an enormous demand for books of all kinds. In several countries the period from the 1880s to the end of the 1930s (excepting 1914–18) was a golden age for publishing. The thirst for knowledge was apparently insatiable. In Britain, France, and Germany the publishers of encyclopaedias and collections of famous works, such as the Everyman editions or the Librairie Plon, enjoyed almost a licence to coin money. There was great demand for fiction, especially in the comparatively new form of the detective story. Serious books, examining important issues, also enjoyed surprisingly good sales. Public libraries, private lending libraries, and travelling libraries testified to a great growth of public interest in the written word. With the knowledge acquired came changed attitudes and new assumptions; these affected both contemporary affairs and life long after 1945.

Until 1914 steadily improving living standards for many Europeans enabled them to use their leisure more profitably. The period before

1914 witnessed a rapid increase in the number of clubs and associations – especially those which required only limited expenditure. Many of these were sporting clubs, of which particular favourites were cycling, fishing, shooting and a whole variety of games. It was not entirely by chance that the Olympic movement was revived in the 1890s. Better and cheaper transport not only enabled these clubs to flourish, especially in Britain and Germany, but they brought people from different areas and backgrounds together. The old ways of using leisure time in consequence declined. Fewer people made their own clothes or cultivated substantial kitchen gardens. The identification of Sundays with religious observance, already in decline, was further reduced; the churches largely ceased to be the centre of village life, as they had long since ceased to be in the towns. Markets, fairs, travelling sideshows, carnivals and charivaris became less frequent, and, where they survived, did not fulfil the economic or social functions of the past.

After 1914 economic difficulties meant that the use of leisure time did not perhaps develop as fast as might otherwise have been expected, but there could be no return to the ways of the past. While the culture of the masses was changing, so too was that of the minority. The enfeeblement of old socio-economic structures reduced patronage but also helped remove some of the constraints on artistic development. The twentieth century was one of a violent acceleration of change in painting, sculpture, drama and music. Picasso, Rodin, Shaw, Strindberg and Stravinsky were modern figures who owed a debt to, but were not bound by, the past. The work of the modernists responded to, and helped shape contemporary events. The arts had frequently had a high, though not always active, political content in the past; this era was one of high political activism. Literature did not remain isolated from this process and the nature of the political debate was much affected by the contributions of writers. The rise of totalitarianism, the conflicts between its exponents, and the dilemma of liberals and progressives as to how they should respond, were the concerns of artists and writers who vigorously expressed their views through their preferred medium. The works of Brecht, Benda, Orwell, Koestler, Picasso, Spengler and Gorky, to cite only a few examples, show how intertwined were the arts and politics. The old culture of a largely privileged minority in Europe, like that of the masses, was subjected to its own earthquakes and avalanches.

It is evident, then, that the divided Europe of 1945 was quite different from that of 1890. Economic supremacy had been ceded to the USA, as had the leadership in science and technology. The huge colonial empires had either been destroyed or were in the process of disintegration. The apparently boundless confidence which had so marked European attitudes during the seventy-five years after Waterloo had been replaced by pessimism. There were signs of this even before the turn of the century. On hearing of the death of William I in 1888 Salisbury observed, 'The ship is leaving the harbour, this is the crossing of the bar. I can see the sea covered with white horses.'[15] Even Salisbury, however, could not have foreseen the tempests which were to assail the European barque and drive her mastless onto the rocks by 1945. Lack of confidence undermined not merely the feelings of superiority which sustained white supremacy, but also the relationships between classes. Economic deprivation did not fall equally upon all, so at the very time when there was less faith in paternalism and in established government, there was also greater pressure for the rectification of grievances – some long-standing but many of recent origin. Thus the temper of the people was different and was reflected in new ideas, groupings, demands, and culture. Established states disappeared and established religions declined. New ideologies came to the fore, and in due course they, too, were found inadequate to meet the diverse challenges of the age.

The instability which characterized this period has posed awkward problems for those who have wished to study it, mainly because of the speed and breadth of developments. This has been true of other periods, for example the Reformation and the French Revolutionary – Napoleonic era, but the scale of complexity and the number of problems of the 1890–1945 period is quantitatively quite different. A further difficulty has been the influence of Marxist analysis of events, now, correctly, widely regarded as redundant. Marxist interpretations of history are not unique to this period, though usually when dealing with earlier periods they only commanded limited support. For this era, however, Marxist analysis has seemed much more relevant, mainly perhaps because of the existence of states, movements and individuals that claimed to be working towards the inexorable victory of Marxism. Furthermore, the undeniable fact that mass movements, organization and culture became more significant than in the nineteenth-century era of *laissez-faire* and robust individualism probably persuaded even non-Marxists to write in terms that favoured grand theories of explanation. In short, determinism of different types, not just the Marxist version, has flourished among those who have studied the history of the period in all its aspects: political, economic, social and cultural.

Acceptance of the assertion that rapid change was the most obvious characteristic of the period would seem to render almost superfluous the search for other overarching themes. Nevertheless, it is still possible to discern, if sometimes rather dimly, the emergence of other patterns. Some of these have already received attention, such as the emergence of a mass franchise, or general economic decline. One theme, however, deserves further mention – the changed relationship between the state and society. The role of the state increased substantially in this period, especially in its scope for intervention and hence its impact upon social and economic life. This means that questions arise as to what constituted the state in this era of flux – how far could it be regarded as the expression of individual or collective wills? how far did it represent oligarchies, vested interests, classes, or ethnic groups rather than the totality of the people? These questions cannot be easily answered, if at all, but need to be asked because it is clear that even before 1914, let alone by 1945, expectations concerning the role of the state were quite different.

In order to attempt to answer these questions it is necessary to look beyond the methods and sources once regarded as sufficient to inform analysis. The changing relationship between state and society demands that attention be paid in particular to the emergence of pressure groups. Among the most important of these in the majority of states may be numbered local or regional forms of government, industrial, trade, and labour organizations, religious bodies, private associations and societies, the movements for female emancipation, the press and other media of information. It is also necessary, of course, to examine the interaction between political parties, ideology and class. The conventional relationships between established institutions, élites, parties and the people need, as ever, to continue to be taken into account. Finally, it should not be forgotten that the new sources – like the old – may be liable to misuse, distortion or suppression, sometimes in the name of a 'higher truth'. Such hazards are, and always have been, inseparable from the study of the past.

The essays in this book attempt in a general and limited way to describe and account for the great changes which overtook Europe in the period 1890–1945. Necessarily, some important developments and issues could only be mentioned briefly and some not at all. The authors would not claim individually, or collectively, to have produced a comprehensive view of the era. Indeed, there are clear differences in perspective and of weighting of issues. This, however, might charitably be regarded as a strength, rather than a weakness of the book, in that different opinions are more likely than conformity to inform debate.

Finally, it is surely not entirely inappropriate if in describing an era of turbulence there should be some disagreement as to what mattered most and why.

NOTES

1　A. J. P. Taylor, *Europe: Grandeur and Decline* (Harmondsworth: Pelican, 1969), p. 373.
2　There is a useful discussion of this question in relation to female suffrage in T. Wilson, *The Myriad Faces of War* (Cambridge: Polity Press, 1986), pp. 724–8.
3　Article 17. Quoted in E. M. Hucko, *The Democratic Tradition: Four German Constitutions* (Oxford: Berg, 1989), p. 153.
4　A useful analysis of the relationship between rights and the state may be found in R. Plant, *Modern Political Thought* (Oxford: Blackwell, 1991), pp. 253–91.
5　A. Offer, *The First World War: An Agrarian Interpretation* (Oxford: Oxford University Press, 1991), p. 14.
6　Lord Newton, *Retrospection* (London: John Murray, 1941), p. 233.
7　Lord Vansittart, *The Mist Procession* (London: Hutchinson, 1958), p. 180.
8　Especially in East Africa. See B. Farwell, *The Great War in Africa, 1914–1918* (London: Viking, 1987).
9　The impact of the enormous demand for manpower is well treated in T. Wilson, op. cit., and the raising of these forces in P. Simkins, *Kitchener's Army: The Raising of the New Armies, 1914–16* (Manchester: Manchester University Press, 1988).
10　F. Thompson, *Lark Rise to Candleford* (Oxford: Oxford University Press, 1984), p. 244.
11　E. Weber, *Peasants into Frenchmen: The Modernization of Rural France, 1870–1914* (London: Chatto & Windus, 1979), p. 302.
12　Germany was probably the country of which this was least true. The case of Britain has been carefully reviewed in C. Barnett, *The Audit of War* (London: Macmillan, 1986). This has been much criticized, but its central thesis seems to me to emerge strengthened, rather than diminished, by the assaults of critics.
13　H. J. Morgenthau, *Scientific Man versus Power Politics*, quoted in W. H. G. Armytage, *The Rise of the Technocrats* (London: Routledge & Kegan Paul, 1965), p. 356.
14　As in the case of British foreign policy. See F. R. Gannon, *The British Press and Germany, 1936–39* (Oxford: Clarendon Press,

1971), and M. Kitchen, *British Policy Towards the Soviet Union during the Second World War* (London: Macmillan, 1986).
15 Lady Gwendolen Cecil, *Life of Robert Marquis of Salisbury*, vol. 4 (London: Hodder & Stoughton, 1932), p. 96.

FURTHER READING

There are enormous numbers of books which might be read with profit. I have tried to limit suggestions to those which are readily available and which try to examine issues or topics in a synoptic way.

The pre-1914 period is well covered in: B. Tuchman, *The Proud Tower* (London, 1966); J. Romein, *The Watershed of Two Eras: Europe in 1900* (Middletown, 1978); A. J. Mayer, *The Persistence of the Old Regime* (London, 1981); O. J. Hale, *The Great Illusion, 1900–1914* (London, 1971); F. S. L. Lyons, *Internationalism in Europe, 1815–1914* (Leiden, 1963); I. F. Clarke, *Voices Prophesying War, 1763–1984* (London, 1966); T. P. Hughes, *The Development of Western Technology* (New York, 1964); D. S. Landes, *The Unbound Prometheus* (Cambridge, 1969); and C. Trebilcock, *The Industrialization of the Continental Powers, 1780–1914* (London, 1981).

For the post-1914 period the abundance of good books is even greater. Well worth looking at are: D. H. Aldcroft, *From Versailles to Wall Street, 1919–1929* (London, 1977); C. P. Kindleberger, *The World in Depression, 1929–1939* (London, 1973); J. M. Keynes, *The Economic Consequences of the Peace* (London, 1919); A. J. Mayer, *Politics and Diplomacy of Peacemaking* (London, 1968); P. Kennedy, *The Rise and Fall of the Great Powers* (London, 1988); A. J. P. Taylor, *The Origins of the Second World War* (London, 1964); C. J. Bartlett, *The Global Conflict, 1880–1970: The International Rivalry of the Great Powers* (London, 1984); F. Gilbert, *The End of the European Era, 1890 to the Present* (New York, 1984); and R. J. Sontag, *A Broken World, 1919–1939* (New York, 1971).

2 France and Germany: Belle Epoque and Kaiserzeit

Paul Hayes

The war of 1914–18 has profoundly affected the way historians have looked at the quarter of a century preceding the events of June–August 1914. It has led to particular attention being paid to those who prophesied doom and disaster for the old European order. As a result, the weaknesses of the pre-1914 structure of both international relations and domestic politics have received much more attention than their strengths. It ought not to be forgotten that late nineteenth-century Europe, especially in the west, was both prosperous and self-confident – even if not all of its inhabitants were rich, and even if not all believed that the future would necessarily be better than the past or the present. Romein summed up the situation neatly when he observed 'the summer of European supremacy was making way for the autumn' but there was also 'an atmosphere of spring and renewal no less than of autumn and decline'.[1] In many aspects of life, especially cultural, scientific, technological and political, the period from 1890–1914 cannot be fairly described as one of decline, decay and tortured uncertainty. Indeed, especially in Britain, there was more commonly a tendency to exaggerate the permanence and the certainties of society as it existed in 1900. As Tuchman put it, 'People were more confident of values and standards . . . than they are today, although they were not more peaceful nor, except for the upper few, more comfortable.'[2]

In France and Germany attitudes were significantly different from those in Britain. Many Britons found it hard to come to terms with the events of the Boer War, but this adjustment was small in comparison with that required of the French after 1871. The twin shocks of defeat at the hands of Prussia and a temporarily successful revolution in Paris produced in many of the French people a deep sense of national humiliation. Despite a remarkably swift economic recovery, and the establishment of a new, if unloved, political system, French self-respect was never entirely restored. As a result, France craved recognition of its status as a force with which to be reckoned; this affected French attitudes towards all kinds of issues and questions. Sometimes manifestations of this anxiety were ephemeral or even absurd; on occasion they could be more substantial or even menacing. The widely-held belief in 1898, at the time of Fashoda, that France could afford to have both Britain and Germany as enemies could easily have led to disaster. The obsession with the recovery of Lorraine produced not only ruin for the literary career of Rémy de Gourmont – 'this new Babylonian captivity leaves me entirely cold'[3] – but, more seriously, encouraged the doctrine of the *offensive à outrance* which came to dominate French strategic planning from 1912 onwards.[4] The lack of realism of adherents to this doctrine was gravely to weaken the effective use of French military resources in the war of 1914–18.

Germany, by contrast, seemed very, perhaps unduly, self-confident. Yet it is almost common ground among those who have studied post-1815 German history that fears, often indefinable fears, profoundly affected the German psyche. The victories of 1864–70, and the growth of the economy from mid-century onwards, did little to dispel individual or collective *Angst*. By 1890 Germany ought not merely to have been a satiated power, but the Germans should have been a satisfied people. The situation was quite otherwise. After 1870 France was sensitive to its perceived loss of status; less understandably, Germany appeared slighted whenever full acknowledgement of its newly-achieved position was not rendered. As in the case of France, this response could be discerned at both trivial and important levels. Little harm was done when William II wrote to Nicholas II, calling him 'Admiral of the Pacific' and signing himself 'Admiral of the Atlantic'.[5] But the attempt to build a fleet able to hold its own against that of Britain, combined with a diplomacy characterized by its lack of finesse, depicted German ambitions in sinister rather than semi-comic colours. Similarly, German imperial ambitions, unlike those of France, added unnecessarily to the list of Germany's substantial opponents. In addition to German clumsiness and ineptitude there existed a habit of presenting German demands in such a way that suggested that Germany was not being fairly treated. This was not well received by other powers; nor was the implied threat that if Germany were not loved then other nations would have to be made to love her. These unendearing impressions were described by Rumbold in 1916 as 'the Rhine-whine';[6] a decade earlier Crowe had characterized the Germans as 'essentially people whom it does not pay to run after'.[7] It is hard to judge the extent to which external opinions about French and German foreign policies affected conditions and attitudes inside those countries, but it seems reasonable to suppose that they had some effect. What was to be increasingly important after about 1890 was simply that France, expected by other powers to be restless and to pursue a policy of *revanche*, seemed to be more prudent than had been anticipated; Germany, expected to be a force for stability, appeared tetchy, nervous, and unduly active. After signing an alliance with Russia in 1894 and an *entente* with Britain in 1904, France recovered much of its self-esteem and confidence (with not wholly benign effects), while Germany became obsessed with breaking free from an encirclement which did not actually exist. Thus it was Germany which was increasingly identified as a source of international instability; this perception certainly affected opinion and behaviour in Germany and France, and in other states too.

It is now necessary to turn to the political and economic structures of France and Germany in order to assess and compare the stability of their societies and governments. Where better to begin than with the people themselves? In 1914 the French numbered just over 39 million, a figure scarcely different from that in mid-century. For much of the period 1890–1914 the birth rate was below that of the mortality rate and it was only an influx of foreigners, usually Belgians or Poles seeking jobs in industry, that enabled population levels to be maintained. By contrast, Germany had a population of 60 million in 1914 – close to double what it had been in mid-century; the population was still growing despite heavy emigration, especially to the USA and Latin America. Germany also was host to immigrants and, as in France, they were concentrated in industrial areas. This was not always productive of social harmony, as integration proved difficult and there was much evidence of chauvinism and xenophobia in both states. Pogroms in Russia led to an exodus of Jews and the growth af anti-Semitism, especially in France, where the infamous Dreyfus Affair disgraced French political life from 1894 to 1906. In Germany anti-Semitism had deeper roots, and there too anti-Jewish sentiments became more widely held as the century drew to a close.[8] As in other states, and other eras, immigration provided an excuse for nationalist excesses and produced therefore a political atmosphere not conducive to stability.

The significance of the disparity in population sizes could be seen in the economic differences of two unequal internal markets – very important in an age of tariffs and protectionism – and in the psychology of status. In fact it was the comparative weakness of the French economy, despite substantial industrialization by 1914, which made it impossible for France to compete on equal terms with Germany. This was accentuated by, but not caused by, a smaller population. But many French citizens saw the problem almost exclusively in terms of there being fewer French than Germans. This led, both before and after 1914, to futile attempts to encourage the birth rate. The concern over relative numbers was based upon recognition of the fact that in 1870 France had lost a war against a Prussia of approximately the same size. How could there be a successful war of revenge in the face of an enemy more numerous by 20 million? No wonder, then, that France also sought to expand its overseas empire (and recruit troops there) and to court Russia as an ally. Furthermore, conscription weighed more heavily on the French than the Germans, especially after the *Loi de Trois Ans* was passed in 1913. In actuality this measure hardly bridged the gap in resources – unless a war lasted only a few weeks – as German reserves were much larger. The concern about manpower and its linkage with the status of France led, therefore, to serious social and economic strains on France which contributed not inconsiderably to that pre-war social crisis perceived by many historians.

The people of France were not only less numerous than those of Germany but were educated differently, did very different jobs and lived in different ways. Even in 1914 the mass of the French population not only lived in small towns (fewer than two thousand inhabitants), villages, hamlets or isolated farms, but were engaged in farming, forestry or fishing. One way or another about five out of every nine Frenchmen were thus employed. In Germany, even on the most generous calculations, only about 35 per cent were engaged in the same occupations and lived in similar communities. Not only were there far more city-dwellers in Germany, Germany was also more industrialized. The strength of service industries in Germany, and the consequently large proportion of white-collar workers, demonstrated how much more advanced was the German economy. Germans, too, were much better educated than the French. Although French education improved very considerably during the period, mainly because of the education reforms of the 1880s, it could not stand comparison with the universality and thoroughness of the German system. Illiteracy was still a serious problem in both France and Britain – as their armies were to find out after 1914 – but not in Germany. In 1908, for example, out of 160,588 recruits for the German armed forces only 39 were illiterate (and these were mainly educationally sub-normal) and another 38 were literate, but in a non-German tongue.[9] The literacy of the German people enabled economic development to be achieved in ways undreamed of by French and British entrepreneurs, manufacturers and politicians.

How different, then, were the economies? France, although still mainly a country of peasants, made great industrial progress during this period. The process had begun during the Second Empire and had continued in the early years of the Third Republic. By 1914 France was a substantial industrial power. Traditional strengths remained – the production of food, wine and many luxury items, especially porcelain, glassware, perfumes and high-quality cloth – but in addition many new industries had been developed and some old or decayed ones revived. Prominent among new industries were those of electricity, automobiles and chemicals. All of these were major employers by 1914. The development of an electrochemical industry and the presence of bauxite, both in France and in parts of its empire, soon enabled France to become the world's largest producer of aluminium; this was to have important consequences in the war. Old industries which gained a new lease of life were coal, iron and steel. In the period 1890–1914 the production of coal increased by about 60 per cent, that of iron ore (as a result of the Gilchrist-Thomas process) by 1,000 per cent, and that of steel doubled. Heavy industry was, as in Germany and the USA, largely cartelized by 1914;[10] where France was so different was that small enterprises continued to dominate. In 1906 nearly half the industrial workers, 49.2 per cent, were employed in workshops with fewer than five wage-earners, and only 10.8 per cent of wage-earners were employed in firms with more than five hundred workers.[11] As one would expect, then, these different industrial conditions were reflected in unique patterns of urbanization, the formation and development of trade unions, affiliation to parties of the Left, and the level of wages.

French industrialization did not narrow the gap with Germany. By 1914 Germany had the most powerful and best-balanced economy in Europe, and this strength was reflected in its industrial production. Germany produced twice as much steel and cotton goods as its nearest European competitors (respectively, Britain and France), as much coal as Britain and more electricity than Britain, France and Italy together. Germany was vastly superior in the production of dyes, chemicals, synthetic materials, lead, zinc, drugs and fertilizers. It was a leader in many industries which demanded advanced technology or high technical skills, including photography, plastics, printing, optics, precision instruments, glassware, paper-making, dynamos, and cables; its success reflected in part its educational advantages. Much of its industry was organized on the grand scale; it was frequently cartelized or so market-dominant as to be almost monopolistic. Some industries, especially heavy industry and shipbuilding, benefited from very favourable government contracts, but many firms held well-deserved international reputations. Among these could be numbered Siemens, AGFA, AEG, Krupp, Bayer, Höchst, Blohm and Voss, Vulkan, and BASF. While there were many small companies, the trend in this period was to large firms and vast factories.[12] In the Ruhr, Alsace-Lorraine, and Silesia were concentrated enormous populations which put great strain upon living and working conditions. After a period of considerable restriction upon trade union activity there was a growth in labour organizations, and after 1895 union membership, especially among the unskilled, expanded quickly. As in France, this had marked effects on industry, government, the political parties and social policy.

Industrialization and the growth of trade led in both countries to the expansion of banking and financial services. French and German firms shared a common reluctance to permit their future to be determined by the banks – an attitude of particular importance in an era when the power and range of interests of banks increased substantially. In France there was only minimal advance towards the merging of industrial and banking capital. The reasons for this were fairly clear-cut. The great banks – whether merchant, joint-stock or regional – were at best limited, more commonly reluctant, investors in industrial enterprises. Joint-stock banks, such as Crédit Lyonnais, or the Comptoir National d'Escompte de Paris, tended to take the line that industrial investment involved an unacceptable level of risk. The regional banks, such as those of the Nord or the Ain, were much more accommodating, and were willing to enter limited partnerships with levels of investment strictly controlled; these banks did not try to determine the policy of those enterprises they supported. The merchant banks were the most adventurous and responded to a perceived market need; some of them, such as Paribas or Parunion, became heavily involved with large industrial concerns. A second consideration was that many banks were themselves operating as businesses. Post-1870 France had a very high savings to earnings ratio and the big financial institutions were cash-rich. Much of this capital went to finance businesses in the empire, in Russia, in the Ottoman empire, in the Americas and in eastern Europe. Large sums also went to financing government spending in France, to public state loans, and to certain very profitable large-scale industries – such as armaments. The survival of many small firms, however, is evidence not only that cartelization was limited but also that investors were prepared to place funds in small-scale enterprises which did not promise exceptionally high levels of return. Many businesses, including some significantly large ones, in effect financed themselves, and in the period 1900–14 over 70 per cent of investment was in the form of reinvestment.[13]

If in France the pattern was generally one in which firms and banks alike were agreed that limited cooperation would best preserve independence from financial control by the banks, the picture in Germany was differently defined. The growing domination of German industry by cartels was mirrored in the banking world, and in the symbiotic relationship between cartels and banks. Apart from the Reichsbank which, like the Banque de France, played a different role, and a handful of other banks (most notably some federal state banks and the Prussian-based Seehandlung) commercial life was dominated by six great banks and their provincial affiliates. The greatest of these was the Deutsche Bank, which held some 32 per cent of the combined capital and reserves of the big six. The banks did not hesitate to use their financial power – especially their large shareholdings and their ability to determine the terms on which capital was advanced – to promote industrial mergers and cartelization energetically. The banks were also active in financing overseas investment, especially in the newly-acquired German colonies, the Ottoman empire, the United States and the colonies of lesser imperial powers such as the Netherlands, Portugal and Italy. In Germany little encouragement was given to the creation of small enterprises, and those firms which were successful were often taken over or placed under the umbrella of a cartel.

The changes in society generated by industrial development were substantial in both countries. In addition to a large increase in the numbers of urban workers there was also a considerable growth in the size, wealth and influence of the middle classes.[14] The greater concentrations of population led to pressure on existing institutions and services, especially the provision of education, health education, transport and power. Traditional family life, rural social organization, religious beliefs, and systems of government, both local and national, were all affected. The collective impact was profound, and was quite visible to contemporaries. Fears of, or conversely hopes for, revolution were widespread in both states. Nor were these the concerns or aspirations of reactionaries or revolutionaries. Many cautious conservatives and liberals feared lest social unrest break out in violent form and sweep away existing social, political and economic structures. For them, as Rebérioux observes, 'It was the shadow of radicalism that hung over not only the great massacre but also the profound crisis in cultural and political values and the social crisis, all the basic elements of which were already present before 1914.'[15] Attitudes in

Germany were essentially the same, though the different political systems produced rather different effects.

Industrialization also heightened social, economic and political tension by adding to the army of the discontented. There were the losers from changes – those whose livelihoods were lost or significantly reduced, especially as a result of modernization or mechanization. Then there were those whose expectations were disappointed. In France and Germany, as elsewhere in Europe, there were many who found that urban industrial life had many drawbacks, not least of which was the absence of a communal spirit of mutual aid which had so often characterized rural settlements. Even among those who had prospered there existed fears of loss of income or status. These very different concerns produced markedly disparate social and political attitudes; collectively they added nothing to social harmony or cohesion. There was an evident breakdown in the traditional structures of society, clear in the cities but by no means invisible in the countryside. Technological and scientific advances led to increased job opportunities, to improved transport and to better communications. All of these factors encouraged migration; their effects were felt too upon those who remained in their hamlets and villages. The old certainties, whether derived from faith, custom, or ignorance, were perpetually under challenge. There was thus a spirit of restlessness which could easily be transformed into discontent, or, perhaps, revolution. It was this that the wealthier and more privileged feared, and there seemed little they could do to control or prevent it.

The part played by education in changing social attitudes is disputed, though it seems agreed that the French were much, and the Germans significantly, better educated in 1914 than in 1870. It has been argued that education was a key factor in change:

> Like migration, politics, and economic development, schools brought suggestions of alternative values and hierarchies; and of commitments to other bodies than the local group. They eased individuals out of the latter's grip and shattered the hold of unchallenged cultural and political creeds.[16]

Others have suggested that a significant effect of education was to reinforce existing structures and assumptions: 'The very organization of the German school system served as a brake upon social mobility and tended to freeze the existing social system.'[17] Are, in fact, such apparently divergent assessments completely irreconcilable? Probably not; both verdicts are true, but only up to a certain point.

It seems clear that in the most general sense better education and increased opportunities for learning produced a more restless society. To suggest that this was not true in Germany or France would imply that the concerns of the rulers and the upper classes in both countries were entirely imaginary. Such an argument seems even more implausible when various social and institutional changes are observed – the decline of religious observance, the search of the Churches for new social doctrines, the development of trade unions, the rise of parties of the Left, the attempts to rig existing electoral systems, and a greater readiness by the state to try to control dissent. More education produced more physical, social, economic and political pressures – though it was, of course, far from being the only cause of these developments. However, education was also used as a method of underpinning the state and society. Education produced conformists as well as rebels and revolutionaries. The higher reaches of education were only attained with great difficulty even among the lower-middle classes; as far as university education was concerned, those who came from non-educated or poor backgrounds probably had more chance of rising in France than in Germany or Britain. Furthermore, because of past controversies, teachers in France were politically more radical (opponents would have said subversive) than in Germany. The *Volksschulen* turned out large numbers of Germans who revered the monarchy, the army and the law; their conservatism and their subservience to appointed authority was legendary. Nevertheless, all German children had a minimum of eight years' education and significant numbers of these either reacted against the values of their teachers or, after release from the school system, used their numeracy and literacy to find new careers and new homes. The new problems they then encountered led to the phenomenon of the educated working-class trade-unionist or political activist. While examples of this type can be found throughout Europe, even in backward countries such as Russia and Spain, they were most common in Germany. If, indeed, education was a brake upon social mobility then it was not always effective when the economy was moving at high speed.

The growth of trade-unionism, socialism and parties of the Left posed problems for employers, governments and the middle classes. There were substantial obstacles to overcome before trade unions could exist freely and socialist parties could function on a basis of equality with other groups. Perhaps the most formidable of all obstacles was public attitudes in both France and Germany, especially the latter. Public attitudes consisted of a mixture between the official position of the established institutions, the opinion of other influential groups or individuals, and folk memory of the past–often inaccurate.

In Wilhelmine Germany official attitudes were hardly likely to be sympathetic to the aims of trade unionists and socialists. Fairly accurately, these groups were depicted as anti-monarchical, anti-religious, egalitarian, and in favour of higher wages and reformed tax and voting systems. Largely incorrectly, they were also said to be unpatriotic, anti-parliamentary, revolutionary, criminal, and desirous of seizing property. While in public few were prepared to admit, as did Waldersee, that military force was the best way of controlling these new groups – if necessary through a *Staatsstreich*, or coup from above – there were many who privately concurred. The not entirely inaccurate belief that William II shared this opinion contrived to lend undue respectability to it among many middle-class Germans. These views were often bolstered by the words and deeds of individuals, firms, and groups who feared they had much to lose from the rise of radicalism in industry, society and politics. Finally, folk memories – especially those of the triumphant nationalism of 1870–1, the horrors of the Commune in Paris, the regular murders of prominent figures in many countries, and the fear of a return to poverty – reinforced public attitudes towards trade-unionism and socialism.

To this psychological obstacle could be added legal restrictions, of which the most important was the 1878 law which rendered impossible most of the activities of the Social Democratic Party of Germany (SPD). As the trade union movement in the period 1870–90 was in essence an offshoot of the party, this law enabled officialdom to attack union activism. In the 1880s this tactic was combined with legislation to alleviate social misery, including health insurance in 1883, accident insurance in 1884, and old-age and disability pensions in 1889. Trade-unionism went into steep decline. Even Bismarck, however, did not dare ban the SPD; renewal of the 1878 law was passed in 1886 only with difficulty, and in 1890, following complicated wrangles within the Reichstag, a new version of the law was defeated. Less than four weeks later the SPD won 35 Reichstag seats and polled nearly one and a half million votes, despite the distortions of the electoral system. The advance of the party, however, continued to be hampered by weak trade unions and the commitment to Marxism, which terrified many potential supporters. Demands for a revision of party dogma became more insistent after 1890, led first by Vollmar and later by Bernstein. While a full revision and abandonment of Marxism was not achieved until the 1950s, by the early 1900s it was evident to many that if the SPD was revolutionary in theory, it was not so in practice. This impression was reinforced by the revival of the trade unions. In 1890 the unions established a new central body, headed by Legien, which campaigned for attainable objectives, such as increases in wages, shorter hours, better working conditions, unemployment relief, improved pensions, the recognition of collective bargaining, and so on. The political profile of the central union organization was also moderate, supporting reform rather than revolution. By 1906 it had forced the party to abandon its enthusiastic advocacy of the general strike as a weapon to achieve political change.

In these circumstances it is hardly surprising that the SPD made further political progress, though remaining encumbered by indifferent leadership and personal and ideological differences between Bebel, Bernstein, Kautsky, Liebknecht and Luxemburg. In 1903 in the Reichstag elections the SPD polled more votes than any other party and in 1912 it won the largest number of seats, 110. The form of government adopted by Bismarck's successors became ever more difficult to maintain as the parliamentary arithmetic changed. The early 1900s also witnessed, as in Britain, France and the USA, an upturn in industrial unrest. The principal causes of this seem to have been low wages, high food prices, some regional unemployment, and frustration with the political system. From 1905 until the outbreak of war in 1914 strikes were so common that on no occasion was the number of days lost annually fewer than five million; in 1910 the figure rose to as high as nine million. The progress of the SPD and the growth of industrial unrest produced near panic among the governing classes.

In republican France trade union activists and socialists seem similarly to have been viewed with little enthusiasm by the governing classes. It is true that the franchise was more equitable in France, but the system of elections virtually ensured after 1889 the return of a large majority of politicians whose views were republican and only mildly radical. Much of the establishment, especially in the Church, the armed forces and the higher ranks of the bureaucracy, held reactionary views little different from those of Waldersee. The Senate was even more conservative than the Chamber of Deputies, so those who ruled were generally unsympathetic towards the Left. Those who were prosperous in France – and these included most of the bourgeoisie and a large number of the peasants – were equally unlikely to support revolutionary doctrines. Recollections of the Commune terrified property owners, and the mass of citizens made nationalist by the desire to wipe out the shame of Sedan did not subscribe to the internationalism of the Left. Although governments changed, the attitudes of the nation's rulers and representatives evolved much more slowly. Instability was only on the surface; quite apart from the trials of the 1880s, French governments in the 1890s were resilient enough to survive the Panama scandal, the Dreyfus Affair and Déroulède's attempted coup in 1899. Yet behind this apparent confidence were deep-rooted fears, as was evident in attitudes towards trade unions and socialism.

French socialists were less well organized and well disciplined than their German counterparts. The French Workers' Party (POF) split into quarrelling groups, and in the 1880s signally failed to forge links with the trade unions. The unions themselves were weak, not least because of the prevalence of small firms. By the early 1890s there were some fifty socialist deputies in parliament – drawn mainly from three areas, the industrial north and north-east, the poorest agricultural regions of the centre and south, and Paris – but these did not form a cohesive group. The existence of significant anarchist and nihilist groups complicated the task of the socialists who were frequently, and usually erroneously, deemed guilty by association. The pivotal import-ance of the Franco-Russian alliance and the demands of the Russian government for the control of revolutionary groups in France created a serious problem for successive French governments. How could such control, demands for which found support among the bourgeoisie, be reconciled with the rather liberal French tradition of political asylum and the fundamental rights of free assembly, speech and belief?

It was impossible to devise a policy which would resolve such a fundamental conflict of interests. In practice stringent methods of control were adopted, especially against avowedly revolutionary groups, based upon the anti-anarchist laws of 1894. However, by the end of the decade it looked as if the government had trained its sights on the wrong targets. The revolutionary groups, despite an abundance of windy rhetoric, seemed less and less likely to pose significant danger. In the meantime links were being established between the socialists and the trade unions, and by 1898 the various socialist parties were polling about three-quarters of a million votes. This process was advanced by some of the worst industrial unrest in Europe, economic change and advance being punctuated by a series of bruising incidents. The most politically significant of these were the exchange of shots at Fourmies in 1891, railwaymen's strikes in 1898 and 1910, strikes at Chalon-sur-Saône in 1900 and Monceau-le-Mines in 1901, unrest among agricultural workers in 1904, 1907 and 1911, and disputes with civil servants in 1907 and 1909.

The growth of the trade union movement was both politically and industrially significant, despite the fact that it was subjected to many different pressures. The most practical aspects of trade union activity were to be found in the *bourses du travail*, the number of which grew rapidly in the 1890s, which acted simultaneously as labour exchanges, centres of information and welfare, and union headquarters. The *bourses* remained independent of the Federation of Trade Unions (where the influence of the Marxist intellectual Guesde was strong), and in 1892 set up their own federation, led from 1895 by Pelloutier (whose opinions were largely anarchist in character) and committed to unification of the trade union movement. This was temporarily made easier by the decision of the Federation of Trade Unions in 1894 to support the idea of a general strike, thus launching workers' organizations on the path of revolutionary syndicalism. In September 1895 the General Confederation of Labour (CGT) was established, though both Guesde and Pelloutier stood out against it; the CGT was firmly independent of all political groups, though plainly socialist in sympathies. In the meantime parliamentary socialism continued to advance under the leadership of Millerand, elected in 1885, and Jaurès, who rose to national fame in 1893.

The response of governments to the growth of socialism and trade-unionism was more flexible in France than in Germany. Restrictive or oppressive policies were pursued; despite the 1884 law permitting the formation of trade unions no government would permit its employees to join a union. When there were strikes the military might be called in; as Romein observed, 'The "good workman" . . . had only to raise his voice and the soldiers of the Republic were rushed to the spot to silence him.'[18] The power of anti-socialist reactions can be seen in the enthusiasm with which astute judges of the political mood, such as Clemenceau, embraced harsh measures. Governments and parties also found other ways of combating the socialist advance. Socialists were taken into administrations, beginning with Millerand in 1899; there they found their radicalism tamed or diluted. Once they had accepted office their status among many left-wing groups was irreparably damaged; this had the effect of reopening the disputes on the Left between those who believed in reform and parliamentarism, and those whose commitments were to revolution and the use of the strike as a political weapon.

In both countries attitudes towards and within the working classes were affected by the growth of pressure for social reform among religious groups. In Germany, despite the conservatism of religious hierarchies, concern about the poor and less privileged was a long-established feature of both Catholic and Protestant churches. Positions on such issues as the length of the working day, child labour, factory conditions, the provision of housing, insurance, and education became more liberal as the century drew to a close. In the early 1900s the leading role was taken by Naumann, who in his *Demokratie und Kaisertum*, published in 1902, advocated policies of social unity and of reconciliation between the state and the workers. Catholics and Protestants hoped, of course, to revitalize religious belief through their work with, and for, the poor. The effects were mixed. There was little sign of a genuine religious revival, and not much of a growth in support for the predominantly Catholic Centre Party at the expense of either socialists or liberals. The Centre Party, in any event, certainly did not challenge the established order of government by crusading for social reform; rather, it sought to protect privileges, especially in education, for the interests it represented. Nevertheless, the existence of Social Catholicism did nothing to advance the cause of working-class solidarity, and the genuine commitment of the religious groups to improving the lot of ordinary Germans eased the plight of the poor and probably reduced the already slim chances of revolution.

The situation in France was more complex, necessarily so as a large part of the Catholic Church remained obstinately committed to reactionary views – thus making reformism hard to adopt as a doctrine. The social conservatism of many devout Catholics spilled over into political and constitutional issues – the Dreyfus Affair, education, taxation, the monarchical movement against the Republic – and hence pointed reform more in the direction of the cautious, conservative reformism of Christian democracy, though even that threatened to split the Catholic Church. Yet there were those who persisted in their attempts to drag Catholicism away from its hostility to republicanism and legitimate secularism, most notably Piou in the 1890s. These bold souls were helped by the papal encyclical of 1891, *Rerum Novarum*, in which it was in effect argued that social activism was a Christian duty. The reformers then proceeded to involve themselves actively in social and economic affairs, founding their own Catholic trade unions, banks, cooperatives, welfare associations, libraries, meeting-places for working men, and publishing their own pamphlets, books, and most importantly, newspapers. In the end these activities did not produce a party of Christian democracy, but they helped ameliorate working conditions and thus, as in Germany, both reduced social tension and made it less likely that revolutionary doctrines would permeate the entire working classes.

If attention has thus far been concentrated upon the poor and the development of political and industrial movements intended to reflect their concerns and promote their interests, it should not be forgotten that this was also a period of great prosperity. There were, as in Britain, small numbers of the immensely rich, though these were less often found in the form of the owners of broad acres. Indeed, in Germany, and especially in Prussia, there were many traditional landowners who feared loss of both wealth and status. In France landholding patterns had been changed by the revolution and the social and political influence of the aristocracy had been substantially curtailed; even so, France was not bereft of either an aristocracy or great landowners. But in both states the influence of land was challenged by the growth of trade and industry. The most astute of the old aristocracy sought to preserve their power, prestige and prosperity by becoming involved in the flourishing sectors of the economy. By 1914 a significant number had succeeded. A new aristocracy of wealth, talent and enterprise had also emerged. This was an age when the captains of industry, the bankers, the leading brokers of Paris and Frankfurt, and the heads of great trading houses were famous for their wealth and influence. In the early 1900s the prominence of this class was remarkable; among its most famous members could be numbered Rouvier, Schneider, Motte, Ballin, Rathenau, Duisberg and the Siemens brothers. The very wealthy had much to lose from social conflict or revolution, and were willing to adopt a variety of measures in order to protect their position.

Prosperity was, however, widely spread among the middle classes. Economic development brought comfortable incomes to a large number of those involved in management and services; those who prospered exceptionally included the managers of firms and factories, engineers, builders, accountants, brokers and lawyers. Perhaps rather more surprisingly, academics, especially in Germany, were both well paid and influential. Certain kinds of suppliers, usually of quality products, and dealers, often in pictures, furnishings and other antiques, also prospered. Their prosperity and their high levels of consumption sustained an enormous class of domestic servants and the economic well-being of hotels, inns and holiday resorts. The middle classes in France and Germany built houses and bought apartments. It is not just in the great cities of Berlin, Paris, and Hamburg that the evidence of this wealth can be seen, but in the traditional provincial centres and in the university towns. Late Victorian and Edwardian prosperity, as exemplified in Oxford, pales into insignificance in comparison with the houses in, for example, Dijon or Göttingen.

The proportion of white-collar workers was increasing rapidly as a result of the growth of both service industries and governmental activity. This was particularly true in Germany where there were large numbers of officials, often ex-soldiers, who enjoyed modest incomes but special status. The railways, the post offices, local government, local courts of justice, the tax office, the bodies dealing with customs, excise, harbours, canals and so on were all major employers by 1914. The loyalties of their employees were to the state, and they rarely identified their interests with those of industrial or agricultural workers, especially when union activities appeared to threaten the established order of things. In France the growth of officialdom in these forms was less marked, though there was a large increase in the number of bureaucrats employed in ministries, local government, and by the prefects. Although administration in the departments was largely efficient and respected, often because of the close relations between local mayors and prefects, it was clearer in France than in Germany that the role of administration was frequently political in character. In other words, administration was not politically neutral but involved taking or implementing decisions with significant economic and social – and hence political – consequences. As a result, civil administration in France did not usually pretend to be 'above politics'. These officials held a slightly different status and were regarded rather differently in France from in Germany. But their own views were, perhaps, only marginally less conservative than those of their German counterparts.

The fact that so many in France and Germany were comfortably off, including some working-class people, meant that there was bound to be more than token resistance to the aims of revolutionaries and, perhaps, even to mild reformists. Yet the fact that the prosperous would resist parties, ideas, and movements in favour of the redistribution of wealth and property did not mean that their interests were entirely identifiable with those of the established authorities. The notion of a structural or social crisis suggests the existence of a situation in which government and society could not deal with social, economic, political, cultural, or ethnic demands without the need for changes which would irrevocably alter the established framework. The crisis might be 'solved' by revolution from below or above, but the existing system would be destroyed. In this sense the existence of class-based or occupation-related hostility to reform or change represented part of the structural crisis, and not a defence against it. If the middle classes did not want to see socialism triumph – which they did not – they had their own interests, which were only partly compatible with those of the existing rulers. The more flexible the political system the better the chances were of its modification; cautious reform would enable governments to harness the satisfied conservatism of the prosperous. To a considerable extent this delicate exercise in political juggling was successful in Britain, less so in France, and still less so in

Germany. It is, therefore, necessary to turn to those aspects of government and politics in France and Germany which led to this failure to produce a political system that matched economic and social structures.

Those who ruled in both countries were not so unintelligent that they failed to see that there were problems which could not easily be solved or disregarded. They were faced with awkward choices – which vested interests should be preserved and which sacrificed; which concessions should be made and which withheld? In retrospect, it may seem that governments stumbled from one crisis to another, concerned only with immediate survival, with no overview of the situation and no long-term plan – in short, a modern version of the Danegeld payments. Alternatively, it may seem as if governments worked ruthlessly to control or eliminate dangerous threats, creating coalitions of interests, albeit at the expense of complicated concessions, to ward off the triumph of the utterly unacceptable. This has been a favoured description for governments in Wilhelmine Germany. It has been argued that *Weltpolitik* was used to prop up authoritarianism, that concessions were made in a number of areas of policy and to a number of interest groups in order to preserve the electoral system and a Reichstag of limited power which permitted such authoritarianism, and that there was a deliberate and consistent attempt to reduce or isolate the influence of the SPD in order to maintain the privileges of important groups. This was certainly the opinion of liberals such as Delbrück, who feared that nationalism and authoritarianism had, by the end of the nineteenth century, almost completely perverted what he saw as the true purposes of unification.

Though it would be wrong to suggest that there was no truth in this description of Wilhelmine government, it is far from being completely accurate. As so often in human affairs, governments were neither entirely devoid of a plan nor agreed on one – still less able to carry out such a plan had it existed. In other words, governments in Germany recognized that there were problems, and that some of these problems were linked, but not that they were structural and hence required comprehensive treatment. If anyone intelligent among the ruling groups held such a pessimistic view it was most probably Bismarck himself, and he left office in 1890. Indeed, there were many, and not just supporters of the new government, who argued that one of Bismarck's most unscrupulous characteristics had been his habit of representing the situation of first, Prussia and later, Germany as one of perpetual and overwhelming crisis from which only his arts could rescue the state. The reaction against Bismarck, especially in the 1890s, was such that his successors took, if anything, a rather optimistic view of both Germany's place in the world and the government's capacity to govern. In due course, following numerous disappointments, there was a reaction against this in the 1900s in the form of a return to neo-Bismarckian pessimism and post-Bismarckian bloc-building in politics.

What exactly, then, was wrong with German government and why did this matter? The most obvious failing was that in a period of economic growth and social change the structure of government, from its electoral base to the attitudes of those at the apex, did not keep pace with these developments. As Jerome K. Jerome presciently observed, 'Hitherto, the German has had the blessed fortune to be exceptionally well governed; if this continues, it will go well with him – when his troubles will begin will be when by any chance something goes wrong with the governing machine.'[19] In fact, a whole series of mistakes and omissions characterized the years from 1890–1914. Changing fashion has at times attributed the debasement of government to the prejudices, folly, and frivolity of William II, to the departure, or, alternatively, the heritage of Bismarck, to the selfishness of the Junkers, to the corruption of big business interests, to the lack of a spirit of liberalism among the middle classes in Germany, and so on. All of these observations contain a substantial element of truth, but none is a sufficient explanation in itself. The principal and overriding fault was that the imperial constitution failed to develop along democratic lines; if anything, Germany was less democratic and more authoritarian, though less consistently efficient, in 1890 than in 1871, and in 1914 than in 1890.

The weakness of democracy was evident at the most basic level, that of the franchise. Ostensibly it was democratic, as long as the existence of women is ignored, since all male citizens aged twenty-five were able to vote by secret ballot. Constituencies were, however, very far from equal in size and this problem grew worse as boundaries were not revised, despite large-scale migration to the cities. By 1912 some constituencies were ten times larger than others. This state of affairs favoured the more conservative parties and the Centre Party in particular. In order to win a seat it was necessary for a party to win an absolute majority in that constituency; thus a second round of voting was quite common, and this enabled deals to be struck. As a result, despite a significant increase in turnout as the years went by (from 50.7 per cent in 1871 to 84.5 per cent in 1912), the SPD was significantly disadvantaged,[20] being grossly under-represented in the Reichstag.

Nor was the Bundesrat, or Federal Council, an effective body in assisting the development of democracy. It had been created to represent the twenty-five states which constituted the German Empire, thus recognizing the fact that unification had in part been achieved through the voluntary surrender of sovereignty by some states. In turn, states' rights were given limited recognition. Certain elements of taxation were dealt with by states such as Baden, Bavaria, and Württemberg; these involved principally customs and excise duties, and revenues from the postal and telegraph systems. But the sums of money involved were not large enough to be able to ensure any genuine independence for the states south of the Main. On paper the rights and duties of the Bundesrat looked impressive; in practice it was a pretty feeble body, unable to assert itself against Prussian hegemony. Prussia held only seventeen of the fifty-eight seats, but its dominance was assured by veto power over all legislation relating to the armed forces, taxation, customs and excise, or any constitutional change. Its position was also strengthened by close association with some small near-absolutist states, such as the Mecklenburgs.

Constitutional arrangements within the states affected not merely the membership of their assemblies (where such bodies existed), but also operation of the federal system. In Prussia the House of Representatives was elected by a 'three-class franchise', voters being assigned to one of three groups of electoral weight according to the amount of tax paid.[21] The lowest of these three classes contained over 90 per cent of the voters; the system thus favoured the wealthy few rather than the numerous poor, and the countryside rather than the towns. Because Prussia contained so many of Germany's citizens and so much of its wealth, its political practices were of special significance. In Prussia administration was firmly in the hands of the emperor, landed nobility, great industrial barons, and high-ranking officials; their conservatism was notorious, and when they were not conservative they were far more commonly reactionary than liberal. As Prussian government was almost synonymous with German government, its lack of accountability became of national importance.

The working head of the imperial government was the chancellor, who also doubled as the minister-president of Prussia. He and other ministers were appointed, or dismissed, by the emperor. They had no real obligation of accountability to the Reichstag or Bundesrat except that which they freely offered, a rare occurrence, or that implied by Article 72, which required the chancellor to present an annual account of expenditure; nor could they be dismissed by the Reichstag or Bundesrat. The emperor also had the power to dissolve the Reichstag, or to prorogue its sittings or those of the Bundesrat. This power was nominally limited but was in practice substantial. Increasingly the emperor was seen by supporters and opponents alike as the real sovereign. There were thus few obstacles to his personal rule, or to that of a chancellor backed by him.

The armed forces remained in effect a state within a state. All German troops were bound by oath to obey the emperor unconditionally in his capacity as commander-in-chief. There was no civilian authority over the military, and the ministers who dealt with military matters were Prussian, and hence accountable not to the Reichstag but to the Prussian House of Representatives which, given that body's composition, meant not accountable at all. Despite recurrent problems over finance and conscription, the armed forces treated the civil authorities with repeated contempt, most notoriously in 1913 at Zabern. The emperor and the armed forces knew that many Germans saw them, rather than parliamentary bodies, as the symbols of unification and greatness, and did not hesitate to trade upon this feeling. Indeed, the army sought to perpetuate its hold upon German citizens by encouraging the growth of veterans' associations, regular parades, the provision of jobs for its loyal servants, and the use of honorary commissions to acquire new allies among civilians. Thus the armed forces, while far from devoid of popular backing, formed part of the ruling system and shared its values rather than being representative of the citizens of Germany as a whole.

A further democratic weakness lay in the inadequacy of the party system. By 1900 there existed numerous parties, some exclusively regional, as in the case of the Danish Party, and others with national status and appeal, but which were often heavily dependent upon a particular section or class of voters, as in the case of the Centre Party. The smaller parties usually won 15 to 20 per cent of seats in the Reichstag and had two adverse effects on the prospects for properly accountable government. First, their appeal siphoned off votes that in all probability would otherwise have gone to cautious, preponderantly middle-class parties. This fragmented opposition to the groupings further to the Left or Right. Second, their tenuous existence and limited objectives made them anxious to do deals with the government. In return for often quite minor concessions their support was secured for measures which preserved the authoritarian character of political life. The larger parties were, equally, interest groups with more substantial followings. During this period five played a significant part in political life – the SPD, the Centre Party, the Conservatives (usually in alliance with the much smaller Reichspartei), National

Liberals, and Independent Liberals (who, usually south of the Main, appeared as the People's Party). The political balance was distinctly right-of-centre in the Reichstag, therefore. Only the SPD stood clearly on the Left; on some issues it might be supported by the Centre Party or the Independent Liberals, but almost never by both. This situation, although not created by Bismarck and his successors, was most agreeable to them, as it provided good prospects of either majority rule or a minority government against which the opposition would find it hard to muster a majority.

These institutional defects, combined with what Meinecke described as 'a levelling habit of conformity of mind which narrowed the vision and also often led to a thoughtless subserviency toward all higher authorities',[22] led to a failure to secure the advance of democracy. Indeed, it is not entirely unfair to suggest that many Germans did not even begin to consider what the implications of this democratic deficit might be in the long term. The preamble to the 1871 Constitution seemed almost to suggest that institutions and rights were in the gift of the emperor, rather than the necessary building blocks of a united, free and democratic state. As long as the economy continued to grow, as long as most Germans became increasingly prosperous, and as long as Germany seemed secure, it is hardly surprising that relatively few Germans saw the risks attached to the perpetuation of an increasingly anachronistic authoritarianism. Those who did often had quite irreconcilable views on how to reform or change the system. Thus the structural crisis grew worse, but its collapse not more imminent.

Bismarck and his successors, naturally enough, were reluctant to leave more than was necessary to chance. They were able to behave much of the time as politicians did elsewhere in western Europe. Quite legitimately they sought to reduce or eliminate dangers, and to consolidate support. These actions took a variety of forms. The social insurance schemes were in part designed to reduce working class discontent. The tariffs on grain pleased the Junkers, and industrial tariffs were popular with many small manufacturers and, initially, with many great industrial barons. Despite the possible benefits from free trade, Germany's outlook was basically protectionist throughout this period. After the experiences of the *Kulturkampf*, governments were prudent enough to rein in their desire to control the Catholic Church. Once the Centre Party became a key element in informal coalitions it could be safely assumed that the government, with the startling exception of Bülow during 1907–9, would leave Catholic interests in education and agricultural protection largely untouched. Even the heavy expenditure on a large navy after 1897 probably ought to be seen as an attempt to placate a number of vociferous groups – steel producers, shipbuilders, international traders, the imperial lobby – rather than a considered attempt to overthrow British naval primacy or to grasp after world power. In undertaking these and other policies German leaders behaved in a way which would have been regarded as normal in Britain, France or the United States. If some of these policies proved unwise, it is not obvious that they were undemocratic or irrelevant to public concerns.

The democratic deficit was present nevertheless. It was present in the sense that many of these policies were never properly debated, unlike, for example, the introduction of tariffs by France and the United States, or their rejection by Britain. It was also apparent in the fact that governments were not in reality chosen by the voters through the party system via a majority in the Reichstag, and that, once chosen, governments were not properly accountable to elected representatives. Censorship, control of the press, abuse of the administrative system and the judicial process showed the authoritarian nature of the government. German citizens were expected to be obedient and to let the government decide what was best for them. The rules of the political game were so arranged that the authorities won even when they lost; short of a revolution it is hard to see how there could have been a real change in the government – a fact which made the exercise of the vote less important than it ought to have been. Finally, the fact that Germany's rulers were prepared to consider the possibility of a *Staatsstreich* – even though they hoped to avoid using this ultimate weapon – is evidence enough that they felt that some decisions were too important to be left to the people. Cut off from their own people by such beliefs, it ought not to be a cause of surprise that Germany's leaders failed to comprehend the concerns of the peoples of other nations. It was this combination of 'national egoism and the state-power idea'[23] which ultimately launched Germany into war and turned the long-standing structural crisis into the catastrophe which destroyed the old system.

Both on and beneath the surface the nature of French politics was very different. France was, albeit as much by accident as design, a republic. Furthermore, its character was firmly bourgeois and individualist. By 1890 the possibility of a monarchical restoration was remote, and by 1914 virtually inconceivable. There was an aristocracy, and aristocrats did play some part in political and administrative affairs, but of a limited nature. The kind of leadership provided by the emperor or chancellor in Germany was almost wholly absent from

French politics until the crisis of 1914. The seven men who held the office of president between 1887 and the outbreak of war were experienced politicians, comfortable with the traditions of republican, bourgeois France and chosen for that very reason by the National Assembly. After MacMahon and Grévy the French preference was for presidents – until the prolonged international crisis of 1911–14 produced Poincaré – who would play a ceremonial, rather than a key political role. In fact, the powers of the president were so limited that in 1895 Casimir-Périer resigned, remarking on the contrast between 'the burden of the moral responsibilities that weigh on me [and] . . . the powerlessness to which I am condemned'.[24] Nor did the heads of the numerous administrations which governed during this period, some twenty-five in all, possess the powers of either their German or British equivalents. Changes of governments did not usually lead to substantial changes in the composition of the ministries, either in personnel or political balance. Right and Left were largely excluded until 1914.

The result of these characteristics was that governments were more often bent upon survival than action. It was not that governments could not act – there are numerous examples of strong policies, boldly pursued, during this period, among them Dupuy's laws of 1894 against the anarchists, Méline's tariffs, Combes's 1904 anti-clerical legislation, and the Rouvier government's 1905 law on the separation of Church and State. Equally, there were other important issues from which a majority of politicians backed away; these included attempts to obtain votes for women, the continuing Dreyfus Affair, the introduction of income tax, and demands for proportional representation. Not only did the formation of governments prove difficult, so did their maintenance – especially if there were ministers who wished to do things, at least on any grand scale. Despite the regular fall of ministries, governing France was, on the whole, a comfortable and tranquil process, though somewhat disguised by the French custom of describing almost all of their politicians as crooks or rogues claiming as issues of national importance even the most minor defects of a ministry. Most politicians were not thin-skinned, which was just as well given the tradition of scathing attacks on them in parliament and in the press.

French governments were so constructed and constrained because of the character and interests of those elected as representatives of the people. The apparent simplicity of adult male suffrage was rendered more complex by the perpetuation of constituencies of unequal size, which favoured the more conservative, generally rural, areas over the more radical, usually urban, districts. The constitutional changes of the 1880s reinforced this conservatism. The 1882 law which gave municipal councils (except Paris) the right to elect their own mayors helped cement the partnership between local politicians, the prefect and the parliamentary representatives which so characterized the Third Republic. The 1884 changes to the Senate electoral law, while abolishing the principle of life senators, left the election of senators to an indirect process, essentially by local notables. Finally, in 1889 the experiment of the *scrutin de liste* was abandoned, and the return to the *arrondissement* system strengthened the position of the independent with strong local connections. The result of this was that power was wielded by a rather large and predominantly bourgeois oligarchy. If the political class was on display in Paris, its roots lay in the provinces. A large proportion, even in 1914, of those who made up the centre of the political spectrum were, in fact, independents rather than party, or even faction, loyalists. Groupings, especially in the Senate, were loose associations of individuals rather than tightly-knit and disciplined organizations. Both senators and deputies respected the power of local opinion within their constituencies, and were generally assiduous in their protection and advancement of local interests. There was a fairly consistent ascendency of local issues over national questions in the bargaining process which led to the formation of ministries. Once a representative was established in his constituency, unless he was foolishly lazy, death or a major scandal were more likely causes of his removal than the swing of the political pendulum.

This form of government made France more obviously democratic than Germany. Elections meant more, and those chosen to represent the people had greater freedom of action. But there was a price to be paid for the way the system worked – the difficulty of achieving coherence in government. Neither the president nor the prime minister could wield strong executive powers without the consent of parliament. The Senate could, and did, act as a counterweight to the Chamber of Deputies; this, as in other bicameral systems in which both chambers are elected, caused problems, especially the risk of deadlock. By 1914 the growth in power of the Senate, accentuated by the long tenure (nine years) of its members, made it an increasingly attractive home for ambitious politicians – unlike the House of Lords, or the Bundesrat. The power of the parliamentary groups in France was certainly not less than in Germany, and that of the individual deputy was much greater. This too had its price. The most important power wielded by the deputy was that of *interpellation*, which was the right to interrupt the order of the day's business by asking a minister to explain some matter involving his department. The results were not infrequently spectacular, and it was not uncommon for ministries to fall as a consequence of a well-judged intervention on a sensitive issue. The cost of this right was an increased likelihood of governmental instability, and hence, perhaps, a reduced possibility of effective legislation or the establishment of a proper programme of government.

The absence of a coherent programme had not seemed to matter until the 1890s. It had seemed enough for governments to assert that their purpose was to regenerate France by means of establishing a strong, secular, participatory republic; this was enough to unite a clear majority. The slowly changing nature of politics was reflected in the gradual shifts in political ascendency between 1871 and the mid-1890s from monarchists to conservatives to opportunists to progressivists. This peaceful evolutionary process was then interrupted in the 1890s in a way which changed the assumptions of both governed and governing. Governments were faced with a series of problems which tested their ability both to govern and to reflect the wishes of the people. They were only partially successful in tackling these problems, and, equally, failed to re-establish that lost consensus of the 1880s in an appropriate contemporary form.

The problems which arose in the 1890s were in some cases new, in others the remains of unfinished business from the past. In the latter category may be placed the church–state and the civil–military relationships. Before the 1890s the process of secularization had advanced as far as it could without a frontal assault upon the redoubts of Catholic education and property. The altered positions of the Papacy and the Catholic Church in France on a number of issues in the 1890s compelled a re-examination of the relationship. The most significant points of conflict were education, laicization, socio-economic issues, and the increasing identification of the Church with the extreme anti-republican Right. These difficulties were much magnified and complicated by the emergence of a coherent anti-republican political movement, led by Déroulède, and given intellectual thrust by Maurras, Barrès and others. If their monarchical enthusiasm was unattractive to many Frenchmen, their nationalism, anti-Semitism, and pro-Catholic positions were powerful counterweights. Their advocacy of an army virtually free from what they asserted to be the corrupting influences of republicanism and egalitarianism seemed to make sense in a period when so many Frenchmen felt that they were hemmed in by enemies on all sides. The Dreyfus Affair proved a catalyst for the revival of a whole range of issues previously regarded as dead or moribund. Worse still, the Dreyfus Affair split the old republican consensus, and it was not until the early 1900s that a new radical, republican bloc was established. Once in power, following the elections of 1902, the bloc took vigorous action against both Church and army. Promotion within the armed forces became a matter for the government, especially in the case of high-level appointments, and not for the previously ultra-conservative and self-perpetuating military hierarchy. The educational and property rights of the Church were fundamentally revised by the legislation of 1904–5.

The renewal of radical, republican opinion in the face of an apparent challenge from the Right brought, however, in its train other political difficulties. In order to resist the Right, concessions had to be made to the Left; yet republican moderates no more wished to aid the triumph of Jaurès and the socialists than Déroulède and the reactionaries. Political necessity had compelled the moderates and the Left to act as partners in resisting the Right, but much that was old and much that was new divided the reluctant associates. The moderates predominantly shared with the Right their enthusiasm for nationalism, imperialism, and the rights of property owners. They were also often anti-Semitic and Catholic. The Left, by contrast, was internationalist (if only formally so in some cases), anti-colonialist, egalitarian, in favour of redistribution of wealth and free-thinking, and was generally sympathetic to the Jews. The growth of an urban working class, a trade union movement, and socialist political ideas were new features of political life in late nineteenth-century France; the moderates had little sympathy for, and virtually no identification with, any of these new developments. Even the Radicals, who bridged the gap between the moderates and the Left proper, largely shared the attitude of the moderates towards these matters.

The purpose of governments, having defeated the Right, then became that of containing the Left. The groups which sustained governments in the decade before 1914 were the Radicals and Radical-Socialists. Their formula obviously enjoyed considerable public support, for in the elections of 1906 they won as many seats as the Left and Right combined. It was thus not difficult for them to make slight adjustments to policy in order to secure the acquiescence of either Left or Right, according to the issue in question, or, as became increasingly common as the years passed, to establish an informal alliance with moderate conservative forces which usually controlled about forty votes in the Chamber of Deputies. Thus by 1913, as the election of Poincaré to the presidency confirmed, governments were generally of a conservative and cautious nature, though plainly not of the Right. From the ministry of Clemenceau (October 1906 to July 1909) onwards, governments dealt harshly with manifestations of left-wing activism. Strikes were vigorously repressed, proposed electoral reforms were rejected, and income tax was only accepted by the Radicals in the Chamber of Deputies safe in the knowledge that the Senate would throw the proposals out. Attempts to control rearmament and the extension of conscription were abandoned. Small wonder, then, that the Left saw the governments as conservative or even reactionary.

The structural and social crisis which faced France in the early twentieth century was thus rather different from that in Germany. Despite the fact that France enjoyed parliamentary democracy, bolstered by a strong local component, there existed a democratic deficit. The electoral system did favour moderately conservative forces, whose core support could be found among the bourgeoisie, wealthier peasants and white-collar workers, at the expense of the old Right and the Left. The nature of political groupings made it easier to push forward specific measures, or to prevent them, than to promote a comprehensive programme. There thus arose, inevitably, the question of what the parties stood for. Right and Left were more or less in agreement that the groups most commonly in government were concerned with the protection of vested interests, including their own hold on power. Right and Left tended to place political, social, economic and cultural issues in a fairly coherent ideological framework. Most politicians chosen by the French people did not hold strong viewpoints, or when they did were simultaneously, for example, strongly nationalist and anti-clerical. They saw nothing inconsistent in allying with the Right on the former, and with the Left on the latter. The chief element, then, in the democratic deficit was the lack of a real alternative in government, as both Left and Right were regarded by the mass of the electorate as not to be trusted. Not only was this absence of alternative dangerous in normal times, being likely to encourage corruption and engender complacency, but in periods of crisis it found governments in power which were in composition and attitude ill-equipped to take hard decisions.

The continuing hold on power of the Radicals and their allies demonstrated the intractability of the problem. Changing economic and social conditions had produced a new poor in France, heavily concentrated and politically under-represented. To avert the spectre of revolution or class war it was necessary to undertake some reforms, but to do so effectively would have required a more comprehensive review of political, social and economic assumptions than the Radicals would have found acceptable. The Radicals were no longer, by 1906, a force for change, yet they were not entirely comfortable when in power. It is hard to know for what principles Clemenceau or Caillaux stood; in any event their uncertainties mirrored those of the groupings that supported them. In the short term the collective inability of the voters to recognize the seriousness of the domestic problems facing France reinforced by the *immobilisme* of the electoral system, was hidden by the demand for national unity in the face of the darkening international situation. Anti-German feeling, as in Britain in the same period, provided a convenient glue with which to stick together an increasingly fragmented society. Politics in pre-1914 France thus already provided, in minor key, a version of *L'Union Sacrée*, though without the outbreak of war it is hard to see how this spurious national unity could have long continued.

France and Germany thus provide an interesting contrast in terms of political systems attempting to adjust to economic and social change. In both countries the preferred answer among those who ruled was to exclude hostile groups from power and influence by means of an electoral system which discriminated against them. The weakness of party, unlike in the United States or Britain, prevented any compensating form of democratic balance emerging. In Germany, if this method failed, the answer was to be sought in increased authoritarianism, to which the alternative would be revolution. In France, dominated by a political class which distrusted state power, the answer to powerful challenges was a mixture of the temporary exercise of strong measures and the reconstruction of a political consensus by limited concessions which would remove some opponents without imperilling core support. Both in theory and in practice the French response to awkward issues was more democratic and sensitive than the German. But by 1914 both countries faced a serious domestic situation because of an unwillingness, perhaps an inability, to control vested interests; if there was one simple cause of this state of affairs, it was that these governments only too accurately represented those interests.

NOTES

1 J. Romein, *The Watershed of Two Eras: Europe in 1900* (Middletown: Wesleyan University Press, 1978), pp. 24–5.
2 B. Tuchman, *The Proud Tower* (London: Bantam, 1966), p. xv.
3 Quoted in G. F. Kennan, *The Decline of Bismarck's European Order* (Princeton: Princeton University Press, 1979), p. 413.
4 See, amongst other works, G. Krumeich, *Armaments and Politics in France on the Eve of the First World War* (Leamington: Berg,

1984), pp. 25–7; and J. J. C. Joffre, *The Memoirs of Marshal Joffre*, vol. 1 (London: Bles, 1932), esp. pp. 83–112.

5 N. F. Grant (ed.), *The Kaiser's Letters to the Tsar* (London: Hodder & Stoughton, 1921), p. 101.

6 M. Gilbert, *Sir Horace Rumbold* (London: Heinemann, 1973), p. 139.

7 G. P. Gooch and H. Temperley (eds), *British Documents on the Origins of the War, 1898–1914*, vol. 3 (London: HMSO, 1928), p. 419.

8 A good account of the cultural context of anti-Semitism in Germany in this period can be found in: G. L. Mosse, *Germans and Jews* (London: Orbach & Chambers, 1971).

9 *Journal of the Royal United Service Institution*, 54 (London, 1910).

10 This did not apply to coalmining, where mergers had been forbidden since the early 1850s.

11 J.-M. Mayer and M. Rebérioux, *The Third Republic from its Origins to the Great War, 1871–1914* (Cambridge: Cambridge University Press, 1989), p. 268.

12 The best brief account of German industrial development can be found in W. O. Henderson, *The Rise of German Industrial Power, 1834–1914* (London: Temple Smith, 1975).

13 See J. Bouvier, F. Furet, and M. Gillet, *Le Mouvement du profit en France au XIXe siècle* (Paris: Mouton, 1965).

14 Neither the German 'Mittelstand' nor the French 'bourgeoisie' accurately conveys the picture conjured up of the British middle classes of the same era. However, the problems of definition are so complex that it seems least unsatisfactory to refer to 'the middle classes', while acknowledging that use of this term begs almost as many questions as it answers.

15 J.-M. Mayer and M. Rebérioux, op. cit., p. 353.

16 E. Weber, *Peasants into Frenchmen: The Modernization of Rural France, 1870–1914* (London: Chatto & Windus, 1979), p. 338.

17 G. A. Craig, *Germany, 1866–1945* (Oxford: Clarendon Press, 1978), p. 189. Curiously, given this verdict, he also quotes with apparent approval Fontane's comment of 1898: 'The workers have attacked everything in a new way; they not only have new goals but new methods of attaining them' (p. 270).

18 J. Romein, op. cit., p. 163.

19 J. K. Jerome, *Three Men on the Bummel* (Harmondsworth: Penguin, 1987), p. 201.

20 The clearest short account of the 1871 Constitution and its working

can be found in E. M. Hucko, *The Democratic Tradition: Four German Constitutions* (Oxford: Berg, 1989), pp. 22–38.

21 A good summary of the way this worked can be found in N. Stone, *Europe Transformed, 1878–1919* (London: Collins, 1983), pp. 167–8.

22 F. Meinecke, *The German Catastrophe* (Boston: Beacon, 1963), p. 11.

23 ibid., p. 21.

24 Quoted in J.-M. Mayer and M. Rebérioux, op. cit., p. 163.

FURTHER READING

There are many good general histories of France and Germany in this period. France is well covered in J.-M. Mayer and M. Rebérioux, *The Third Republic from its Origins to the Great War, 1871–1914* (Cambridge, 1989); R. D. Anderson, *France 1870–1914: Politics and Society* (London, 1977); S. Hoffmann, *France: Change and Tradition* (London, 1963); and the old, but invaluable, D. Brogan, *The Development of Modern France, 1870–1939* (London, 1967). Extremely well informed, but difficult to digest, is T. Zeldin, *France, 1848–1945* (Oxford, 1973 and 1977). Also of interest, though now greatly dated by its Marxist perspective, is R. Magraw, *France, 1815–1914: The Bourgeois Century* (Oxford, 1983). For Germany the best starting-point is G. A. Craig, *Germany, 1866–1945* (Oxford, 1978). Other very useful works include H.-U. Wehler, *The German Empire, 1871–1918* (Leamington Spa, 1984); A. Ramm, *Germany, 1789–1919* (London, 1967); H. Holborn, *A History of Modern Germany, 1840–1945* (London, 1969); and R. J. Evans (ed.), *Society and Politics in Wilhelmine Germany* (London, 1978).

Social and economic issues have received an enormous amount of attention. I have found these works, some of which have received mention in the footnotes, particularly helpful: W. O. Henderson, *The Rise of German Industrial Power, 1834–1914* (London, 1975); D. S. Landes, *The Unbound Prometheus* (Cambridge, 1969); P. Gay, *The Dilemma of Democratic Socialism: Edward Bernstein's Challenge to Marx* (New York, 1962); F. Stern, *The Politics of Cultural Despair: A Study in the Rise of the Germanic Ideology* (Berkeley, 1961); A. J. Mayer, *The Persistence of the Old Regime* (London, 1981); E. Weber, *Peasants into Frenchmen: The Modernization of Rural France, 1870–1914* (London, 1979); B. H. Moss, *The Origins of the French Labour Movement, 1830–1914* (Berkeley, 1976); J. Merriman (ed.), *Cities in Nineteenth-century France* (London, 1981); J. Howorth and P. Cerny (eds), *Elites in France: Origins, Reproduction and Power* (London, 1981); F. Caron, *An Economic History of Modern France* (London, 1979); R. Rémond, *The Right Wing in France from 1815 to de Gaulle* (Philadelphia, 1969).

Other works dealing with more general political, military or religious issues which the reader is likely to find helpful include: D. Johnson, *France and the Dreyfus Affair* (London, 1966); J. McManners, *Church and State in France, 1870–1914* (London, 1972); M. Larkin, *Church and State after the Dreyfus Affair* (London, 1974); J. J. Sheehan, *German Liberalism in the Nineteenth Century* (London, 1982); G. Eley, *Reshaping the German Right* (London, 1980); D. S. White, *The Splintered Party* (Cambridge, Mass., 1976); G. A. Craig, *The Politics of the Prussian Army, 1640–1945* (Oxford, 1964); D. Porch, *The March to the Marne* (London, 1981); G. L. Mosse, *Germans and Jews* (London, 1971).

3 Russia and Austria-Hungary: empires under pressure

Paul Hayes

During the war of 1914–18 the Romanov and Habsburg empires collapsed. Though the timing and circumstances of their fall were different it is, nevertheless, evident that the principal cause was that of the effects of the war upon the political and economic systems of the two states which eventually rendered their governments helpless. Widespread agreement on the existence of a relationship between the strains of war and imperial collapse masks profound disagreement concerning the strengths and capacities of the two states in the quarter-century preceding 1914. It has been argued that both states were strong, or that both were weak, or that Russia was strong but Austria-Hungary weak and vice versa. Historians have adduced evidence from all aspects of life: the economy, society, culture, religion, nationalities, political representation, the legal and administrative systems, and, perhaps most significantly, the conflicts between traditionalism and modernization. Contemporary opinion in the two states was similarly unagreed on their actual and relative strength and, in addition, was often characterized by wishful thinking, national interest or prejudice, rather than by observation and rigorous analysis.

The impression of impending collapse was widespread in the West, among both allies and enemies of the two states. In March 1914 Jagow disparagingly remarked of Austria-Hungary: 'the want of cohesion in the Monarchy ... was becoming more marked every day.'[1] Acute British and French observers, such as Wavell and Langlois, were similarly concerned about the fate of Russia. Inside the two empires the advocates of bombastic expansionism vied for attention with the prophets of gloom and doom. In the Western democracies ludicrous optimism and deep despair were also not unknown, but the nature of political life perhaps encouraged the peoples and governments of those states to take a more dispassionate and less apocalyptic view of the future than in the two great empires of eastern Europe. Those who predicted the imminent demise of the French or British empires were certainly treated less seriously than their counterparts in Austria-Hungary and Russia. The fact is that the development of the economy, society and government posed very different challenges to institutions and beliefs in eastern Europe. It is these developments and challenges to which it is now necessary to turn.

Any examination of basic facts about the two empires reveals important similarities and differences. Neither state possessed overseas territories, unlike the other great powers, but both had large minority populations mainly concentrated in territories on the periphery. Only about 45 per cent of Russia's population in 1914 was Russian; in Austria-Hungary Germans and Magyars between them comprised about 44 per cent. According to the 1897 census the population of Russia was almost 129 million; fairly accurate estimates suggest that the figures for 1890 and 1914 were, respectively, 117.8 million and 178 million. Most of this population lived west of the Urals. Austria-Hungary was much smaller in size and population. In 1890, including Bosnia-Hercegovina, the population was about 43 million, rising to 51.4 million by the census of 1910; by 1914 it stood at about 52.5 million. In Russia attitudes towards non-Russians were complex. Pan-Slavism coexisted rather uneasily with the contempt and distrust exhibited towards, among others, Poles and Ukrainians. Among the better-educated non-Russian groups the Balts were often influential, Georgians and Armenians much less commonly so. In the remote provinces of the east and south-east the inhabitants were dominated in high imperial style. Anti-Semitism was a strong force, as it was in Austria-Hungary, especially in Vienna. In the Habsburg domains the treatment of the smaller ethnic groups – Poles, Czechs, Slovaks, Ruthenes, Romanians, Serbs, Croats, Slovenes and Italians – varied enormously. The situation differed markedly from that in Russia, however. In Austria-Hungary the ruling élite was principally drawn from two distinct peoples, roughly equal in number – Germans and Magyars. To complicate matters these very different peoples often held incompatible opinions and sought irreconcilable objectives.

These basic differences influenced the ways the empires were ruled, the development of their societies, the claims of nationalities, the progress of education, trade, industry and agriculture, and the evolution of their legal systems. Furthermore, the 1879 alliance between Germany and Austria-Hungary and the 1894 Franco-Russian alliance imposed external disciplines and demands. These associations required sacrifices as well as conferring benefits and, not infrequently, cut across the internal needs of the empires. The possession of great power status added to existing strains and pressures, a matter of particular importance in the absence of satisfactory representative institutions to absorb or channel dissent and discontent. Yet, important though these external connections were, they were of marginal significance in comparison with the influence of rapidly changing internal conditions upon the governments of the two empires.

In Russia the tsar was perched at the apex of government. The two tsars in this period were poorly trained in duties of government and administration. Worse still, both the nasty and brutish Alexander III (1881–94) and his gentler, but equally stubborn, son Nicholas II (1894–1917), had hardly been educated in any broad sense of the word. As a result neither was able to comprehend ideas and attitudes beyond those existing within a narrow section of society, nor were their personalities suited to the tasks which confronted them. Not unfairly they have been thus characterized: 'Alexander III ... was distinguished only by his bulk, meanness and uxoriousness',[2] and Nicholas II 'was armed only with a knowledge of languages, a love of military ceremonial, and the reactionary creed dinned into him by his political tutor'.[3] Nicholas II was also preoccupied with the problem of the succession, as his only son, Alexei, born in 1904, was a haemophiliac and unlikely, therefore, even if he survived to adulthood, to make an effective ruler.

The incapacity of the tsars was not corrected in the lower tiers of government. Ministers were appointed by the tsar; those at the head of important departments such as foreign affairs, finance, war, or the interior, often spent as much time intriguing against rivals as they did on formulating, explaining and implementing policy. This dismal situation was made worse by the lack of a real system of collective evaluation of policy. There was a ministerial committee but, unencumbered by any notion of collective responsibility, its consultations were not binding on individuals. Its chairman had no special authority, nor had he privileged access to the tsar. The ministers were automatically members of the State Council, the bulk of whose membership consisted of notables – such as provincial governors, generals, admirals, ambassadors and academics – usually appointed for life at or towards the end of a long career in the service of the state. The State Council was supposed to advise on legislation by examining draft laws. This was achieved by dividing its business into three sections: the state economy, general legislation, and civil and religious administration. Following the reform of 1899 a fourth section was added to deal with trade, industry, science and technology. Many of the bureaucrats serving these sections were men of intellect, education and experience.[4]

The effectiveness of this body was reduced because its fifty or so members were all directly appointed by the tsar. Criteria which had little to do with professional expertise thus often determined membership. The State Council dated from 1810, but its potential for political development had been destroyed by the Fundamental Laws of 1832 which had reaffirmed autocracy. Until the changes of 1906 all imperial decrees, commands, and even oral instructions, had the force of law. Tsars did not hesitate to ignore advice from the State Council if it conflicted with their views, though the State Council's own profile was habitually conservative. As late as 1913, for example, it rejected a Duma proposal to define bureaucratic responsibilities more exactly in order thus to open the way for prosecution of officials suspected of having broken the law.

The relationship between government, administration and the rule of law was less clear in Russia than in most contemporary states. The highest court of review was the Senate – whose members were bureaucrats appointed by the tsar. Consequently, it was only intermittently effective as a watchdog, and the exemption from its jurisdiction of state agencies and many key ministries further attenuated its authority. The lack of a proper code of administrative law promoted an impression of corruption and arbitrariness; even just decisions based on a wise exercise of discretionary power were often attributed to sordid motives. This was politically disastrous, as it ran counter to the desire of many bureaucrats in the Ministry of Justice who 'had been exposed to the teachings of law professors committed to the creation of a legal order in Russia, not to mention the provision of fair, equal and incorruptible justice for all Russian subjects'.[5] The reforms of 1864, making the judiciary independent, were not very effective in establishing the rule of law or the principle of accountability. This failure stemmed not from the self-interest and corruption of a bureaucratic élite, but from the absence of an effective framework of political responsibility within which the legal reforms could operate. As one historian observed, the bureaucrats 'were responsible to no constitutional body and subject only to arbitrary recall by the Czar, who . . . exercised it constantly'.[6]

The effectiveness of the bureaucracy was also limited by its size. Acute and experienced foreign observers frequently believed that there was an excess of government at the top levels matched by an insufficiency of personnel lower down. This made local administration seem particularly inefficient and arbitrary. It is hard to judge how many were employed in the public service as contemporary estimates varied wildly. If the definition is restricted to those who appeared in the various classes of the Table of Ranks, then the number 'employed in central government was approximately 23,000 in 1880 and 52,000 in 1914, those serving in the provinces numbered, respectively, about 12,000 and 16,000'.[7] Many high-ranking bureaucrats were of good education and generous sentiment, but the minor officials with whom regular contact was made by much of the population – railway and postal clerks, policemen, tax collectors, forest wardens and so on – were widely disliked for their self-importance and petty officiousness. The reputation of public servants was probably largely determined by the favouritism of a few at the top and the *amour-propre* of many at the lowest levels.

Of necessity there was some devolution of power at local level. In 1890 Russia was divided into 97 separate administrative areas.[8] Each was headed by a governor whose powers and duties were extensive. This was illustrated by the widespread use of an originally temporary regulation of August 1881 which enabled governors to suspend many of the forms of protection for citizens offered by the legal code. The regular abuse of this power and the misuse of other privileges made the office of governor highly unpopular among all ranks of society, thus making cooperation with local representative bodies more difficult. The creation of the *zemstvo* system in 1864, followed by that of municipal councils six years later, aroused expectations of wider public participation in local affairs, though this system never extended to the non-Russian territories, where military and bureaucratic absolutism reigned. After 1881, especially during Tolstoy's years as Minister of the Interior (1882–9), many local councils found their powers reduced rather than developed. More liberal areas, such as Tver, were predictably offended, but there was also a more general resentment even among the conservative gentry. Koshelev, the famous Slavophile, even remarked that the appointment of Tolstoy mocked all that was best in Russian society.[9]

The executive of the *zemstvo* had many responsibilities but lacked executive authority over the lower levels of provincial administration. Each province was subdivided into districts (*uezdy*), these into cantons (*volosti*); at the lowest level was the peasant village commune (*obshchina*). The ability of the governor and officials to obstruct or overrule *zemstvo* decisions prevented reform and inhibited the evolution of democracy at the grass roots. The influence of Tolstoy and Pobedonostsev also proved detrimental to the evolution of representative and responsible local government. Under Durnovo, Tolstoy's successor,

(1889–95), a series of measures to limit *zemstvo* power was implemented. The principal effects were to increase the already substantial
proportion of noble deputies, and to eliminate the direct election of
peasant representatives at *volost* level by transferring the power of
selection to the governor. These measures provoked resistance both
from the gentry and the professionals employed by *zemstvo* boards at
local level. In the municipalities there was generally less independence
of spirit, and the very gentle pace of growth of representative government was hampered by the introduction in 1892 of higher property
qualifications, thus reducing the electorate almost to vanishing-point.
During the last years of peace less than one per cent of the population
of Moscow and St Petersburg was able to vote. Furthermore, mayors,
local officials, and even whole boards of elected councillors, could be
removed at the instance of the governor or the Minister of the Interior.

These problems were shared at the lowest level of government, the
commune. During the late nineteenth century there was a rising tide of
unrest among the peasantry. There were many causes, among them
lack of skills and knowledge which could have improved agricultural
output, natural disasters, the strains imposed by complex rules of
inheritance and land tenure. But administrative problems played their
part too. Abuse of power, corruption, embezzlement, and misallo-
cation of rather slender resources were regular features of rural administration. Local officials were often unpopular, especially and
predictably the tax collectors, the police, the notaries, and those
connected with enforcing conscription – even though the manpower
requirements of the army were surprisingly modest.[10]

Tolstoy recognized the defects of the system and responded in 1889
by creating the office of land commandant. This new official was
required to be a member of the local hereditary nobility and was given
wide powers over the commune and canton. By the early twentieth
century the land commandant was firmly established as the most hated
official. He was able to ignore or cancel local elections or nominations,
and from 1905 was specifically required to weed out those deemed to
be politically unreliable from any post of responsibility or organ of
representation. The post was strongly disliked by much of the gentry as
it exacerbated already difficult class relationships in many localities.
Administration probably did become more efficient and certainly less
corrupt, but at a high political price. After 1905 the office was no
longer restricted to the hereditary nobility, being more commonly
given to bureaucrats and ex-officers. Representative government at
local level was effectively derailed, thus making *zemstvo* achievements
all the more remarkable.[11]

The alternative of a representative constitutional body was, of course, not adopted. Pressure for a parliamentary institution had surfaced regularly during the first half of the nineteenth century. By the 1880s fears of revolution and of accompanying loss of property and privileges had driven many more of the gentry and middle classes to support at least some reform of the political system. This process was intensified by a growing awareness among an enlarged class of professional people that the importance of their services was not matched by an equivalent political responsibility. Some of the privileged in Russia reacted to the rapidly changing situation by advocating a harsher autocracy, but by 1900 these were probably a minority of the non-peasant classes. Those of this opinion were, however, strongly represented in court circles. The tsar needed little encouragement to resist calls for a popular assembly, as he had shown in January 1895 when he referred to 'senseless dreams about participation by representatives of the zemstvo in the affairs of internal government'.[12] This remained, in essence, his position until the end of his reign. Events in 1905 obliged Nicholas II to accede to demands for representation by accepting the election of a state assembly, the Duma. But his true feelings were shown by his strong resistance to its creation, his attempts to reduce its powers then and subsequently, his attitude towards its members, his encouragement of exercises in gerrymandering, and his resentment towards those, like Witte, whom he believed had helped force his hand. In 1917, at the time of his abdication, the tsar refused to trust those who were reputed to enjoy public confidence, and on 3 March, referring to his brother's acceptance of demands for a Constituent Assembly, noted in his diary 'I wonder who advised him to sign that filth'.[13] Nicholas II neither would nor could accept the part of constitutional monarch; neither autocracy nor representative democracy thus seemed plausible systems of government in Russia by the early twentieth century.

Even if these difficulties had not existed there were others which might well have sabotaged the development of good government. The morale of government servants was often poor, particularly as many were very conscious of the inadequacies of the system they were paid to administer. The peasantry further complicated their task by being both suspiciously obstructionist of most changes and yet disliking the existing state of affairs. The identification of government with demands for men, money or time, rather than with the provision of benefits, was obviously not conducive to its popularity. The result was much ill-focused unease and unrest; the possibility of a largely illiterate[14] peasantry clamouring for democratic institutions as an alternative to autocracy could be safely disregarded, but the risk of mass revolt could not. Political activists among the intelligentsia often found the peasantry unresponsive, though the peasants had little sense of positive identification with the existing regime. In truth, the educated and the uneducated understood each other very badly, if at all.

Governments were also chronically short of money, despite large gold reserves held to protect the value of the rouble. Demands on state finances increased markedly in this period. Revenue was limited by the undue reliance on indirect taxation rather than direct taxes on income or property;[15] nor were the methods of collection invariably efficient. Certain claims, such as those of the army and the secret police, received very favourable attention when resources were allocated. It is not, perhaps, too inaccurate to suggest that external and internal security were thus in part maintained at the expense of better government. Paradoxically, perhaps fewer police would have been needed if less had been spent on them and more elsewhere, though the perception that 'the regime was based upon an ant-heap of secret police'[16] seems exaggerated. However, it does appear likely that contemporary opinion was correct in believing that both the governments and the administration of Russia were poor at identifying and solving problems; money alone could not have cured many of the ills.

Russia, therefore, had an administrative structure with some potential for good government. This remained largely unfulfilled despite a civil service that was more energetic and enlightened than has often been suggested. Several obstacles to good government were particularly important as they were to play significant roles in the collapse of tsarism. It is plain that the system demanded either enlightened direction from the tsar, or an effective constitutional system which would exercise authority on the basis of public consent. After 1894, if not before, it is evident that the tsar was incapable of taking command or making decisions in anything other than a notional sense. The result was that at the very top levels government tended to be either chaotic or non-existent. The confusion over the purposes and implications of Zubatov's 'police-unionism' after 1901 provides perhaps the best-known example of counter-productive governmental and administrative infighting. The well-documented incapacity of Nicholas II, made worse by his inability to distinguish good public servants from bad, produced a laterigrade system of government in which ministers advanced their policies (if they had any) at their own speed, and in the direction of their choice, virtually oblivious, deliberately or unknowingly, to the actions of supposed colleagues. As the autocratic system was by definition a pyramidal hierarchy this version of autocracy was not a success.

However, the most important problem facing the Russian state was its lack of social and political cohesion – the absence of a 'well-established sense of community, comparable with that to be found at this time in the nation states of Western Europe'.[17] The lack of such cohesion would in itself have posed a threat to the continued existence of the empire; matters were made worse by the refusal of many, particularly the reactionaries, to recognize openly this lack of cohesion. Privately, of course, many did and thus favoured coercion in various forms as a method of producing the required cohesion – at least on the surface. This was what so often struck the casual observer: 'A traveller to Russia in 1900 might be forgiven for concluding that the autocratic regime was as strongly entrenched as ever. One of a population of nearly 130 millions no more than a few thousand actively sought its overthrow.'[18] The reality was otherwise; the strength of the autocracy was superficial, the bonds which held society together were tenuous. The political solutions put forward were, by and large, utterly unrealistic and were in most cases known to be so. Conrad wrote perceptively of this cynicism being

> the mark of Russian autocracy and of Russian revolt. In its pride of numbers, in its strange pretensions of sanctity and in the secret readiness to abase itself in suffering, the spirit of Russia is the spirit of cynicism. It informs the declarations of statesmen, the theories of her revolutionists, and the mystic vaticinations of prophets to the point of making freedom look like a form of debauch.[19]

Events were rapidly overtaking the system as the century drew to a close. The long-term stability of the regime was threatened by the rapid growth of the economy, population and industrialization and the related problems of modernization. The multinational character of the empire, encompassing great differences in language, religion and culture, was intensified by expansion. Instead of the sensitivity which was needed to respond to nationalism, a policy of Russification was pursued, albeit inconsistently and erratically. Indeed, the temptation in governing circles was often to attribute problems merely to the malevolence of non-Russian groups in the empire. Crude anti-Semitism became a staple government response to unrest; pogroms and show trials, such as that of Beilis in 1913, were used by the authorities as a safety-valve. The concentration of Jews in the towns (by 1914 about 85 per cent lived in urban areas), and in the Pale of Jewish Settlement in particular, facilitated both repression and resistance.

The defective policy of the regime entirely omitted to take into account that many complaints made by Jews derived from their occupations, their class and the conditions of life, rather than from their Jewishness. To have admitted this fact would have forced the authorities to abandon some of their most cherished assumptions about Russian society and the relationship of the Russian people to the tsar and to autocracy. If the Jews were singled out for restriction and persecution, other groups were also badly treated. Sometimes compromises were forced upon the autocracy – as in the cases of Finland and the Baltic administrative areas – but in Poland, the Ukraine, and many remote areas of the south and east, Russian rule was characterized by repression, intolerance and contempt.

At the heart of government concern about the preservation of the system was the question of the peasantry,[20] comprising about three-quarters of the population in 1900. In most areas the peasants were very vulnerable to adverse circumstances such as those of 1891, which produced agrarian distress on a grand scale. Despite famine, disease, migration and some emigration, the rural areas were overpopulated. There was a shortage of land, though it is clear that at least since 1880 the peasants had held more than half the arable land; by 1905 the nobility had sold 20 million more acres to the peasantry.[21] Another important factor was the failure to secure a growth in productivity to match the rise in population. The backwardness of agriculture was notorious and apparently incurable. The commune system actually perpetuated out-of-date methods and antiquated attitudes. It did help prevent the emergence of a large class of landless peasants but at a great price: mass poverty, immobility of labour, low yields, wastage of land and the inadvertent encouragement of a belief among the peasantry that what they needed was more land (which could only come from lands held by the nobility, the Crown, the Church or some municipalities), rather than higher productivity. The inevitable result was social tension, directed especially at local landowners, coupled with demands for the distribution of estates; these attitudes conflicted head-on with the conservative tsarist policy of seeking to prop up the position of the gentry. The commune system thus conspicuously failed to act as a force for stability as so many reactionaries believed.

As well as trying to control the rising flood of discontent governments also attempted to divert it. In March 1891 established policies on migration were reversed and in 1896 an agency for resettlement was created, thus permitting and aiding settlement in Siberia. Attempts were made to prevent the alienation of peasant land through sale or mortgage, and to encourage peasants to improve their land by prohibiting partial redistribution and by extending the intervals between total redistributions in the commune. In March 1903 the collective responsibility of the commune for the payment of taxes and redemption dues was abolished. Throughout this period the Peasants' Land Bank, founded in 1883, provided funds for communes and individuals to purchase land – a task made more difficult by the existence of the Nobles' Land Bank after 1885. But, despite all efforts, by about 1900 even conservative figures were beginning to doubt the value of the commune as a means of preserving social stability or promoting agricultural prosperity.

In 1905, under the strain of war, the situation exploded. There was widespread looting and arson, taxes and rents were withheld, promises to abolish redemption payments fell on deaf ears. In some parts unrest continued for almost a year, and was particularly persistent in a number of border areas (where ethnic factors exacerbated the situation), and in the fertile areas of Poltava, Kursk, Tambov and Orel (where population pressures had been strong for many years). These events terrified a large proportion of the propertied classes and many of the previously liberal-minded bolted into the welcoming arms of the reactionaries. The failure of the commune was now patent, and between 1906 and 1911 the new prime minister, Stolypin, set about the task of reform. Not only were peasant freedoms widened, by reducing the powers of the land commandant, but the peasants were encouraged to leave the communes or at least to consolidate their holdings within them. The effect of these changes was that by 1914 about half the peasant households held their land by hereditary private tenure. In addition about another 31 million acres were purchased by the peasants, mainly from the nobility.[22] Migration to Siberia and other thinly populated areas was also encouraged. By 1914 the agrarian problem, while not solved, was certainly less pressing.

In the urban centres unrest was also developing towards the end of the century. Here the state was, perhaps, a victim of economic success as well as political rigidity. Despite attempts to control migration, peasants had poured into the towns. By 1914 the urban population had risen to about 27 million, approximately double that of 1890. Urban life had, in the meantime, declined in quality. Working conditions were mainly deplorable and those of housing were even worse. Schools, hospitals and transport were all in short supply. The provision of gas, water and electricity was erratic at best; there was a great deal of industrial pollution and a perpetual risk to health from inadequate treatment of sewage and waste. In short, conditions were grim, though in many areas not much worse than in the industrial black spots of western European countries at an equivalent stage in their development. But government concern about the way of life of city-dwellings and private philanthropy were less in evidence than in the West. Yet still the peasants poured into the towns. Many, of course, were seasonal workers who returned to the countryside at important times, such as harvesting. This ebb and flow of the population was made easier by the lack of specialized forms of industrialization and the continued ownership of land, even among those working in the cities. But this process both limited the extent of industrial advance and reduced the effectiveness of government control over its citizens.

Successive governments tried hard to influence the development of the economy, especially by encouraging foreign investment and by raising import duties. Witte, who was Minister of Finance from 1892 to 1903, put the rouble on the gold standard in 1897, and there was a series of laws passed to protect industrial labour, including the introduction of a maximum working day of eleven and a half hours in 1897. But trade unions were prohibited, and both employers and employed frequently found that the Ministry of the Interior, on the grounds of the need to maintain public order, nullified the progress instituted by the Ministry of Finance. Despite all difficulties the economy grew rapidly, and trade with Germany, France and Britain became particularly important. Coal, petroleum, textiles, the metallurgical industries and wood pulp contributed to a huge growth in exports. Describing the period after 1900, Gerschenkron was moved to observe that 'as far as the general pattern of its industrialization . . . was concerned, Russia seemed to duplicate what had happened in Germany in the last decades of the nineteenth century'.[23] The influence of the banks, and the development of cartels and monopolies also grew apace, often promoted by a political system unamenable to democratic control. The advantages of large-scale industries in terms of profitability and numbers employed were counterbalanced by their impersonal nature, and by the xenophobia encouraged by apparent dependence on foreign loans, expertise, technology and even management.

The growth of industry and the increase in population mobility, despite an internal passport system and a poor transport infrastructure, intensified pressures on the system. The inability of the regime to respond to the social needs of the industrial workers and to the political claims of the professional classes created a potentially explosive situation. The folly of the Russo-Japanese War further diminished the reputation of the government at home and abroad. Revolutionary propaganda became both more widespread and secured more of a response. Russian political life had always been punctuated by violence, assassinations and riot. By the early twentieth century the violent overthrow of the system was increasingly seen as the only answer to autocracy. The failure of successive Dumas to make any headway in the struggle for constitutionalism disillusioned democrats and moderate reformers, and strengthened the hand of extremists at both ends of the political spectrum. In the last few years before 1914 political strikes became much more common, and the use of force to suppress economic demands was only temporarily adequate as a response. Similarly, the Western influences to which Russian society was necessarily exposed as a result of increased trade, could not be suppressed by censorship or arbitrary arrest or exile. Illegal presses flourished, a sub-culture of radical and revolutionary societies grew up, and the enlightened bureaucracy became ever more exasperated with and frustrated by the absurdities of the doctrine of autocracy. If Russia was not on the brink of revolution in 1914 it was, nevertheless, an empire in which strong support for the existing system was very limited indeed.

How comparable were events and trends in Austria-Hungary? In fact, despite exposure to many of the same forces which influenced the evolution of Russia, the empire of the Habsburgs was throughout this period a very different creation. This is readily seen at the top level of government, in the person of the ruler himself. In comparison with the tsars, Franz Josef (1848–1916) seems enlightened and perceptive. He was better educated, though some historians have argued that he was too much influenced by his mother's autocratic beliefs. Nevertheless, it is evident that he understood the processes of politics better than his Russian counterparts and worked harder at being emperor. The effect of this was, however, probably reduced by his addiction (like Philip II of Spain) to clerical drudgery, rather than to the examination of evidence and the relating of this evidence to political strategy. In any event, by the turn of the century Franz Josef was an old man, worn down by the tragedies involving his wife, his son and his brother. After 1889 he found relations with the new heir, Franz Ferdinand, just as difficult, if for different reasons, as those with Rudolf had been. The intertwined questions of the existence of the state and the succession were as much a problem to the emperor as to the tsar, and in 1914, when Franz Ferdinand and his wife were assassinated at Sarajevo, Franz Josef had only very slender reserves of energy and emotion upon which to draw.

The existence of Franz Josef

> was a guarantee against a catastrophe – the break up of this state –
> which appeared likely after his death, though few of his subjects
> really wanted its total dissolution . . . the only person in his domin-
> ions whose interests were general in the sense that they were con-
> cerned with the Empire as a whole.[24]

This state of affairs was the product of the *Ausgleich* (compromise) of
1867 between the Germans and the Magyars. The *Ausgleich* had
created a strange and potentially unstable political structure. The
Austro-Hungarian state consisted of two parts, sharing a ruler, an
army, and three joint ministries: foreign affairs, war and finance. To
complicate matters further, there existed two separate assemblies, in
Vienna and Budapest. When matters involving both parliaments
needed to be discussed these were dealt with by their appointed
'delegations' (in effect executive committees, each of sixty members)
which met annually alternately in the two cities. They communicated
normally only in writing; only if they could not agree was a plenary
session held when decisions could be reached by majority vote. In the
absence of a majority the decision was left to the emperor. This
cumbersome and elaborate system was an attempt to meet Hungarian
fears that any changes to the 1867 system would be disadvantageous to
their interests.[25] The existence of, in effect, a Hungarian veto on
change had produced by 1890 an inability to respond to social and
economic developments which required modified political structures.
The emperor's conservatism made him an unlikely reformer and by the
close of the century, despite an accumulation of prestige and authority
during his long reign which might have enabled him to risk some
political initiatives, he was vigorous only in his defence of executive
powers over military and foreign affairs.

  The system of joint ministries also failed to act as a focal point for
effective and accountable government. Ministers were appointed and
dismissed by the emperor. Because politicians with national standing
were rare, ministers were usually drawn from the nobility or the higher
echelons of the bureaucracy. Even then they only reported to the
'delegations', rather than to the parliaments of Austria and Hungary.
No cabinet existed, so collective government was conspicuous by its
absence. A Crown Council existed, consisting of the three joint ministers, the minister-presidents of Austria and Hungary, and such other
important figures as the emperor saw fit to summon, but it met intermittently.[26] Inevitably, this lack of cohesion made political developments and political management in the separate parliaments more
important. By 1890 the consolidation of substantially different

interests in Vienna and Budapest was well advanced, especially as a result of the long domination of Taaffe's government in Austria (1879–93), and that of Tisza in Hungary (1874–90).

Financial arrangements also reflected, as well as promoted separatism. As a result of the *Ausgleich* the national budget consisted only of that part of the finances needed to sustain the activities of the joint ministries. These expenditures were to be reviewed every ten years; originally the Hungarian kingdom paid 30 per cent, though this rose in the 1890s to 34.4 per cent of common expenditure and later still to 36.4 per cent. Nevertheless, this remained 'far less than would have been appropriate on the basis of Hungary's economic resources and potential'.[27] These arrangements, already less than ideal, were further complicated by contrasting attitudes towards tariffs and taxes. Even the customs union, partly because of the different levels of economic development, was often the target of vitriolic criticism. The individual parliaments also inspected their own budgets, presented to them by their own governments. This, again, proved to be a recipe for particularism and obstruction. It seemed more prudent to put the interests of Austria or Hungary above those of the dual monarchy; at times of great tension this attitude appeared to be a prerequisite for political survival. Inevitably, then, the functions of the joint ministries were consistently under-funded, while particularist and local projects received a more liberal endowment.

The malfunctioning of the representative system produced in practice a transfer of power to the bureaucracy. Political and administrative functions were intertwined and were not uncommonly identified as one and the same. The custom of appointing legally qualified civil servants to the most important judicial offices impaired the process of obtaining redress against maladministration. Almost all the aspects of government were increasingly regarded as the business of officials. The civil service of the dual monarchy became an attractive career as it seemed to offer both security of tenure and the prospect of wielding power almost untrammelled by any external form of review. By 1914 well over three million bureaucrats managed the affairs of Austria-Hungary. A large proportion of the taxes they raised was spent on their own employment, rather than on projects the state might usefully have undertaken. The bureaucracy became increasingly concerned to protect its privileges and to preserve its status; its individual members were similarly preoccupied with their own advancement through the elaborate and stylized system of grades and ranks. The bureaucracy developed its own archaic language, style and practices which became so notorious that they were the subject of harsh criticism and comic invention.[28] Lest it be imagined that these lampoons were exaggerated, it should be borne in mind that in Vienna twenty-seven officials handled each tax payment.[29]

As well as being stifled by bureaucracy, democratic pressures were also faced with a constitutional and legal structure of a highly conservative kind. Under the terms of the *Ausgleich* certain legal rights were guaranteed, though, characteristically, the texts used in Austria and in Hungary were not identical. Broadly, citizens of the dual monarchy were deemed to be equal, to have freedom of expression, to have the right to use their own language and to be educated in it at the primary level. The linked questions of language and education were so important that they were specifically recognized in the Austrian version of the constitution in 1867: 'the public schools shall be organized in a way that every ethnic group receives the necessary funds for training in its own language without being compelled to learn the second language of any land.'[30] As no fewer than seventeen territories were represented in the Reichsrat (Imperial Parliament), with some ten languages spoken within them, this was a substantial commitment. The results were very different from those suggested by a narrow reading of the constitution. There was no formal definition of what was meant by an ethnic group, and in any event, it was not always easy to determine whether, for example, an area was predominantly German or Czech. The desire to advance a career promoted the learning of German among non-Germans; many German speakers felt that their children's interests would be helped more by learning French or English than a Slav tongue. At a local level, however, this led to a non-German domination of the bureaucracy in the lower ranks. The failure to define legally the status of an ethnic group also meant that those who sought redress against unjust discrimination were deprived of the protection, however feeble it might have been, of the Reichsgericht (Imperial Court), as such questions were deemed outside the competence of the court. The issues of education and the use of languages repeatedly led to crises within Austria during this period, causing, for example, the fall of its government in 1895 and again in 1897.[31]

The situation in Hungary was rather different, though no better. The Magyars were obsessed by the need to maintain independence and their own status within the kingdom of Hungary. This developed to such an extent that maintenance of their language became an important goal that overrode pragmatism. In 1889 there was serious opposition to the use of German as the language of command in the armed forces levied in Hungary, and in 1903 the same issue provoked a constitutional crisis. In 1907 Apponyi pushed through an Education

Act which in effect prevented the nationalities having their own private schools, and in the same year Kossuth made Magyar the only language to be used on railways throughout the kingdom. In this atmosphere the minority ethnic groups in Hungary became increasingly discontented with their lot. As unrest grew, so oppressive measures were adopted, and these in turn fuelled demands for autonomy or independence, especially in Croatia, the Banat and Transylvania.

It was political discontent among minorities in both sub-states that highlighted the lack of an adequate representative system. In Austria a real attempt was made to come to terms with demands for representation and voting rights. After 1873 deputies were directly elected, but by four groups of unequal number and wealth (the towns, the rural communes, the trade associations and the large landowners). In 1882 the property qualification was reduced from ten to five guilders. In 1896 Badeni modified the existing system substantially. The number of deputies rose from 353 to 425, and a fifth group (general franchise, based on literacy and tax-paying qualifications of a modest kind) added.[32] The voting power of the propertied classes was hardly affected, however, and it was not until 1907 that adult male suffrage was introduced. The smaller national groups gained from these reforms, but the effects of this shift were relatively slight as the complex arrangements between national groupings in the Reichsrat remained almost undisturbed.

The issues of the franchise and ethnic representation were naturally closely linked. In Austria a reasonably successful method of containing the nationalities problem had been adopted before this period. Each of the seventeen units had its own diet or assembly and, as many grievances could be treated best at a local level, this eased pressure on the Reichsrat. Where it was felt appropriate quite wide powers were granted to these local assemblies and their governments. After 1869 Galicia, inhabited mainly by Poles, enjoyed considerable autonomy. As a result the Polish bloc in the Reichsrat, usually about seventy strong, could normally be relied upon by the government. The Czech-inhabited areas, however, posed a much more difficult problem – partly because of different social structures, educational attainment and economic development, and partly because in much of Bohemia and Moravia Czechs and Germans were not settled on fairly distinct ethnic lines. In 1890 an attempt was made by Thun-Hohenstein to solve the conflict over education and language in Bohemia. His failure led to a massive victory by the Young Czech party at the polls in 1891. In 1897 Badeni made a further effort, promulgating ordinances which put Czech and German on an equal footing in the administration. These decrees produced a violent response from the Germans, who both resented them and feared lest they be duplicated in other Slav areas of Austria. Matters became so desperate that parliamentary rule was temporarily abandoned and rule by the cabinet, according to Article 14 of the constitution, was adopted. After several changes of government the Badeni decrees were eventually withdrawn. An attempt to divide Bohemia and Moravia into different administrative districts, in order to alleviate the problems, foundered on both Czech and German opposition. Even the suffrage reform of 1907, introduced partly in the hope of outflanking middle-class nationalists, failed to ease the problem. The Reichsrat now found itself overflowing with parties (more than thirty after the elections of 1911), as well as with national blocs. It was a recipe for paralysis.

The situation in Hungary was slightly different. In 1868 two important laws had been passed which influenced political behaviour in the kingdom for the next three decades. The nationality law was, in some aspects, more liberal than the equivalent legislation in Austria. However, the domination of the Hungarian parliament, and government by politicians of a distinctly Magyar nationalist hue meant that failure by the bureaucracy and the courts to protect the rights of individuals and groups was permitted to remain uncorrected. The Hungarian – Croatian compromise of the same year also failed to meet expectations, at least among the Croats. Croatia was in theory granted considerable autonomy, with its own assembly, but the delegates Croatia sent to the Hungarian parliament were habitually outvoted by the Magyar majority, and the head of administration in Croatia was usually a Magyar whose influence was, in practice, exercised in the cause of Hungarian hegemony.[33] In any event the limited autonomy given to Croatia was not extended to the rest of the non-Magyar areas, so that by the end of the century there were strong nationalist movements in Slovakia, Ruthenia and Transylvania. Even the two million Germans who lived in the kingdom felt sufficiently threatened to form their own party in 1905. They, however, were able to look to the emperor and to fellow German-speakers in Austria for some protection against Magyar excesses. Other minorities were less well placed and were increasingly inclined to think in terms either of genuine autonomy or of secession; the Romanians in Transylvania naturally looked to union with Romania.

These problems were exacerbated by the narrow franchise and the corrupt and manipulative system of government. Elections were rigged, and political differences were subsumed in the interest of preserving Magyar hegemony. By 1903 this system was in decay as radical and clerical parties emerged to fragment Magyar unity. Two prime ministers – Bánffy (1895–9) and Szell (1899–1903) – failed to check the rising tide of demands for constitutional and electoral reform. Magyar nationalists responded by reasserting their claim to primacy in the kingdom and to absolute equality in the dual monarchy. Their weapon was to refuse to pass joint defence legislation unless German was abandoned as the sole language of command in the armed forces; in effect calling for a separate Hungarian army. After several years of conflict, beginning in 1897, the emperor made it evident in September 1903 that this was unacceptable to him, and a new premier, Tisza (1903–5), pushed the legislation through. Elections followed, which the pro-nationalist groups won. Failure to reach agreement led to an interim government operating without strong parliamentary support under Fejérváry (1905–6). The situation rapidly deteriorated; censorship was introduced, public meetings restricted, the parliament was first prorogued and then dissolved. Chaos was only avoided by an astute imperial démarche. Franz Josef caused a bill to be introduced which would have led to universal suffrage in the kingdom. A wide franchise would not only have promoted non-Magyar representation, but would also have enfranchised industrial and agrarian workers and many smallholders. Thus the privileged position of the existing political classes would have been utterly undermined, as already seemed to be the case in Austria. Attitudes were rapidly revised and, in return for abandonment of the franchise reform, under Wekerle (1906–10), the military quotas were agreed and attempts to modify the *Ausgleich* were abandoned. The fundamental problem of a very unrepresentative system, however, remained.

In a state already prey to ethnic conflict the rise of anti-Semitism produced further strains. Many Jews fled Russian persecution only to discover that integration and acceptance were difficult to achieve in Austria-Hungary. By 1914 there were large Jewish communities in both parts of the dual monarchy, amounting to almost 5 per cent of the population. In Hungary anti-Semitism was more a problem of rural than urban life, and was the product of suspicions about city-dwellers as much as religious or cultural differences. In Austria the tide of anti-Semitism was both stronger and more overt. Two leading politicians, Schönerer and Lueger, peddled a mixture of Pan-Germanism, anti-liberalism and anti-Semitism. Lueger became mayor of Vienna in 1897 (despite three imperial vetos between 1895 and 1897), an office he held until his death in 1910. The prominence of Jews in Viennese intellectual, cultural and business life made them easy targets, culminating in the 1905 riots when Jewish students were physically prevented from attending the university. Lueger, far from discouraging attacks on Jews, was a regular contributor to Wolf's *Wiener Volkszeitung*, a rabidly anti-Semitic newspaper with a large circulation among the poorer middle-class and working-class Viennese. Yet matters could have been worse, as they were in Russia where official persecution was the order of the day.

While the constitutional and ethnic problems of the dual monarchy were obvious sources of tension, economic and social change also played a large part in threatening the antiquated compromise. As in Russia, economic development created great pressures which were reflected in the decline of traditional forms of employment, shortages of housing, schools and hospitals, and serious strains on the transport infrastructure. Agriculture remained the largest employer even in 1914, though there had been a significant decline from the two-thirds of the working population so engaged in 1900. In less-industrialized Hungary the social and economic structure was slower to change than in Austria, but, even so, considerable readjustment took place. Increasing production of cereals for export in Russia and North America compelled the consolidation of estates and the investment of capital in machinery and fertilizers. Many smallholders were squeezed out and, despite migration to the towns, already in 1900 landless labourers represented 40 per cent of those employed in Hungarian agriculture.[34] Austria was less badly affected, though there were serious problems of a similar kind in some areas, especially in Bohemia and Galicia. Peasant unrest became a regular feature of political life, especially as real wages declined. In 1897 there were widespread strikes by farm labourers in Hungary, and a decade later there was very serious unrest in Transylvania. Although productivity increased substantially during this period, it was largely at the expense of living standards and social stability in the countryside.

Industry developed remarkably in this period, especially in the Austrian half of the state. Heavy industry underwent a transformation from being a peripheral activity to having a central and profitable role in the economy. Coalmining in Bohemia, Moravia and Galicia, iron and steel industries in Bohemia and Styria and other smaller metallurgical industries, such as lead, tungsten, uranium, nickel and copper, all expanded enormously. By 1914 Austria-Hungary produced more coal than all other European states except Germany and Britain; iron and steel manufactures had increased so quickly that the dual monarchy had become the fifth largest producer in Europe. Many other industries boomed, especially those of textiles, brick-making, brewing, chemicals, electrical goods, glass, paper and wood pulp, timber and petrochemicals. Sugar-refining expanded, though wine-making declined – principally because of phylloxera. In order to meet the demands of agriculture, enterprises producing fertilizers and agricultural machinery were founded. Although the areas enjoying the greatest industrial advances were Bohemia, Galicia, Moravia, Upper and Lower Austria, there was also considerable development in the Hungarian heartland, including Budapest, and the Adriatic ports. By 1914 Austria-Hungary exported 7 per cent of its Gross National Product; still only half that achieved by Germany, but a considerable expansion since 1890.

As might be expected, industrial growth was accompanied by improvements in transport. By 1914 there were 40,000 kilometres of railway, and there had also been some attention paid to road-building and bridge construction. All of these changes required capital, much of which came from foreign investors who continued to invest heavily until 1914, though the increasingly tense situation in the Balkans after 1908 produced a more cautious assessment of the political risks involved. The state itself made major commitments to industry, transport and housing, and concessions were made to entrepreneurs and developers to encourage investment. The banking system expanded, with Vienna as its centre, though the price of involvement of the banks in industrial expansion was the development of cartels and near-monopolies. Prague became a secondary financial centre in the early 1900s and, as industrialization took place in Hungary, Budapest began to assume greater importance as a financial market. Economic growth and prosperity, however, were impeded by policies of protectionism, especially on foodstuffs, and the absence in practice (as distinct from theory), of a truly free internal market.

During this period the towns and cities expanded very quickly. By 1914 Vienna had a population of about 1.8 million, Prague about 400,000 and Budapest about 900,000. Other cities, such as Trieste, Pressburg, Brunn, Cracow, Graz, Lemberg and Klausenburg grew substantially, both in size and as centres of regional trade. Migration produced demands for housing, schools and hospitals on an unparalleled scale, as well as a need for improved communications and transport. The state itself invested heavily in communications and education – 24 per cent and 3 per cent respectively of the Austrian national budget in 1913.[35] The Hungarian government was slower to act, but by the early 1900s was giving help in the tasks of urban reconstruction and development. Private benefactors, particularly the much-maligned Jews, played their part by donating money for hospitals, libraries and other public buildings.

Urbanization and greater mobility stimulated new political, social and industrial demands. New ideas threatened existing social and economic assumptions made by the ruling élites. The spread of new ideas was greatly aided by the advance of literacy and by the emergence of a largely uncensored press. By 1914 about 80 per cent of the population was literate; in some areas, especially Bohemia and Moravia, illiteracy was a rarity. The rapid growth and multiplication of parties hugely complicated the process of debate and the tasks of government. By 1914 parties representing specific religious, ethnic, economic, cultural and social interests had been established, vying for votes and influence with broader groupings. The pre-1890 political pattern changed significantly. The most significant gains were made by the Young Czechs, the Christian Socials, the Socialists and the Agrarians. After *c.*1900 the Nationalverband (National Association), a Pan-German organization with a large middle-class membership, steadily increased its influence behind the scenes. In Hungary the groups which profited were the Socialists, the People's Party, and the various ethnic movements. Complicating politics at every level was the tendency, even of parties of the Left, to split into national factions. In 1911, for example, the Czech Social Democratic Party formally separated itself from its sister party in Austria proper. These developments naturally hindered the achievement of goals common to all socialist and most radical parties.

As in the rest of Europe, the process of industrialization led to the creation of labour movements. Conditions of work were often poor, though rarely as bad as in Russia, except, perhaps, in Budapest where the pressures on housing, transport, sanitation, schools and medical services were not dissimilar to those in St Petersburg. A mass movement among industrial workers already existed when, in 1890, the May Day parade in Vienna terrified the prosperous and the propertied.[36] While living conditions remained poor in many towns, and dreadful in the slums of the cities, there were some improvements, and by 1900 the worst examples of industrial confrontation were already in the past. In 1887 laws had been passed which required insurance against accidents and sickness, and in the 1890s there were further advances with legislation against child labour and excessive hours of work for women. Sunday was established as a day of rest, and the use of police and troops to break strikes declined. While some limited rights of combination had been established in Austria as early as 1867, and in Hungary a few years later, there was no official acceptance of trade-unionism even in 1900; though the authorities turned a blind eye to the fact that by that date trade unions had a membership of about half a million. If there was no industrial peace, neither was there industrial war. Fear of unemployment helped keep wages low in the cities, and in the country-side the workers were less well organized. Farm labourers and those employed in cottage industries did not receive the protection offered by the legislation previously mentioned. Gradually, therefore, there was a rise in unrest in rural areas and a growth of peasant associations with both political and economic goals. The potential threat to the political system posed by rural discontent was very serious, and no solution to the problem was in sight when war broke out in 1914.

What, then, were the prospects of imperial Russia and Austria-Hungary on the eve of war in 1914? Both governments were trying to grapple with a broad range of problems – social, economic, ethnic, religious, administrative and constitutional – without having a repre-sentative structure capable of absorbing some of the shocks generated by rapid change. Democratic institutions would not, of course, have solved all the problems, though some would have been eased. But it is hard to see what democratic government would have meant to a largely illiterate Russian peasantry, or to those in Transylvania who wanted only to be united with their fellow Romanians. More import-ant than fully democratic political institutions would have been en-lightened administration which respected the rights of citizens and was properly accountable. Maladministration, inefficiency and the ab-sence of clearly defined goals were as damaging to governments as tyranny or repression. Unrest and dissent in the form of sullen obstruc-tiveness, wildcat strikes or non-cooperation represented a more seri-ous threat than the more spectacular activities of anarchists and nihilists. The ruling élites were largely composed of those who lacked both perception and political flexibility. Those who saw more clearly responded in different ways. Some advocated reformism, others revol-ution; some resorted to the cynicism of *après moi le déluge*,[37] others abandoned politics to engage their energies in commerce or study, or in attempts to ameliorate distress directly.

There was thus no clear, cohesive and agreed response in either state to the most important challenges posed by internal developments after 1890. Worse still, much energy was exhausted in the pursuit of goals in foreign policy of, at best, a questionable desirability. Resources were poured into armies and navies which would objectively have been much better spent elsewhere. Revolution or disintegration might have been avoided in both states, but radical change could not be, and for the majority of the ruling élites revolution, disintegration and radical change were, in effect, the same undesirable process.

Finally, is it possible to give a verdict on the comparative potential for survival of the two imperial systems? Austria-Hungary had the advantage of being ruled by a more intelligent and better respected emperor. Its population was better educated than that of Russia, though this carried with it disadvantages as well as advantages. In terms of representative institutions it was also better equipped than Russia, though the eccentricities of the *Ausgleich* made political advance more difficult than it might otherwise have been. On the other hand, the problem of the nationalities was more acute, and carried with it wider international implications for Austria-Hungary than for Russia. In Austria-Hungary too there was a widespread belief that the death of Franz Josef would be the signal for the breakup of the state. In Russia the economy had a much greater potential than in Austria-Hungary, but its more rapid advance had produced a more general misery of living conditions. Russian relations with Germany, the most obvious source of improved technology and expertise, were obviously much worse than those between Germany and Austria-Hungary. The problems of ruling vast territories without resorting to autocracy and over-centralization were plainly worse in Russia. Revolutionary movements were more active in Russia, though the police were more energetic in their attempts to repress unrest. In liberal, western Europe, both regimes were widely seen as anachronistic and seriously defective – enthusiasm for them being largely the product of what was seen as military and strategic necessity. The difficulties of reform were rarely correctly assessed in the West, as was to become apparent in 1917. The verdict, then, must be that both systems looked doomed, but the answer as to which in peacetime conditions was the more likely to collapse remains hidden in a cloud of Delphic ambiguity.

NOTES

1 G. P. Gooch and H. Temperley (eds), *British Documents on the Origins of the War, 1898–1914*, vol. 10, part 2 (London: HMSO, 1938), p. 773: Goschen to Nicolson, 27 Mar. 1914.

2 N. Stone, *Europe Transformed, 1878–1919* (London: Fontana, 1983), p. 201.

3 A. Summers and T. Mangold, *The File on the Tsar* (London: Fontana, 1978), p. 33.

4 For an excellent and up-to-date analysis of the State Council see

D. C. B. Lieven, *Russia's Rulers under the Old Regime* (London: Yale University Press, 1989).

5 Lieven, op. cit., p. 178.

6 B. Tuchman, *The Guns of August: August 1914* (London: Constable, 1964), p. 79.

7 H. Rogger, *Russia in the Age of Modernisation and Revolution, 1881–1917* (London: Longman, 1983), pp. 49–50.

8 The terms used do not easily translate into obvious English equivalents, but there were 78 provinces (*guberniya*), 18 districts (*oblast*) and 1 zone (*okrug*). The forms and nature of the administration differed slightly in each case. By 1914 three additional administrative areas had been created.

9 Rogger, op. cit., pp. 30–1; T. Emmons, *The Russian Landed Gentry and the Peasant Emancipation of 1861* (Cambridge: Cambridge University Press, 1968); pp. 171–2; and in Lieven, op. cit., pp. 163–4.

10 For a thorough description of this issue for the period before and during the war of 1914–18 see N. Stone, *The Eastern Front, 1914–17* (London: Hodder & Stoughton, 1985), pp. 212–18.

11 For an interesting and informative discussion of the achievements of the *zemstvo* see T. Emmons and W. S. Vucinich (eds), *The Zemstvo in Russia: An Experiment in Local Self-government* (Cambridge: Cambridge University Press, 1982).

12 H. Seton-Watson, *The Russian Empire, 1801–1917* (Oxford: Oxford University Press, 1967), p. 549.

13 G. Katkov, *Russia 1917* (London: Fontana, 1969), p. 473. There is much solid evidence regarding the tsar's attitudes towards the Duma. See especially the memoirs of Polivanov, Witte, Trubetskoy and Izvolsky, as well as the pen-portraits of keen observers such as Seraphin. The overall effect shows that the tsar's understanding of political issues was usually weak, but his response to political challenge was a mixture of obstruction and devious dishonesty.

14 According to the 1897 census only 25 per cent of the men and 10 per cent of the women in non-urban areas were literate. See J. L. H. Keep, *The Rise of Social Democracy in Russia* (Oxford: Oxford University Press, 1966), p. 4.

15 Although there were slight variations the relationship between indirect and direct taxes was, on average, about 85 : 15 in yield during this period.

16 Tuchman, op. cit., p. 79.

17 Keep, op. cit., p. 1.

18 ibid., p. 1.
19 J. Conrad, *Under Western Eyes* (Harmondsworth: Penguin, 1987), p. 105. Originally published in 1911, this novel provides important insight into the nature of contemporary Russia.
20 Peasants had a certain legal status, which they did not necessarily change by moving into cities; thus in St Petersburg a clear majority of its inhabitants were 'peasants' in 1914.
21 Seton-Watson, op. cit., pp. 506–17, provides a concise account of the main changes in landholding patterns.
22 A detailed analysis of these changes may be found in G. T. Robinson, *Rural Russia under the Old Regime* (London: California University Press, reprint, 1973).
23 A. Gerschenkron, *Economic Backwardness in Historical Perspective* (London: Harvard University Press, 1962), p. 138.
24 Sir Llewellyn Woodward, *Prelude to Modern Europe, 1815–1914* (London: Methuen, 1972), p. 231.
25 For a succinct and clear description of these arrangements, see R. A. Kann, *A History of the Hapsburg Empire, 1526–1918* (London: California University Press, 1977), pp. 333–5.
26 This point is well illustrated in the accounts given by Stone, *Europe Transformed*, pp. 305–6, and Woodward, op. cit., pp. 235–6.
27 Kann, op. cit., p. 334.
28 For example in Karl Kraus's contemporary attacks on 'bureaucretinismus' and the later (1921) classic by Jaroslav Hasek, *The Good Soldier Schweik*.
29 W. M. Johnston, *The Austrian Mind: An Intellectual and Social History, 1848–1938* (London: California University Press, 1983), p. 48. This is an excellent and invaluable study of the period.
30 Kann, op. cit., p. 339.
31 There is a useful discussion of these problems in R. Okey, *Eastern Europe, 1740–1985* (London: Hutchinson, 1986), pp. 138–47.
32 Kann, op. cit., p. 425.
33 See the articles by C. Jelavich and B. Krizman in the *Austrian History Yearbook* vol. 3, part 2 (Houston: Rice University Press, 1967).
34 See D. Good, *The Economic Rise of the Hapsburg Empire, 1750–1914* (Berkeley: Berkeley University Press, 1984), for a well-documented account.
35 Okey, op. cit., p. 114.
36 B. W. Tuchman, *The Proud Tower* (London: Bantam, 1966), p. 477. Contemporary evidence of the shock of the parade and of

Adler's calls for a general strike was recorded in S. Zweig, *Die Welt von Gestern: Erinnerungen eines Europäers* (Stockholm: publisher unknown, 1942).
37 A. J. Mayer, *The Persistence of the Old Regime* (London: Croom Helm, 1981), esp. chs 4–5.

FURTHER READING

A number of works already referred to in the footnotes are of considerable help. Good general accounts of Russia in this period are to be found in H. Rogger, *Russia in the Age of Modernisation and Revolution, 1881–1917* (London, 1983); H. Seton-Watson, *The Russian Empire, 1801–1917* (Oxford, 1967); R. Charques, *The Twilight of Imperial Russia* (London, reprint 1974). Equivalents for Austria-Hungary are more difficult to find, but the relevant part of R. A. Kann, *A History of the Hapsburg Empire, 1526–1918* (London, 1977), or A. Sked, *The Decline and Fall of the Habsburg Empire* (London, 1989), are very useful.

Economic issues are well treated. Notable among the many good books are: T. Emmons, *The Russian Landed Gentry and the Peasant Emancipation of 1861* (Cambridge, 1968); G. T. Robinson, *Rural Russia under the Old Regime* (London, reprint 1973); A. Gerschenkron, *Economic Backwardness in Historical Perspective* (London, 1962); W. S. Vucinich (ed.), *The Peasant in Nineteenth century Russia* (Stanford, 1968); M. E. Falkus, *The Industrialization of Russia, 1700–1914* (London, 1972); D. Good, *The Economic Rise of the Hapsburg Empire, 1750–1914* (Berkeley, 1984); I. T. Berend and G. Ranki (eds), *Economic Development in East-Central Europe in the 19th and 20th Centuries* (New York, 1974); J. Komlos, *The Habsburg Monarchy as a Customs Union: Economic Development in Austria-Hungary in the Nineteenth Century* (Princeton, 1983).

Political and social issues are covered in the following: D. C. B. Lieven, *Russia's Rulers under the Old Regime* (London, 1989); J. L. H. Keep, *The Rise of Social Democracy in Russia* (Oxford, 1966); L. Kochan, *Russia in Revolution, 1890–1918* (London, 1966); R. E. Pipes, *Russia under the Old Regime* (London, 1974); E. C. Thaden, *Russia since 1801: The Making of a New Society* (New York, 1971); D. Balmuth, *Censorship in Russia, 1865–1905* (Washington, DC, 1979); G. L. Yaney, *The Systemization of Russian Government* (London, 1973); P. Pomper, *The Russian Revolutionary Intelligentsia* (New York, 1970); R. H. McNeal (ed.), *Russia in Transition, 1905–1914:*

Evolution or Revolution? (New York, 1970); A. J. Mayer, *The Persistence of the Old Regime* (London, 1981); C. E. Schorske, *Fin-de-siècle Vienna: Politics and Culture* (London, 1980); W. M. Johnston, *The Austrian Mind: An Intellectual and Social History, 1848–1938* (London, 1983); I. Banac, *The National Question in Yugoslavia: Origins, History, Politics* (Ithaca, 1984); R. Pearson, *National Minorities in Eastern Europe, 1848–1945* (London, 1983).

Other books also likely to be of use include: N. Stone, *Europe Transformed, 1878–1919* (London, 1983); B. W. Tuchman, *The Proud Tower* (London, 1966); E. Crankshaw, *The Fall of the House of Habsburg* (London, 1970); R. Okey, *Eastern Europe, 1740–1985* (London, 1986); and E. L. Woodward, *Prelude to Modern Europe, 1815–1914* (London, 1972).

4 Intellectual and cultural revolution, 1890–1914

Michael Biddiss

The way in which, today, we tend to view and discuss many areas of human experience is still deeply influenced by crucial changes in perception and expression that developed in Europe during the quarter-century before 1914. The changes embraced the worlds of nature and of mind, the sphere of the spiritual as well as that of secular social and political analysis, and not least the domains of literary and artistic creation. The range and significance of this transformation, originating in the context of 'high culture', compel us to treat it as nothing less than an intellectual revolution. It has indeed been rated amongst 'those overwhelming dislocations, those cataclysmic upheavals of culture, those fundamental convulsions of the creative human spirit that seem to topple even the most substantial of our beliefs and assumptions'.[1] This is a high claim. But how else can we do proper justice to the achievements of an epoch that is associated with such figures as Einstein and Freud, Nietzsche and Lenin, Durkheim and Weber, Ibsen and Proust, Picasso and Stravinsky?

The full span of their dates of birth – from that of Ibsen in 1828 to that of Stravinsky in 1882 – encompasses those central decades of the nineteenth century during which European intellectual and cultural life was most strongly affected by a climate of confidence. Wider social and political developments contributed much to this mood. Particularly over the two or three decades after 1848, Europe experienced the remarkable economic and industrial expansion of its 'railway age'. As critics like Karl Marx and Friedrich Engels stressed, the financial and other benefits were very unevenly spread. Even so, an increasingly large number of Europeans were coming to enjoy either the actuality or the fairly imminent prospect of richer and more varied habits of consumption.

Advances in fields such as communications and food supply, urban sanitation and health care, and education and literacy were all readily packaged together as facets of a single master-image of 'progress'. The variety and interdependence of its manifestations were never more strikingly displayed than at the 'Crystal Palace', which in 1851 housed at Hyde Park the 'Great Exhibition of the Works of Industry of all Nations'. Victorian Britain was prominent not just in these matters of material improvement, but also as a source of progressive inspiration in politics. Indeed, the economic prosperity which apparently stemmed from applying the principles of *laissez-faire* served naturally to enhance the prestige of other liberal commitments – especially those supportive of parliamentary institutions elected on a broadened franchise. Under these circumstances, the rebuffs to European liberalism suffered in 1848–9 could appear all the more temporary. It became plausible – though not invariably correct – to regard the new Italian kingdom of 1860–1, or Tsar Alexander II's measures of the 1860s, or the Austro-Hungarian *Ausgleich* of 1867, or Britain's Reform Act of that same year, or universal manhood suffrage for the new German Reichstag of 1871, or the eventual ascendency of republicanism in France as each forming part of one great force, relentlessly advancing against the enemies of freedom, democracy, and happiness.

Much of this naively optimistic spirit survived into the new century. For example, even while economic growth was slowing in the relatively depressed circumstances of 1873–96, many countries became involved in a burst of colonial expansion more explosive than any previously recorded in the long annals of European imperialism. The motivations behind this 'scramble', into Africa and eastern Asia especially, were complex. Simpler, however, was its principal intellectual consequence – a tendency to reinforce familiar beliefs about the naturalness and permanence of Europe's hegemony in political, technological, cultural, and even racial terms. In domestic settings too, the ruling classes were over-reliant upon the stability of old assumptions and established structures: a perilous complacency surrounded, for instance, the elegance and glitter of Viennese society as it danced the last waltzes of the Habsburg age. Regarding the wider bourgeoisie, Alan Bullock writes:

> With light taxation, no inflation, cheap food, cheap labour, a plentiful supply of domestic servants, many ordinary middle-class families with modest incomes lived full and comfortable lives. No wonder that so many who came from such families and survived the War, looking back, felt that there was a grace, an ease, a security in living then which has since been lost for ever.[2]

Nowadays, equipped with hindsight and haunted by indelible images from the battlefields of 1914–18, we can more readily grasp the significance of certain anxieties which undoubtedly did surface during the pre-war epoch, even if they also remained underrated at that time. Among them were fears about the disruptive dynamics of mass social-ization, and about the violence associated with the anarchist, socialist, and nationalist challenges to an old order whose own rulers had already locked themselves into a potentially destructive arms race. The horrors soon to occur along the Marne and the Somme, at Ypres and Verdun, would give a whole continent much more urgent cause to question the doctrine of progress and much else that the nineteenth century had tended to take for granted. But how far, even before 1914, had intellectuals and imaginative artists themselves embarked upon their own dissolution of confident expectations and familiar former certainties?

Changes within the natural sciences form a fundamental part of any proper answer. Here, seemingly, had been the very paradigm of progress. Much of that material advance which helped to inspire the nineteenth-century faith in human betterment had been dependent upon the practical exploitation of scientific knowledge, as exemplified by the use of Louis Pasteur's germ theory in combating disease, or that of electromagnetic principles in refining the dynamo. Indeed, so strik-ing seemed the capacity of scientists to harness their understanding of nature to the purposes of social improvement, that their discipline was well on the way to winning the kind of dominant intellectual status once occupied by theology or philosophy. Increasingly, science appeared destined not just to supply firm answers to its own traditional questions, but even to bring other domains into the sphere of its methods and achievements. That expectation was central to the nineteenth-century cult of 'positivism' – a secularizing belief that science (as distinct particularly from theology) could provide the supreme model for all real knowledge. It followed that the insights claimed by other disciplines might be valuable only in so far as they incorporated or imitated scientific habits of enquiry, observation, testing, and commit-ment to rational causality. At the core of the cultural upheaval of the years around 1900 we find not simply a revolt against such positivistic insistence upon science as intellectual lodestar, but also a shattering of the established image of the physical world itself.

During the generation before 1890 the liveliest debates had sur-rounded biological issues, especially those tackled so controversially by Charles Darwin in *The Origin of Species* (1859) and its main sequel *The Descent of Man* (1871). His achievement was not to discover the evolutionary transformation of species – a familiar topic in itself – but to explain its principal way of operating through a new theory of 'natural selection'. This presented a relentless struggle for existence, occurring within and between species against the broader setting of a potentially hostile environment; in this situation, the inherited variations which chanced to be most favourably adapted to the relevant circumstances would tend to be preserved at the expense of others less favourable to the organism in question. The randomness of such variations seemed to negate conceptions of ideal form and purposeful direction within nature. Thus the creation even of the remarkable human species need no longer be explained by reference to a separate and special act of God. Men and women were being invited, rather, to accept their own evolution from certain less highly organized forms, according to a pattern of kinship which revealed the ape as their distant cousin.

Between 1890 and 1914 such biologists as William Bateson, Hugo de Vries, and Thomas H. Morgan filled important gaps left by Darwin's own theory, especially regarding the matter of explaining how variations are transmitted over generations. Pre-eminent here was the founding of a new science of 'genetics', involving belated recognition of Gregor Mendel's pioneering studies from the 1860s on particulate inheritance, and the pursuit of related work on the theory of 'mutation' as applied to evolutionary leaps. Yet, in another vital sense, Darwin's structure was actually looking less complete by the early twentieth century. Before his death in 1882 he had certainly managed to achieve not just a remarkable synthesis of human, zoological, and botanical studies, but also the integration of these with the geological and palaeontological discoveries of the earth sciences. On that basis many had been confident about all of this soon becoming subsumed into an even broader unifying theory of physics. It was, above all, this early expectation of still more ambitious synthesis which got plunged into doubt by certain scientists as the century turned.

The nub of the matter is the occurrence around 1900 of a revolution in physics which matched in scope, and challenged in substance, the upheaval achieved by Isaac Newton two hundred years before. His was still the overall framework that nineteenth-century scientists sought to refine. They continued to treat the universe as being composed of material bodies existing in separate dimensions of time and space; to view the basic units of matter as billiard-ball atoms of fixed weights capable of being variously lumped together; and to describe the dynamic forces (such as those of gravitation) operating between these units in terms of a mathematics whose own neatness crystallized the regularities supposedly essential to external reality. The principal achievements of the period from the 1840s to the 1880s – especially in the fields of thermodynamics, chemical elements, and electromagnetism – served simply to confirm the emerging tidiness of things. This was the harmonious structure about which biology also seemed increasingly destined to supply confirming testimony. Such order, potentially consistent from microcosm to macrocosm, offered even the eventual prospect of total description and explanation. As more of the master blueprint was unrolled, science – rather like that supreme technological symbol, the Eiffel Tower of 1889 – would surely reach its own symmetrical pinnacle. Accordingly, whatever remained presently unknown was merely that which happened to be as yet undiscovered, rather than anything which might be in principle unknowable. Such confidence in the progressive unfolding of a systematic reality had provided nineteenth-century positivism with its chief sustenance. Equally, it was this same faith which a new physics would now imperil.

Among the advances most crucial in triggering off a challenge to conventional explanation was Konrad Röntgen's identification of X-rays, widely publicized in 1895 as a form of fluorescence stimulated by discharge tube and capable of penetrating certain solids. This led Henri Becquerel and Marie Curie to discover other kinds of radiation, emanating spontaneously from such elements as uranium. It was soon recognized, especially through J. J. Thomson's work at Cambridge, that the huge amounts of energy involved in these 'radioactive' transformations of matter must stem from processes operating within the structure of atoms hitherto deemed indivisible. Investigation of these unheralded sub-atomic levels, where scientists had suddenly to confront the electron and other elementary particles, thus became central to physics as further refashioned by Ernest Rutherford and Niels Bohr in the years down to 1914. Within their strange new world, the orbit of electrons – and much else besides – was characterized by a jerky unpredictability, utterly at odds with the traditional assumption that some regular pattern of continuity and determinacy must reign through all the causal relationships of nature. The foundations for a very different view had been laid in 1900 by Max Planck. His ideas about 'the quantum' were pivotal to his formula for gauging the discrete discontinuities involved in the emission of energy, and in 1905 they were similarly central to Albert Einstein's extension of the argument into a particulate theory of light.

The range of Einstein's contribution to scientific revolution stretched further still, through the special and general theories of relativity propounded in 1905 and 1915–16 respectively. In the former, he presented time and space as interdependent aspects of a single fourth-dimensional continuum; insisted that light had a constant velocity whatever the movement of its source or observer; argued for the mutual convertibility of mass and energy, which were to be viewed as different ways of expressing a single process; and concluded that each particle of matter held energy (E) equivalent to its mass (m) multiplied by the square of the velocity of light (c^2). Thus was generated the famous formula $(E=mc^2)$, through which Einstein expressed the vast power contained within the atom. As for the general theory, this focused on problems of celestial motion that resisted convincing solution along Newtonian lines. According to Einstein's very different model, such movement did not confirm to the 'flatness' of Euclidean geometry. Instead, it must be understood as an expression of the qualities of 'curved' space-time at successive points, with allowance made for distortions by the electromagnetic fields surrounding large bodies. Just as Planck's work highlighted discontinuity and indeterminacy, so Einstein's relativity amounted to a denial of any absolute frame of reference. By such means the nature of scientific laws themselves had been called into question. Could they still be viewed as operating consistently across all the levels, from microcosm to macrocosm? And what sort of objective existence might they still possess independently of the constructs framed by the scientist's own imagination? It was plain, at the very least, that the new physics was dealing with phenomena less predictable, more mysterious, than the old. Here was a vast leap in knowledge – yet it was one which raised even more problems than it solved, and thus opened up vast vistas of uncertainty far beyond anything anticipated by nineteenth-century positivists.

No less perplexing was the work of Sigmund Freud, a Viennese specialist in nervous ailments whose creation of 'psychoanalysis' in the 1890s well exemplified the ambiguities to be encountered along the borderlands between scientific and imaginative endeavour. He had no need to discover the fact of the subconscious. What he claimed to reveal was its *power*, as an active force embracing concepts and memories literally too terrible to contemplate. Freud's patients were encouraged to engage in relaxed narration. This served them as a means of therapy, yet also provided him with material that he could analyse (through rather speculative procedures of verbal association), for the purpose of probing into the depths of the mind. As his experience widened, particularly into self-analysis, Freud incorporated the evidence of dreams. They were illusory as keys to the future, but as 'a disguised fulfilment of repressed wishes' they could be central in unlocking an individual's past. Here, he argued in the epochal *Interpretation of Dreams* (first edition dated 1900, but issued in the previous year), was 'the royal road to a knowledge of the unconscious activities of the mind'.[3] What guaranteed Freud's notoriety, however, was his further insistence on the extent to which, even from infancy, such activity was dominated by sexual concerns. He came to view his female patients' tales of childhood seduction by their fathers not as being literally true, but as something that might look even more shocking to respectable society: recollections of the girls' *own* wishful fantasies. This conviction was then incorporated into a broader theory of sexuality which stressed every child's passion for the parent of opposite sex. Freud argued that its thwarting produced in all of us a measure of 'neurotic' guilt and anxiety which was the more powerful for being uncomprehended, and that the degree to which such strain was successfully accommodated through unconscious processes of repression conditioned society's perceptions of the essentially hazy frontiers between 'normality' and 'abnormality'.

While the physicists were putting curves into time and space, the more dubious 'science' of psychoanalysis appeared to be warping the customary categories for discussion of sanity, morality, and rationality too. However, despite his enemies' claims to the contrary, Freud was never intentionally a wrecker bent upon compelling civilization to dissolve itself amidst a morally irresponsible riot of primal urges. True, on the map of mind which he was replotting, the domains of reason were much reduced. Yet he believed that the revised chart, covering even the logic of the dreamily illogical, would reflect reality far more accurately. Thus he aimed to help preserve rationality in human affairs precisely by exposing the more uncritical positivistic exaggerations of its effective scope.

It was all the easier to misinterpret Freud's intentions because his efforts coincided around the turn of the century not just with the physicists' own challenge to familiar patterns of intellectual order, but also with two forms of major reorientation amongst philosophers, each of which seemed to reinforce moral confusion. One of these affected the best of those who, especially in the Cambridge of Bertrand Russell, and the Vienna of his younger associate Ludwig Wittgenstein, continued to develop the positivist tradition. They now abandoned many of its previous aspirations towards generating grandiose systems not simply of intellectual synthesis but of ethical prescription too. The refined positivism of the twentieth century would stake out, instead, a more self-absorbed and precisely limited concern with the specific mathematical, logical, and linguistic mechanisms operating within philosophical activity itself. The second brand of reorientation, which had even greater influence during the generation before 1914, did not really constitute an alternative line of comparable retreat from philosophy's traditional engagement with ethics. Rather, it promised the revolutionary triumph of a new morality aimed at radical subversion of the old.

Here, the figure who made most impact on the early twentieth century was Friedrich Nietzsche, notwithstanding the fact that he himself was irrecoverably insane by 1890 and dead by 1900. Who better than a mad philosopher to inspire 'the new irrationalism'? This aspect of the revolt against positivism drew deep from the wells of romanticism in its challenge to the assumption that reason must provide the primary criterion of philosophical truth. Instead, it assigned higher value to unconscious instinct and vitalistic intuition. Upon that basis, and through the medium of aphoristic semi-poetical prose, Nietzsche had launched his 'attempt to philosophize with a hammer'.[4] Among the received ideas that as a cultural critic he sought to shatter was the cosy assumption that advances in literacy and the diffusion of ideas, in reason and supposed intellectual refinement, would serve to improve humanity. For him, such nineteenth-century progressive illusions amounted simply to a capitulation before herd values. History, if conceived as linear ascent, became meaningless; it must be grasped, rather, as a cyclical process of 'eternal return'. And just as it denied relentless secular progress, so too it confounded all hopes of religious fulfilment. 'God is dead!', Nietzsche famously declared. 'God remains dead! And we have killed him! How shall we comfort ourselves – we who are the greatest murderers of all?'[5] The profoundest challenge thus set for posterity was that of accepting, and then benefiting from, the loss of illusions secular and sacred alike. Nietzsche sought to replace the Christian 'pity-ethic' with his own 'Will to Power', which operated in such a way as to give meaning to virtue only within the context of whatever served towards the purposes of quasi-Darwinistic survival. Those converted to this insight might spearhead a revaluation of all values, taking humanity 'beyond Good and Evil' as hitherto conceived. They alone might aspire to the cherished title of *Übermensch*, or superior being. All this was indeed heady stuff, and by 1914 Nietzsche's legacy had become a focal point of cult and controversy amongst academic, literary, and popular moralists everywhere. In the last resort, what mattered most was not their agreement or disagreement with him. Rather, it was their experience of catalytic engagement with a figure who, like Freud, had scourged the complacencies of a whole era.

For those analysing society and politics during this climax of Nietzschean debate around the turn of the century, there were two other individuals who had also left a posthumous challenge which needed to be confronted. The first was the English naturalist whose biological work (already mentioned) became moulded, indeed often distorted, by others into forms of 'social Darwinism'; the second was Marx. Certain important points of similarity between them were readily evident. Both had laboured during the heyday of positivism, each invoking science to underpin theories of social development which were at odds with religious orthodoxy, which laid emphasis upon group struggle (whether between species or classes), and which raised awkward questions as to how human destinies might be governed far less by conscious choice and rational effort than by impersonal forces operating under the determining imperatives of biological or economic materialism. It was Engels himself who, speaking at Marx's funeral in 1883, only a year after Darwin's own death, quite explicitly bracketed together their supreme achievement as discoverers of the general laws controlling organic nature and human history. However, such a specifically Marxist reading of what Darwin's theory implied for social and political development never went uncontested, and subsequent controversy was all the more vigorous precisely because others besides Engels were keen on benefiting from the same scientific cachet.

What actually emerges as the outstanding feature of social Darwinism by 1900 is its very plasticity: the application of its discourse to multiple, and often mutually inconsistent purposes. Might not, for example, the anti-socialist version of progressive politics championed by liberals draw strength from those parts of Darwin's rhetoric which seemingly endorsed evolutionary rather than revolutionary transformations, or which allowed 'struggle' to be decoded as individualistic competition within the free market of capitalism rather than as war between the classes? Even more significantly, by the century's turn Darwinistic modes of argument were permeating debates concerning the dynamics and likely outcome of contemporary national and racial rivalries. The broad convergence between liberal and nationalist objectives, so characteristic of the generation before 1848, had now dissolved. Nationalism had become a fiercer animal, more aggressively adapted to the quasi-Darwinian jungle of *Realpolitik* where right was derived from might, and morality was assessed only in terms of its contribution towards increasing the chances of survival. The schism from liberalism ran all the deeper as the vogue developed – most markedly, but far from exclusively, in Germany – for treating some concept of racial essence as the principal defining criterion for nationhood. Darwin's phrase about 'The Preservation of Favoured Races in the Struggle for Life'[6] strengthened assertions not just about differentiation between peoples, but also about inequalities of worth which were so fundamentally rooted in biology as to defy any swift erosion through the processes of cultural assimilation. Such racism, in so far as it made the biological constitution of each individual the overwhelming determinant of his social value, plainly aspired to be the ultimate embodiment of a scientific politics. Yet, as matters actually developed towards and beyond the Great War, it proved equally capable of flourishing as part of the broadly Nietzschean and anti-positivistic cult of instinct and intuition, hospitable as that was to the mystical and irrational side of the racist habit of 'thinking with the blood'. This whole potent mixture of gut feeling and rationalization through misconstrued science manifested itself in a variety of contexts during the generation before 1914. One prime example was the rapid intensification of racial anti-Semitism, associated with such developments as Alexander III's pogroms in Russia, and the Dreyfus Affair in France. Another was that pervasive faith in the superiority of the white races over the 'coloured' stocks which accompanied the explosive enlargement of European colonial dominance during this same epoch.

This imperialism was less problematic to social Darwinists than to those who were now extending the Marxist tradition. The latter needed to ask whether the colonial ventures were merely the final symptoms of capitalism's terminal decay or whether they were something more troubling to a revolutionary – that is, a means of postponing collapse by transferring overseas much of the burden of economic exploitation, from the European proletariat to a new horde of the oppressed beyond. The adaptive capacities of Marxist theory during the epoch of the Second International (launched in 1889) were also challenged by other developments which might be interpreted as bids for capitalistic self-protection, including extensions of franchise, state-sponsored welfare schemes, and legal recognition for trade unions. In the British case, for example, pioneering leadership of the industrialization process had not, as anticipated, laid firm bases for revolutionary socialism. The 'gradualist' alternative which prevailed most decisively there, through the Fabian Society and the emerging Labour Party, also remained influential in certain other countries, like France and Germany, where Marxism did take stronger root. The dilemmas were such that towards 1914 the largest of all the parties championing Marxist theory – the German Social Democrats, now inspired by Karl Kautsky – still seemed unable, in actual practice, to escape from the gradualism for which the 'revisionist' Eduard Bernstein (author of *Evolutionary Socialism*, 1899) had been so roundly denounced.

In autocratic Russia, where by 1917 the chaos of war would eventually stimulate a Marxist triumph, much of the western debate had seemed irrelevant, especially because parliamentary institutions were absent before the revolt of 1905 and only feebly present thereafter. However, even while broadly agreeing about some measure of resort to violence, the left-wing intelligentsia could still hotly dispute issues of leadership and timing, as well as the relative roles assignable to peasant and proletarian. Thus it was against the 'populists', and their belief that the key to success resided with the rural masses, that V. I. Lenin, Marx's most renowned revolutionary heir, directed much of his early work on *The Development of Capitalism in Russia* (1899). A sequel, *What Is To Be Done?* (1902), further elaborated his preference for relying chiefly upon the industrial proletariat, despite its far fewer numbers. Nor was that the limit of his élitist propensities, for he also insisted that these oppressed urban workers themselves needed an additional stimulus: an injection of heightened Marxist consciousness from a tightly disciplined cadre of professional revolutionaries charged intellectually to enlighten and politically to command the wider mass. By seeking to demonstrate that any political or economic concession which might come from the tsarist regime would simply render revolutionary militancy more rather than less urgent, Lenin was attacking the very core of the gradualist case. The Russian Social Democratic Labour Party's split of 1903 into Bolsheviks and Mensheviks was occasioned by the latter faction's resistance to his organizational élitism. The divide was then deepened by his conviction that the Menshevik inclination to collaborate with liberal-bourgeois elements would serve only to delay revolution. Of all his fellow Marxist opponents none was more perceptive than Rosa Luxemburg, a Pole prominent within the German movement. She had been particularly scathing about Bernsteinian gradualism, yet she warned also against the general direction in which Leninism seemed to be driving. Was it not threatening to crush all the spontaneity and initiative of the exploited populace beneath the over-centralized dictatorship of a vanguard Bolshevik Party, and thus effectively serving to dispossess the working class even of its most fundamental entitlement to full revolutionary experience?

Fears about the authoritarian potential of the communist movement had been even more broadly expressed within anarchist circles. From that base, Mikhail Bakunin had precipitated the collapse of the First International in 1872 through his attacks upon Marx as the devaluer of spontaneous action, and as a figure keener to exploit than to destroy state structures. The principal anarchist work of the succeeding generation was Peter Kropotkin's *Mutual Aid: A Factor in Evolution* (1902). This argued that Darwinism's most vital lessons pointed towards human cooperation rather than struggle; that men's natural goodness had been corrupted only by flawed institutions; that the true evolutionary goal concerned the attainment of an ethic generated from within, rather than one dictated by forces of external compulsion, such as the state; and that, once conditions of common possession and absolute equality were achieved, this 'morality without obligation or sanction' would come necessarily and spontaneously into existence. Kropotkin believed that, until then, violence must be regarded as a legitimate weapon against economic and political repression. These years around the turn of the century proved to be, in thought and deed alike, the heyday of European anarchism. Though actual bomb-throwers were always a minority, the movement's ideas attracted a remarkably large measure of sympathy amongst intellectuals. Its endeavours to expose the capacity for moral suffocation deeply entrenched within the bourgeois order were both uncompromising and timely. No less so were its pleas for revolt through that mode of seemingly irrational violence which, as the expression of an individual's unique spontaneity, allegedly restored his freedom, identity and dignity. Thus anarchism, when interpreted as a critique of rational constraints and as a philosophy of will given political application, becomes sharply relevant to those strange new worlds of the mind being explored by Freud or Nietzsche.

Similar concerns also confronted sociology, which in these years began to establish itself as a significant academic activity. The term had been coined by Auguste Comte, and many of the subject's central issues had been identified and explored by Marx himself. Their mid-nineteenth-century efforts to expound the 'laws' governing the operation of human communities had reflected a positivistic confidence in grand systems of scientific explanation that looked more questionable by 1900. Even before the revolution in physics exploded many previous notions about the character of the natural sciences themselves, certain distinguished champions of the social ones (such as Wilhelm Dilthey) were reasserting the distinctiveness of these latter domains by virtue of their engagement with all the human complexity of 'lived experience'. As the twentieth century began, the new sociology was coming to appreciate that the sources of action might be far more mysterious than previously thought. Assisted by anthropological studies, it was also tending to undermine any simple belief in the self-evidently progressive evolution of societies from 'primitive' to 'advanced' forms. It questioned, more radically than before, whether

European experience alone could provide adequate criteria for judging the value or necessity of particular social phenomena. For example, despite the complacent belief of the white races in their supremacy, there was evidence concerning alien 'primitive' cultures which succeeded well in satisfying complex needs and in sustaining harmony on bases that were seemingly instinctual and remote from the supposedly more rationalistic constructs of the West. Thus it was timely to ask just how shallow had been previous European assumptions about the conditions under which societies might – or might not – hold together, elicit loyalties from their members, and confer legitimacy on their rulers.

Reconsideration was all the more urgent amidst the unprecedented circumstances associated with the rising influence of the masses. If Marx saw their approaching triumph as a welcome fulfilment of an inevitable historical process, other social analysts could beg to differ and to offer ideas about containing or even redirecting the forces of change. Two Frenchmen were particularly notable for their pioneering, and disturbing, studies of mass behaviour. In *The Crowd* (1895) Gustave Le Bon showed how the apparently rational individual was liable to behave irrationally once placed within a herd context and there exposed to processes of 'mental contagion' productive of credulous unanimity; and the criminologist Gabriel Tarde issued a similar warning, particularly about 'imitation' of superior by inferior, in his widely-read *Opinion and the Crowd* (1901), which investigated the impact of mass communication. Such works raised doubts as to whether, despite all the nineteenth-century talk of democratic and egalitarian fulfilment, a gullible populace could ever really liberate itself from dominance by skilful élites. The role of these was further explored by three celebrated contributors to the early development of political sociology. Here, in *The Ruling Class* (1896), Gaetano Mosca suggested that an élite could successfully perpetuate its authority over the mass simply by purveying astutely-chosen 'political formulas', almost regardless of their empirical truth. From Robert Michels there came *Political Parties: A Sociological Study of the Oligarchical Tendencies of Modern Democracy* (1911), a work whose title amply suggests the drift of its argument about an 'iron law' working towards a professionalization of leadership, and thus towards élitist expertise and dominance. Then, in *Socialist Systems* (1902), and in the more general treatise translated as *Mind and Society* (1916–23), Vilfredo Pareto explored how élites 'circulated', with success going to whatever group that might, from time to time, devise the most appropriate rhetorical structures based upon its grasp of the complex interplay between rational and non-rational behaviour.

Among all those who were at this epoch setting sociology's future agenda, pride of place is shared between a Frenchman and a German, Emile Durkheim and Max Weber. The works of the former included *The Division of Labour in Society* (1893), a refutation of Marx's negative interpretation of this as being inevitably an 'alienating' process; *The Rules of Sociological Method* (1895); *Suicide* (1897), a study of the social dysfunctions conditioning a type of behaviour commonly regarded as supremely individualistic; and *The Elementary Forms of Religious Life* (1912), in which gods are deemed to be the symbolization of social interests, of a felt need for community. Durkheim remained enough of a positivist to seek a truly scientific basis for identifying the form of morality most conducive to harmony within a mass society which was now (rightly, in his view) rejecting Christianity. He believed that the price of failure would be the growth of *anomie* – a pathological absence or confusion of norms. Weber claimed less for sociology (which he treated as an illuminator rather than a determinant of choices that remained ultimately expressions of subjective value judgment), and thereby achieved even more. His *Protestant Ethic and the Spirit of Capitalism* (1904–5) countered Marx not simply by showing how religious factors might rival economic ones as influences on social development, but also by suggesting the inadequacy of any kind of monocausal explanation. Other writings expanded his account of the process of 'rationalization' which he had discerned in capitalism and Calvinism alike, and which was now evident also in the spread of bureaucracy. Here, like Michels, he feared that the linkage between expertise and power might endanger individual freedom. Weber then agonized about whether men would, and should, react to this threat by relying on the emergence of heroic 'charismatic' figures deemed to possess exceptional, almost magical, qualities. Would their leadership provide psychological compensation for what otherwise seemed, under secularized conditions, a diminished sense of purpose and a soulless demoralization? These anxieties stemmed from Weber's view that 'rationalization' also involved 'disenchantment' – a liberation from magic which is nonetheless accompanied by a feeling of loss, indeed by 'disillusionment' as commonly conceived. The ebbing of traditional belief, the crisis of disorientation, and the value of some functional substitute for religion remained, for him as for Durkheim, central issues. No less than Nietzsche or Freud, Weber was querying just how much stark reality humankind could bear.

Such radical questioning of previous assumptions is something which we have encountered across all the fields so far surveyed. It also characterizes the achievements of this epoch in a final broad domain – the sphere of artistic creativity, particularly as expressed through imaginative literature and painting. Here, again, positivism had left a firm imprint on the three or four decades before 1890, during which 'realism' and 'naturalism' dominated the scene in their pursuit of what the French novelist, Emile Zola, called 'the exact study of facts and things'.[7] His own twenty-volume sequence entitled *Les Rougon-Macquart* (1871–93), a family saga detailing the interaction of heredity and environment, was the greatest literary monument to this inclination towards dignifying art by converting it into a documentary supplement to science. It was largely by movement against and beyond such positivistic constraints on creative methods and objectives that the culture of 'modernism' took shape as the nineteenth century drew to a close. Among the most seminal writers in this process was Henrik Ibsen, a Norwegian famed throughout Europe by the century's turn, whose plays first embodied and then transcended naturalism. For example, his treatment of female revolt against the asphyxiating conventions and hypocrisies of male-dominated society becomes subtler – especially in its evocation of those inner forces most defiant of capture by quasi-scientific description – as between *A Doll's House* (1879) and *Hedda Gabler* (1890). The latter set the tone for the consummate psychological and spiritual exploration which pervades Ibsen's final achievements, such as *The Master Builder* (1892), and *When We Dead Awaken* (1899). A similar shift is evident in the case of the German novelist Thomas Mann, and at a far earlier stage within the span of his own career. 'Naturalistic' was the term which he himself applied to *Buddenbrooks* (1902), his first major work, wherein he traced the fortunes of a Hanseatic merchant family similar to his own. Yet, even here, Mann's treatment of the tensions between the values of bourgeois society and those of the artist was hinting that introspective exploration of the nature of individual creativity might properly take precedence over any more mundane concern with mere social documentation. He developed this theme in the novellas *Tristan* and *Tonio Kröger* (both 1903), and his growing preoccupation with it was most memorably confirmed by *Death in Venice* (1911).

That story, where the author-hero Aschenbach dies amidst his obsessive contemplation of the golden boy Tadzio, prompted questions concerning not just the corruptive power of art, but also the degree of frankness permissible in matters of sexuality. As Freud knew, and as writers and artists far more rebellious than he and the similarly ambivalent Mann had eagerly grasped, here was the realm in which the respectable bourgeoisie could be most readily shocked and its hypocrisies most explosively punctured. Attacks on the 'normal' sexual conventions of polite society thus became a central motif within that wider revolt against established assumptions, which is so characteristic of creative activity during this era. The call of 'art for art's sake' was increasingly heard. Did this mean that it could now aspire to impose its own terms and supplant bourgeois values by offering society some counter-morality, Nietzschean or otherwise? Or, more radically, did such slogans imply that art must renounce all social and moral engagement whatsoever? Advocates of the latter course turned inward to concentrate upon a private world of symbolic expression and pure form, accessible only to the limited circle of their chosen peers. They found beauty not in raw nature, but in the artifice that must transcend it. This cult of 'aestheticism' involved making one's own life into a work of art, capable of proclaiming the delights of the extravagant, the useless, and the effete – the allure of the exotic, the occult, and the perverse. Jean des Esseintes, the neurotic and hypersensitive hero of Joris-Karl Huysmans' *A Rebours* (1884, sometimes translated as *Against Nature*), offered a whole generation its main fictional model for a lifestyle that writers and artists such as Oscar Wilde and Aubrey Beardsley might actualize. To condemn this as 'decadent' merely encouraged its practitioners to convert that very label into a badge of pride.

Whereas prose had been the obvious vehicle for expressing the positivistic pretentions of naturalism, it was often poetry that best reflected the more introspective concerns of *fin-de-siècle* writers. Pre-eminent here was the 'symbolist' movement which, while limited to no single country or medium, became most celebrated for the thematic and technical innovations which it brought to French verse during the last decades of the nineteenth century. Outstanding contributors in that language were Arthur Rimbaud, Paul Verlaine, Stéphane Mallarmé, and the Belgian Emile Verhaeren; and their wider influence was apparent also from the work in German by such poets as Stefan George and the Austrian Rainer Maria Rilke. The kind of truth sought by the French symbolists flowed not from science, but rather from what Rimbaud called a 'disordering of all the senses'.[8] Thus inspired, the creative spirit could liberate itself from the imperfections of the mundane and explore far deeper levels of reality. In their concern to evoke atmosphere and to convey intensity of feeling, the symbolists contributed to that heightened interest in the mystical and the irrational that we have already observed elsewhere. They immersed themselves in the flow of language and conjured with the magical properties of sound. The late poetry of Mallarmé (who died in 1898) becomes, indeed, so 'hermetic' and obscure – contorted in grammar and syntax, experimental in typography – as to suggest that the pursuit of artistic insulation from a philistine world had reached the point where the power of words to communicate beyond the self was in peril of exhaustion.

By the start of the Great War no author had managed better than Marcel Proust to encapsulate in a single volume most of that range of concerns which we have seen moulding literature's contribution to the cultural revolution of this epoch. Such was his achievement in *Swann's Way* (1913), the opening novel within a large and long-planned cycle. Especially in its minuteness of observation, this account of French society since the closing decades of the nineteenth century drew upon the techniques of naturalism. Yet it also went beyond them – reflecting, for example, the symbolists' sense of fragile language under strain, and their concern with the stresses imposed upon the introspective artist by his exposure to the everyday world. Here fiction was being used to explore areas that, independently, Freud too was probing: all that was mysterious about levels of consciousness, and about the memory processes through which we recapture something of *le temps perdu*, experience past and forgotten. Proust illuminated especially the evocative power of casual sense-association, most splendidly instanced by the famous dunked madeleine whose savour unleashes for his hero a flood of childhood recollection. Such remembrance is here an active, not passive, force. It gives us our sense of identity, releasing from the prison of the subconscious something of our own past that then becomes vital to our present. Indeed, with Proust, contentment stems only from the recapturing of time gone, from the recontemplation of paradises lost. This is a world where memory is the substance of reality, where the multiple refractions between past and present warp all ordinary chronology, and where every perspective upon persons and places endlessly shifts. Thus, while the Proustian project was never directly inspired by science in the way that Zola's had been, it possessed vertiginous and disorientating qualities which seemed to be curiously congruent with the new physics and to offer similarly 'the picture of a relativistic universe, expanding and contracting in a curved space-time continuum'.[9]

In painting, as in literature, much of the urge towards innovation during this period stemmed from revolt against the naturalistic limitations besetting most orthodox art. Even when Claude Monet and Auguste Renoir launched their own seminal challenge in the mid-1870s, it was upon the quasi-scientific merits of the new 'impressionism' – as 'this study of light in its thousand decompositions and recompositions'[10] was known – that Zola based his influential support. These artists were certainly concerned about accurately conveying the complexity of optical experience, especially in the open air where colours and tones incessantly altered. But, over the longer run, the more specifically scientific pretensions associated with this endeavour were scarcely sustained. Paradoxically, the success of impressionism and 'post-impressionism' resided not in an ability to complete an experiment but in a capacity to suggest mood and atmosphere. Here again, objective description was becoming secondary to subjective evocation. In his great 'series' paintings of the 1890s – repeatedly exploring such subjects as the west front of Rouen cathedral under changing conditions of light and weather – Monet himself was repudiating any idea of definitive version or final answer. He was affirming, instead, that 'reality' is the sum of countless different appearances, each spatially and temporally personal.

A hundred years – and millions of reproductions – later, the works inspired by impressionism over the epoch from the 1870s to 1914 are so familiar and popular that we have to make an effort to remember just how radically they challenged old ways of seeing. By the early twentieth century the European avant-garde was deepening its curiosity about unfamiliar codes of perception and representation. What could be learned, for instance, from the forms through which children, or the insane, or those living in primitive and exotic cultures depicted external reality, or indeed from those through which they expressed their own internal worlds of feeling? The last point, in particular, helps to highlight the most fundamental issue of all: a rethinking of what art itself should aim to be *about*. This is the problem most pervasive during those final pre-war years – perhaps the most stimulatingly hectic decade in the whole history of European art – when the movements known as 'cubism', 'futurism', and 'expressionism' made their mark.

The towering figure amongst cubists was Pablo Picasso, whose *Demoiselles d'Avignon* (1907) constituted the first great statement of their style. While its mask-like faces reflected his debt to African and other exotic art, the depersonalization of its female figures was even more deeply rooted in the angular and fragmented manner of their presentation. As with Proust, a multiplicity of viewpoints was accentuating an uncertainty of identity; as with Einstein, space itself was being conceptually remodelled. Soon Picasso, and his closest associate Georges Braque, were repeatedly shattering the rules of single-point perspective. They superimposed planes, used lines to suggest rather than to define boundaries, and flouted the conventions of opaqueness and transparency. Their splintering of form became such that by 1910–11 it seemed as though cubist art was destined to lose all identifiable contact with those objects from the external world which were still alleged to be its point of departure. Then, relatively suddenly, Picasso and Braque turned to collage, and in a sense hesitated about imminent entry into a fundamentally non-representational realm of painting. Towards 1914 futurism, too, was probing these borderlands between the perceptual and the conceptual, form seen and form thought. Originally launched from Italy in 1909 as a literary movement, it penetrated various genres with its call for an aesthetic focused on the dynamism of the city and machine, the habit of energy, the beauty of speed, and the pursuit of danger and struggle (with war as the supreme manifestation of a mechanized culture). Those painters who soon adopted futurist ideas tended, significantly, to base themselves upon industrial Milan. There the central challenge which they tackled was that of simultaneously freezing and expressing rapid motion. Umberto Boccioni and Carlo Carrà were prominent as refiners of a technique, already used by the cubists, analogous to multiple or continuous exposure in photography. Indeed with Giacomo Balla, who was particularly stimulated by the new physics, one encounters pictures (most notably those of 1913, titled *Abstract Speed*) where the conversion of matter into dynamic light and colour has, yet again, almost reached the point of negating any representation of objects as such.

This was the issue upon which expressionist painting went furthest of all, in its preoccupation with inner feeling and a laying bare of the soul, in its assertion of spirit and imagination against the crushing forces of materialism. Within its pedigree there is a significant place for the Dutchman Vincent Van Gogh (who killed himself in 1890), and the Norwegian Edvard Munch, both of whom superbly communicated states of mental anguish. By the early twentieth century expressionism was developing with particular reference to two artistic circles, one formed as 'Die Brücke' (The Bridge) at Dresden in 1905, and another as 'Der Blaue Reiter' (The Blue Rider) at Munich in 1911. It was one of the latter's protagonists, the Russian Vasily Kandinsky, who spearheaded the breakthrough to a radically non-representational version of art. His consciousness of the revolutionary nature of this process is apparent from his commentary of 1911, *Concerning the Spiritual in Art*. It pleaded for a creativity that would shatter the limits imposed by excessive concern with external phenomena, and would instead stimulate art as 'an expression of a slowly formed inner feeling, which comes to utterance only after long maturing'.[11] Such was the philosophy behind a series of paintings which Kandinsky entitled *Compositions*, in which between 1910 and 1913 he explored the communicative qualities inherent within colours and forms to the point where any residual features from the world of external objects were merely incidental. As an expression of the interior forces of the mind operating at different and interactive levels of consciousness, the work of art in itself now constituted 'reality'.

A few years earlier, in Vienna around 1908, Arnold Schoenberg had begun to write atonal music, pieces abandoning that relationship between keys which had long been fundamental in Western classical composition. The fact that he was also a painter and an associate of the Blue Rider circle again exemplifies the point that the intellectual and cultural revolution of this epoch flowed across all conventional boundaries of genre. In the pre-war tours of Sergei Diaghilev's Ballets Russes, elements of radical innovation from a number of spheres came together with particularly startling effect. That was never more obviously the case than in May 1913, when the Parisian première of *The Rite of Spring* provoked scenes of riot amongst many of its audience. The shocked reaction had much to do with the allegedly unsuitable 'savagery' of Igor Stravinsky's musical score, fiercely percussive and irregular in its rhythms. The uproar stemmed also from the culmination of the ballet's plot, where a maiden dances herself to death in propitiation of the god of spring. By the end of the following year such a climax in human sacrifice had come to seem like a mark of the immediacy, not the remoteness, of the work's applicability to the contemporary condition. A decade later we find the novelist Virginia Woolf looking back across the hideous cratered divide formed by '1914–18', to the period of Edward VII's death and of the first major London exhibition of post-impressionist art. Concerning this epoch, she observed: 'In or about December, 1910, human character changed.'[12] This judgment of hers was, no doubt, unduly precise and altogether too simple. Yet everything we have surveyed here suggests that many far-reaching changes of attitude and perception were rapidly developing even before the guns began to fire, and that somewhere within her own conclusion there surely remains an important element of truth.

NOTES

1　M. Bradbury and J. McFarlane, 'The name and nature of Modernism', in their co-edited *Modernism, 1890–1930* (Harmondsworth: Penguin, 1976), p. 19.

2 A. Bullock, 'The double image', in Bradbury and McFarlane, op. cit., p. 62.
3 S. Freud, *The Interpretation of Dreams*, in *The Pelican Freud Library*, vol. 4 (Harmondsworth: Penguin, 1976), pp. 244, 769.
4 F. Nietzsche, *Ecce Homo: How One Becomes What One Is* (Harmondsworth: Penguin, 1979), p. 37. This work was written in 1888, and first published in 1908.
5 F. Nietzsche, *The Joyful Science* (1882), in W. Kaufmann (ed.), *The Portable Nietzsche* (New York: Viking, 1954), p. 95.
6 This forms the subtitle to *The Origin of Species*.
7 Quoted in L. Nochlin, *Realism* (Harmondsworth: Penguin, 1971), p. 41.
8 Rimbaud to Paul Demeny, 15 May 1876, as quoted in R. Stromberg (ed.), *Realism, Naturalism, and Symbolism: Modes of Thought and Expression in Europe, 1848–1914* (New York: Harper & Row, 1968), p. 188.
9 G. D. Painter, *Marcel Proust: A Biography*, vol. 2 (Harmondsworth: Penguin, 1977), p. 329.
10 E. Zola, 'The Impressionists' (1880), as quoted in Stromberg, op. cit., p. 156.
11 V. Kandinsky, *Concerning The Spiritual in Art* (New York: Dover, 1977), p. 57.
12 V. Woolf, 'Mr Bennett and Mrs Brown' (1924), reprinted in *Collected Essays*, vol. 1 (London: Hogarth, 1966), p. 320.

FURTHER READING

The themes pursued in this chapter can best be followed up by reading the various 'primary sources' which it has cited. Perhaps the most useful collection of extracts from them has been compiled by R. N. Stromberg (see n.8). As for secondary works, nearly all those that follow contain detailed bibliographies of their own.

The best recent attempt to integrate intellectual and cultural developments into a textbook of 'general' history is E. H. Hobsbawm, *The Age of Empire, 1875–1914* (London, 1987). Outstanding among items of general reference literature are P. P. Wiener (ed.), *Dictionary of the History of Ideas*, 4 vols (New York, 1973–4), and J. Wintle (ed.), *Makers of Nineteenth-century Culture, 1800–1914* (London, 1982). Broad surveys of ideas during this epoch include G. Masur, *Prophets of Yesterday: Studies in European Culture, 1890–1914* (London, 1963); M. D. Biddiss, *The Age of the Masses: Ideas and Society in Europe since 1870* (Harmondsworth, 1977); and J. Romein, *The Watershed of*

Two Eras: Europe in 1900 (Middletown, Conn., 1978). The remarkable cultural contribution of the Habsburg capital is examined in C. E. Schorske, *Fin-de-siècle Vienna: Politics and Culture* (London, 1980); and that of the French one in R. Shattuck, *The Banquet Years: The Origins of the Avant-garde in France, 1885 to World War I,* revised edn (London, 1969), and E. Weber, *France: Fin de Siècle* (Cambridge, Mass., 1986).

The role of science is well covered by J. Bronowski, *The Ascent of Man* (London, 1973); C. C. Gillispie, *The Edge of Objectivity: An Essay in the History of Scientific Ideas* (Princeton, NJ, 1960); and S. Kern, *The Culture of Time and Space, 1880–1918* (Cambridge, Mass., 1983).

There is a prolific literature concerning social and political ideas. The most stimulating of these works is H. S. Hughes, *Consciousness and Society: The Reorientation of European Social Thought, 1890–1930* (London, 1959). Other interesting contributions are W. M. Simon, *European Positivism in the Nineteenth Century: An Essay in Intellectual History* (Ithaca, NY, 1963); the first part of K. D. Bracher, *The Age of Ideologies: A History of Political Thought in the Twentieth Century* (London, 1985); R. Aron, *Main Currents in Sociological Thought,* vol. 2 (London, 1968); J. Joll, *The Anarchists* (London, 1964); L. Kolakowski, *Main Currents in Marxism: Its Origins, Growth, and Dissolution,* vol. 2 (Oxford, 1978); and N. Harding, *Lenin's Political Thought,* 2 vols (London, 1981).

A broadly based guide to the European literary scene is the volume cited in n. 1, edited by M. Bradbury and J. McFarlane. The first of these authors has also written a series of stimulating essays entitled *The Modern World: Ten Great Writers* (London, 1988). A particularly useful national study is R. Pascal, *From Naturalism to Expressionism: German Literature and Society, 1880–1918* (London, 1972). Among the older classics of secondary commentary, E. Wilson, *Axel's Castle: A Study in the Imaginative Literature of 1870–1930* (New York, 1931; regularly reissued) deservedly retains a leading place.

The art of this period is usually well represented in those galleries that have major modern collections, among which the Tate and the Courtauld in London can be recommended for particular attention. The general field is well surveyed in G. H. Hamilton, *Painting and Sculpture in Europe, 1880–1940* (Harmondsworth, 1967), and one vital part gets brilliantly illuminated in P. H. Tucker, *Monet in the '90s: The Series Paintings* (London, 1989). Good studies of specific 'movements' include J. Rewald, *Post-Impressionism: From Van Gogh to Gauguin,* 3rd edn (New York, 1978); J. Willett, *Expressionism* (London, 1970);

R. Cardinal, *Expressionism* (London, 1984); D. Cooper, *The Cubist Epoch* (London, 1971); and, for futurism, E. Braun (edn), *Italian Art in the 20th Century* (London, 1989).

Among the good biographies dealing with leading participants in this whole revolution, the following works are especially rewarding: M. Meyer, *Ibsen,* abridged edn (Harmondsworth, 1974); G. Painter, *Marcel Proust,* 2 vols (London, 1959–65); and two studies by R. W. Clark: *Einstein: The Life and Times* (London, 1973), and *Freud: The Man and the Cause* (London, 1980).

5   Origins of the war of 1914

Philip Bell

THE OBSESSION

The search for explanations of the war which began in 1914 has been almost obsessive. A reader who commanded a knowledge of the main European languages could spend a lifetime on the books and articles which have been produced on the subject without getting near the end; and the stream shows no sign of drying up. Why has it mattered so much, and why has the debate not been stilled by the passage of time?

One answer lies in the interests of historians and the nature of historical study. The coming of war in 1914 presents a tremendous challenge to historical explanation. The amount of evidence available is enormous. Historians have laboured on the subject for more than three-quarters of a century, using every tool and approach known to the profession. Students of diplomacy, military and naval affairs, politics, economics and society have all made their contribution; so have those concerned with the human psyche, modes of thought and states of feeling. The six weeks between the assassination of Archduke Franz Ferdinand at Sarajevo, and the British declaration of war on Germany on 4 August, have been subjected to the most minute scrutiny, with events traced day by day and hour by hour. At the same time, the underlying forces which may have influenced men's actions (for example, alliance systems, arms races, nationalism, imperialism) have been examined with equal diligence and intensity. With all this material and effort, it is incumbent upon historians to produce some results.

But we are far from dealing merely with the concerns of professional historians. The war of 1914–18 has weighed heavily on the minds of western European peoples, not least in Britain, where it was long (and surely rightly) called simply the Great War. There has been a profound sense that the war was a true turning-point in European history, the end of the nineteenth century and the age of progress, and the beginning of our own catastrophic era. Through the scale of the fighting and the numbers of casualties, the war has also left its mark on folk memory, which persists even though the generation of those directly involved has almost completely died out. An event of such magnitude, which left so deep an impression, cries out for explanation.

There is a further reason for the obsession with the origins of the war. Remarkable to relate, the question has never ceased to be a part of contemporary politics. During the war itself, the question of its origins was an essential element in the struggle. Among the belligerents, morale depended to some degree on a conviction of the rightness of one's cause; and appeals for the support of neutrals (especially the United States) were often based on the same claims. In the Treaty of Versailles in 1919 a view of the origins of the war – crudely summed up as German war guilt – was made the basis for the demand for reparations to make good the loss and damage suffered by the victors during the war. For the next few years the Germans put a great effort into attacking the 'war guilt' thesis, for reasons which had more to do with undermining Versailles than with a search for strict historical truth. At the same time, a great deal of work was concentrated on how war came about in 1914, with the understandable objective of preventing the same thing happening again. The causes of war (not just of a particular war) were diagnosed so that they could be eliminated. During the Second World War the political outlook on the events of 1914 changed, but remained very much alive. Churchill telegraphed to Roosevelt in the night of 4–5 August 1941: 'It is twenty-seven years ago today that the Huns began the last war. We must make a good job of it this time. Twice ought to be enough.'[1] Views on the conduct of Germany in 1914 – that is, on the origins of the First World War – were thus closely connected with the politics of the Second World War. After that war was over, the question of the continuity or otherwise of the two World Wars became a part, especially in West Germany, of the crucial issue as to whether Hitler and Nazism were a complete aberration in Germany's history, or were part of an essential continuum. The same question is far from being forgotten in 1992, when the views of many people on the unification of Germany are coloured by opinions as to whether or not Germany began the wars of 1914 and 1939.

The problem of the origins of the war of 1914 has thus remained politically alive, and has become part of wider issues like the causes of war in general, and the nature of Germany. It is not surprising that the obsession retains its power. We still puzzle away at the old question:

why did the wealthy, civilized, sophisticated countries of Europe in 1914 become involved in what proved to be so desperate and disastrous a struggle?

INTERPRETATIONS: THE EVENTS AND THE HISTORIOGRAPHY

To examine the interpretations which have been offered as to the origins of the war means looking at two sets of problems, posed respectively by the events and by the historiography.

In looking at the events, the conventional division into long-term and short-term causes of the war serves well. Long-term surveys start at different points according to the issues being placed at the centre of discussion. Some start in 1871, with the end of the Franco-Prussian war and the annexation by the newly-created Germany of the French provinces of Alsace and Lorraine. This point of departure places Franco-German rivalry in the forefront of the picture, and other elements have their prominence decided by this perspective. Other accounts take the Balkans as the centre of attention, and begin in 1878 with the Treaty of Berlin and its temporary settlement of Balkan frontiers. Others again lead off in the 1890s, either with the making of the Franco-Russian alliance between 1892 and 1894, or with imperial rivalries in Africa and Asia throughout the decade.

Whichever starting-point is chosen, accounts of the distant origins of the war describe the building up of the alliance system which dominated European affairs in the years before 1914. Germany and Austria-Hungary were linked in the Dual Alliance, signed originally in 1879. These two powers were also linked with Italy in the Triple Alliance, signed in 1882; but by 1914 this arrangement had grown very uncertain, with Italy becoming increasingly detached from it. France and Russia were associated in an alliance which was concluded in 1894; and they were also attached to Britain by the loose arrangements often referred to as the Triple *Entente*. The terminology was important. Alliances were, in principle, binding agreements, under which the partners would go to war in certain circumstances. *Ententes* (the Anglo-French *entente* of 1904 and the Anglo-Russian one of 1907) involved no such commitment, being limited to provision for consultation and promises of diplomatic support. The Austro-German and Franco-Russian alliances formed solid, opposing elements in the European political system. This alliance system carried within it the danger that a dispute anywhere in the continent might draw in the great powers through their alliance commitments; and the *ententes* made British involvement also a possibility.

Long-term surveys also describe a series of European crises during the ten years before the outbreak of war in 1914. In 1905–6 the first Moroccan crisis saw a Franco-German confrontation over French claims on the then independent state of Morocco. During the period of tension, and at the conference at Algeçiras which resolved the crisis, the Anglo-French *entente* was consolidated and assumed a clear anti-German aspect. In 1908–9 there was a severe and prolonged crisis in the Balkans, set off by the Austrian annexation of the Ottoman province of Bosnia-Herzegovina. This was territory which was also coveted by Serbia, and the danger of the situation lay in the confrontation between Austria on the one hand and Russia, acting in support of the Serbs, on the other. With Germany offering ostentatious backing to Austria, there was outlined with ominous clarity the threat of a conflict between three great powers arising out of a comparatively minor Balkan incident. If such a conflict had come about, France would surely have been drawn in. The lines were drawn for a European war, which at that point did not come about because the Russian government decided it could not take the risk, and so withdrew support from Serbia. In 1911 the second Moroccan crisis brought another sharp dispute between France and Germany, in which Britain again supported France. In 1912–13 there occurred two series of wars in the Balkans, in which the independent Balkan states first combined to defeat the Turks, and then fell out among themselves over the division of the spoils. The greatest single consequence of these wars was that Serbia emerged with enlarged territory and heightened self-confidence, which was now turned against Austria.

These repeated crises produced three dangerous consequences. The most acute was a 'never again' mentality in Russia and Austria. The Russians felt that they could not afford to give way again in face of Austrian and German pressure. If they were in future called upon to support Serbia, they would have to make that support good. The Austrians felt that they had stood aside during the Balkan wars and allowed changes which were to their disadvantage. In another crisis, they would not be able to abstain, but would have to act. The second development was a sharp rise in Balkan nationalism, and particularly in Pan-Serb sentiment, posing an obvious threat to the multinational Austro-Hungarian empire. If nationalism pursued its logical course, then Austria-Hungary was heading for disintegration. Naturally, the Austrian government saw powerful reasons to take drastic action – probably against Serbia – in self-preservation. Third, during the two

Moroccan crises the Anglo-French *entente* developed in such a way that France expected British support in the event of war, and Britain was implicitly committed to such support. In these ways, a scenario emerged which presaged that of 1914, and lines were drawn which in 1914 were followed to their logical conclusions. On the other hand, in all four crises a way out was found; by a conference, by diplomacy behind the scenes, or by one participant backing down rather than risking war. The European system was producing dangerous crises, but it was also working well enough to resolve them without a war between great powers.

So much for long-term accounts. When we move to the short-term causes of the war we are faced with the six weeks between 28 June 1914, when Archduke Franz Ferdinand, heir to the throne of the Habsburg empire, was assassinated at Sarajevo, and early August. The events of these six weeks have been traced in minute detail; the Italian historian Luigi Albertini devoted two massive volumes solely to this short period.[2] To take such trouble is, in itself, an act of historical interpretation; an assertion that the detailed record of those six weeks is crucial in explaining how the war came about. What stands out among the events and decisions of this brief period? First, the Austrian government held Serbia responsible for the death of the archduke, and delivered an ultimatum demanding Serbian compliance with a number of demands, including Austrian participation in the investigation of the crime. Serbia refused some of these demands. In this, Russia supported Serbia, and on this occasion (unlike in 1908–9) was prepared to mobilize, and ultimately to fight. Germany supported Austria to the hilt – 'signing a blank cheque' is the analogy often used. The likelihood of a local war involving Austria and Serbia thus opened out into the possibility of an eastern European war involving Austria, Germany and Russia. At that point the alliance system and military plans came into play. If Russia was at war with Germany, then France would be obliged to join in; and in any case, German military plans had been prepared to deal with the Franco-Russian alliance. Germany's Schlieffen Plan was designed to cope with a war on two fronts by attacking France first and defeating it in six weeks, leaving the German army free to mop up the slow-moving Russians at leisure. The Schlieffen Plan provided the link which was certain, whatever else happened, to turn an east European war into a general one. That left Britain and Italy to decide their course. The British government hesitated for a long time, but was eventually pushed by the German invasion of Belgium (another part of the Schlieffen Plan) to declare war on Germany. Italy declared its neutrality.

During the six weeks, events moved at a gathering pace, and it is easy to see why contemporaries used the metaphor of a river coming to rapids and ultimately a waterfall.[3] The archduke was assassinated on 28 June. On 5 July the German Kaiser Wilhelm II gave Austria a 'blank cheque', offering unconditional support, in the full knowledge that this might involve war with Russia. But then the Austrians took several days to draft and approve their ultimatum to Serbia, which was not actually delivered until 23 July. The Serbs replied on the 25th, accepting most of the terms but not all. On the 28th Austria-Hungary declared war on Serbia, and fired the first shots by bombarding Belgrade. In a sense the die was cast there and then: the crisis was over almost as soon as it really began. By the time another week was up, virtually the whole of Europe was at war. Russia ordered general mobilization on 30 July, Austria on the 31st. Germany, on 1 August, declared war on Russia, on 2 August delivered an ultimatum to Belgium, and on the 3rd declared war on France. On 4 August Britain declared war on Germany. Everything was done in due form with ultimatums and declarations of war properly delivered and received. The diplomatic etiquette of the old Europe was observed for the last time.

These were the events which historians have laboured so hard and long to explain. It is time to turn to the interpretations which have been put forward over the years. The first set of interpretations emerged in the era characterized by the debate on war guilt and the publication of diplomatic documents, stretching from 1914 to the Second World War. The period was dominated by two divergent themes: an attempt to allot responsibility – or,in a harsher word, guilt – for the outbreak of war; and a search for underlying causes of the war, which, if successful, would replace the concept of responsibility with the neutral idea of causality.

Anxiety about blame for causing the war was present before the war itself began, because nearly all the governments were concerned to convince their own peoples that a conflict, if it came, was a defensive one forced upon them by others. When battle was joined, the belligerent governments continued the process of casting blame upon their enemies by publishing carefully selected anthologies of diplomatic documents, designed (indeed, occasionally doctored) to demonstrate their own innocence. The Germans sought mainly to shift responsibility onto Russia, both generally in terms of Russian ambitions in the Balkans, and specifically because the Russians had been the first to mobilize and had thus taken a key step towards war. In France and Britain, Germany was presented as the main culprit; again, both generally, through denunciation of German militarism, and particularly, as a result of the German attack on Belgium. Such views, which attained the status of beliefs, were of great importance in sustaining the will to fight through an unexpectedly long and costly war. The same arguments were also used to appeal for the sympathy of neutral countries, and the allied insistence on German war guilt gradually gained acceptance in the United States.

The war ended in 1918, and in 1919 the major victorious powers – France, Britain, Italy and the United States (these last two belligerents from 1915 and 1917 respectively) – prepared the terms of peace to be imposed on Germany. They embodied in the Treaty of Versailles the acceptance by Germany of the responsibility for forcing the war upon others by her aggression; namely Article 231, commonly called the 'war guilt clause'. This assertion set the pattern for much of the historical discussion during the next twenty years. Some historians, particularly in France, continued to maintain that Germany bore either the whole, or at any rate the major, part of the blame for the war.[4] The German government, on the other hand, threw itself into a campaign to disprove the war guilt clause, and so to undermine the validity of the peace treaty, especially its reparations section. The Germans published a massive series of diplomatic documents, *Die grosse Politik der europäischen Kabinette* ('The High Policies of the European Governments'), which appeared in forty volumes between 1922 and 1926 – a remarkable feat in itself. German historians devoted much care and energy to editing these documents, and also produced books and articles to reach a wider readership. The burden of much of their argument, as set out, for example, in Max Montgelas's *The Case for the Central Powers* and Erich Brandenburg's *From Bismarck to the World War*, was that Germany had not sought war; if it had, there had been better opportunities in 1905 or 1909 than in 1914. On the other hand, Russia and France *had* wanted war: Russia for the control of the straits into the Mediterranean, France for Alsace-Lorraine; and the president of France, Poincaré, and the Russian ambassador in Paris, Iswolski, had actually conspired to bring war about.[5] This conspiracy theory, directed against France and Russia, was also taken up by 'revisionist' writers in France, Britain and the United States. The debate on war guilt thus crossed national boundaries, becoming a general discussion in which the German case gained wide acceptance.

At the same time there developed a very different strand of thought. The British historian, G. P. Gooch, argued in his *Recent Revelations of European Diplomacy* that in 1914 all the belligerent states had good reasons for their actions. Serbia sought to unite the South Slavs;

Austria-Hungary wished to save itself from disruption; Russia could not abandon Serbia; Germany had to support Austria, its one safe ally, just as France had to stand by Russia; Britain could not afford to watch France be defeated and then face a victorious Germany alone. If each country had sound reasons for going to war, then the question of guilt became virtually meaningless, and attention should move to a diagnosis of the *causes* of the war – a very significant change of emphasis.[6]

This search for the causes of the war of 1914 became closely linked with a movement to discover the roots of war itself, with a view to eliminating them. This had long been a concern among utopian thinkers, but the catastrophe of the Great War brought a new urgency to what had often been a somewhat abstract discussion. Several diagnoses commanded attention. Socialists argued strongly that war was the product of capitalism, and of imperialism which Lenin had described as the highest stage of capitalism. There had been a struggle for markets, raw materials and fields for investment, which had led to competition to seize parts of Africa, eastern Asia and the Middle East. Such arguments gained considerably in force when Lenin was no longer an obscure scribbler in a Zurich library, but the ruler of a great state. Moreover, socialism was a growing force over much of Europe in the 1920s, and its views commanded much respect. The case against imperialism fitted closely with that against secret diplomacy. Wars, notably that of 1914, were caused by the machinations of professional diplomats, usually (if not exclusively) aristocrats, who wove their webs of alliances irresponsibly, outside the control of parliaments, the press or public opinion. This case had a strong appeal in Britain, where there was a widespread (and well-founded) belief that the true extent of British commitments to France had not been revealed to Parliament, or even to the Cabinet. This again was bound up with another general explanation of the war: that it was the result of the alliance system, which had bred mistrust and hostility, and in 1914 had transformed what might have been a local conflict into a European war. The next step was a simple one. The alliances had taken the form of armed camps, and war was the result of armaments and arms races. The evidence for this thesis was readily to hand in the Anglo-German naval race, in which the two countries had built battleships in open competition with one another; and in the Franco-German rivalry in the size and equipment of their armies, which came to a head with the German Army Law of 1913 and the French three-year conscription law of the same year. All these explanations could be rolled together in the general assertion that the whole system of conducting relations between states had been wrong. Lowes Dickinson summed the whole view up in the title of his book, *The International Anarchy*.[7]

This flood of discussion and research on the origins of the war was, as we have already seen, motivated as much by political as by historical concerns. It none the less resulted in a vast work of historical elucidation, not least in the establishment of the precise chronology of events during the six weeks of the war crisis. A classic example of this kind of work is the masterly exposition by Luigi Albertini on the dates of the Russian and Austrian mobilizations, which finally laid to rest the long controversy as to which had been first – not a negligible matter when it was plain that mobilization was a crucial step towards war. In this way, even the often arid 'war guilt' controversy could produce enlightenment; and the search for general causes inspired excellent books on, for example, the diplomacy of imperialism and the Anglo-German naval rivalry.[8]

The Second World War brought a pause in speculation about the origins of the First. Many historians served in the forces or in other forms of war work; nearly all had pressing demands on their time and energies. But this distraction was only temporary. The second war was bound to revive questions about the first. Were the two in fact separate? Did the almost unquestioned German responsibility for the events of 1939–41 cast any light on the issue of war guilt in 1914? Among Germany's enemies there was a strong tendency to believe that it did. Even Soviet historians, firm in their assertions that 'imperialism' was to blame for the war of 1914, came to think that the German imperialists were probably more to blame than others. The next great wave of historical debate about 1914, associated primarily with the name of the German historian Fritz Fischer, took shape in the shadow of questions raised by the Second World War.

In 1961 Fischer published a substantial book, *Griff nach der Weltmacht* ('Grasp for World Power'), which was translated into English in 1967 under the feeble title of *Germany's Aims in the First World War*.[9] However, what the English title did make clear was the fact that the book was mainly about Germany's aims during the 1914–18 war, and only its introductory section was devoted to the pre-war period and the question of the origins of the war. Yet this section contained enough explosive matter to set off shock waves: first in Germany, and then among all who were still concerned with the events of 1914. What did Fischer have to say? First, he declared that Germany bore a large part of the responsibility for the outbreak of the war – which was scarcely new for many people in other countries, but was dynamite in German historical circles. Second, he argued that important groups within the

German ruling élite (the general staff, landowners, industrialists, bankers, leaders of the Pan-German League, and university professors) had long held expansionist views, and were willing to go to war to fulfil them. Third (and here Fischer followed the Italian historian Albertini very closely), he maintained that in the July crisis the German government was prepared to risk a general European war arising out of a local war between Austria and Serbia, and that Germany had systematically encouraged Austria to go ahead with an attack on Serbia even when it became clear that the conflict could not be localized. This transformed the analogy of the blank cheque: Germany had not given Austria a blank cheque, but had actually written the amount itself. And the amount meant European war.

Fischer based his arguments on a mass of research in the German archives, penetrating beyond the published collections of diplomatic documents which had been the basis of earlier accounts. He also broke from the usual pattern, which had halted examinations of the origins of the war when fighting began. Because Fischer was essentially concerned with the war, and only partly with its origins, he used material from after the outbreak of hostilities to illuminate the situation before they began. He discovered a particularly explosive piece of evidence in a memorandum by the German Chancellor, Bethmann-Hollweg, dated 9 September 1914, setting out a draft programme of war aims which amounted to complete German domination of Europe, west and east. Fischer claimed that this document was not simply the result of euphoria at a moment of apparent victory, but was in fact the crystallization of views which were common in German ruling circles before the war began, and indeed represented Bethmann's own aspirations. Bethmann, in fact, emerged from Fischer's book not as the well-meaning but inadequate statesman of inter-war history, but as a fully-fledged advocate of German expansion.

Fischer's book thus reopened the war guilt issue, which with the passage of time had been moving into the background in favour of an examination of causes; and he also provoked a sharp reassessment of Bethmann-Hollweg, one of the prominent personalities of 1914. He thus breathed new life into old controversies. But he also opened up a new way of looking at the whole problem. In 1969 he followed up *Griff nach der Weltmacht* with *Krieg der Illusionen* ('War of Illusions'), dealing in detail with the years 1911–14, and trying to make good his earlier summary assertions that the German war aims of September 1914 were not mere improvisation but were the product of expansionist aims which had been present for some time. In this process, Fischer developed the argument that foreign policy had been largely decided by *internal* issues. He analysed the tensions between the old ruling groups in Germany, represented by the monarchy and the landowning aristocracy (the Junkers), and the newer industrial and commercial groups, such as the industrialists of the Ruhr and the shipping magnates of Hamburg. The extraordinary economic growth of Germany at the end of the nineteenth and the beginning of the twentieth century strengthened the position of the newer groups, stimulated demands for a world policy, and brought about a naval competition with Britain which the more conservative elements would never have contemplated. Both these groups were hostile to (and often afraid of) the rising force of socialism. The German Social Democratic Party was the largest and best organized in Europe, and came to be the largest single party in the Reichstag. Its language was anti-militarist, and it attacked the Prussian constitution, which preserved a parliamentary system based on the 'orders' of the eighteenth century, thus retaining a privileged position for the aristocracy. Fear of socialism caused many in the ruling groups to consider war, either as a means of uniting the nation against a foreign enemy, or alternatively as providing an opportunity to crush the socialist party.

In developing this argument, Fischer attacked a long-standing tenet of German historical writing, summed up in the phrase 'the primacy of foreign policy'; the view that foreign policy was essentially decided according to the external interests of the state, and not by internal factors. But this was not an attitude confined to Germany. Most writing about the causes of the war in the inter-war period had been based on diplomatic documents and had used the methods of diplomatic history. It was true that a number of historians had asserted in rather general terms the significance of economic forces; and the internal tensions within the Habsburg empire had long been recognized as one of the forces leading to war. But the main focus had been on the embassies, foreign ministries and chancelleries of Europe, with an occasional glance at the general staffs. To assert the primacy of *internal* politics, and to claim that the war had come about for mainly domestic reasons, was to open a new angle of vision upon events.

To examine this assertion became the work of another generation of historians. An American writer, Arno J. Mayer, started the ball rolling by proclaiming the need for a concentration of research on the internal causes and purposes of war. He, like others before him, thought in terms of the causes of war in general, though referring particularly to the war of 1914. Broadly, his thesis was that decisions for or against war in all the major belligerent capitals were essentially part of internal tensions and struggles between the forces of order (or conservatism) and those of change (or revolution). Mayer accepted that sometimes these tensions were so acute that governments would take a cautious line, for fear that war might be fatal to the existing order of things; but he asserted that the opposite was more often the case. Internal tensions, he claimed, tended to incline governments to go to war to strengthen their own position – which chimed in with Fischer's arguments about the rulers of Germany going to war in 1914 to bring about national unity and preserve their own authority.[10] The whole interpretation presupposes a high degree of far-sighted calculation on the part of ruling groups. How far can it be demonstrated?

The strongest case is also the oldest and most obvious: that of Austria-Hungary. The Habsburg empire had grown up over many centuries, and preserved many of the characteristics of a past era. Its principle of legitimacy was dynastic, and the empire in effect consisted of the long-inherited lands of the Habsburg family. The force of nationalism, which developed so strongly in the nineteenth and early twentieth centuries, threatened its very existence. The empire lost territory, and suffered dangerous damage to its prestige, through the unification of Italy and Germany. In 1914, the most dangerous threat seemed to be from the South Slav movement for union between Serbs, Croats and Slovenes. There was much talk of Serbia becoming 'the Piedmont of the South Slavs'. Such a union would at once detach important territories from Austria-Hungary, and would almost certainly give such encouragement to other nationalities within the empire as to lead to its rapid dissolution. It was this fear of the disintegration of the Austro-Hungarian state, arising from its nature as a multinational empire, which impelled the government in Vienna to strike at Serbia in 1914 in the desperate hope of cutting away external support for internal dissension.

This is the clearest case of internal tensions leading a government to undertake a foreign war in 1914. Its basis was understood perfectly well even in 1914, and modern historiography has added little to the essential argument. At the other end of the scale stand Britain and France, where domestic affairs appear to have played little part in decisions for war. In Britain there were indeed grave domestic problems, notably in Ireland, where there was a danger of civil war arising out of the conflicting aspirations of Irish nationalists and Ulster Unionists. But there is no evidence that the Prime Minister, Asquith, or the Foreign Secretary, Grey, sought to involve Britain in European war to escape from domestic crisis. On the contrary, the Ulster problem absorbed so much energy and attention that the European war crisis came as a bolt from the blue for most of Asquith's cabinet. Grey worked hard to preserve peace. His own thoughts were dominated by the position of France; and the mind of a divided cabinet was finally clarified by the German attack on Belgium which provided a simple moral imperative. In France, there were of course long-term internal divisions dating back to the revolution of 1789, and much sound and fury over the three-year military service law of 1913. But France had lived with such long-term dissensions and sharp political storms for a long time, and there is no sign that French politicians saw European war as a way out of them.

Somewhere between these two extremes lie the cases of Russia and Germany. In Russia there were many influences at work within an ill-organized system of decision-making. One school of thought looked back to the disastrous experience of the war against Japan in 1904–5 which had led to revolution in Russia, and argued that in order to achieve stability at home it would be best to keep out of war abroad. Others, however, held that the regime needed to restore its prestige, both at home and abroad, by a success in foreign policy in Russia's traditional sphere of interest in the Balkans and the straits. Another powerful influence was that of the Pan-Slavs, who believed strongly that Russia must support the Serbs in 1914, especially since it had let them down in 1908–9, during the Bosnian crisis. Between these various pressures upon the tsar, whose own actions seem often to have been governed by a cloudy but sincere belief that both he and his country were in the hands of God, there seems to have been little scope for rational long-term calculation. War might stave off revolution, by drawing people into a common effort, or it might have the opposite result, as it did in 1905. There was no agreement. As for Germany, Fischer undoubtedly makes a very strong case that internal pressures were leading towards war, as a means of resolving differences between the old Prussian ruling classes and the new industrial and commercial élites, and also as a means of forestalling the socialist threat. But it is hard to demonstrate the precise links between such pressure and the actual decisions taken in 1914.

Only in Austria, therefore, is there a clear case for the primacy of internal political calculations in the decisions for war in 1914. In the other countries it is hard to find any single pattern of explanation that fits them all – which is hardly surprising in view of the wide differences between their political systems and circumstances.[11]

The line of approach based on the internal causes and purposes of war has proved valuable in broadening the concept of what is relevant to the origins of the war, but less productive in substance than the efforts put into diplomatic history, which tells us more about actual decision-making. There has been, in fact, some return to the study of the small élites which conducted foreign policy. Zara Steiner in her book on Britain and the origins of the war, and John Keiger in his similar study of French policy, both conclude that the Foreign Office and the Quai d'Orsay had much more influence on decision-making than other bodies, and that the main calculations involved were those of national interest and prestige, as understood at the time by the groups of ministers and officials closely concerned with foreign policy.[12]

Both the diplomatic and the 'internal causes' approaches to the problem rely essentially on the view that politicians and officials make decisions based upon calculation, whether of national interest or of the long-term security of a ruling group. This presumption was challenged in one of the most original contributions to the debate on 1914, made by James Joll in his inaugural lecture at the London School of Economics in 1968, entitled '1914: The Unspoken Assumptions'. His thesis was that statesmen, when under extreme pressure, in circumstances which they do not fully understand, and when they cannot foresee the consequences of their actions, act not upon calculation but on instinct. 'In moments of crisis, political leaders fall back on unspoken assumptions', which are themselves drawn from deep layers of tradition, upbringing, and education. The trouble for the historian is that because such assumptions are unspoken, and for that matter unwritten, they are uncommonly difficult to ascertain. Taking Edward Grey, the British Foreign Secretary, as a key example, Joll argues that it is a mistake to try to make a sophisticated analysis of his policies. His guiding principle was a schoolboy sense of honour; and not just any schoolboy, because Grey (like Joll himself) was a product of Winchester, and his unspoken assumptions were those of a self-conscious Wykehamist. This is a highly specialized diagnosis. We have some remarks made by Grey about his days at Winchester which partly bear it out, though unhappily Grey tells us that only fellow Wykehamists can really understand what it means to be a Wykehamist, which rather narrows the circle of comprehension. To extend the approach to others, we need to know a great deal about the family background and education of the men of 1914, and also about the general climate of opinion and sentiment within which they grew up.[13]

This is a fascinating speculation, whose implications spread out much more widely than the boundaries of the 1914 debate. But, as Joll is well aware, it is an approach that is hard to follow through. True, Grey was a Wykehamist. He was also a long-serving Foreign Secretary, who worked closely with very able and strong-minded Foreign

Office officials. His memoranda show that he thought in terms of the balance of power and British strategic interests, as well as in terms of honour, in the shape of his personal word to the French. In the crisis of 1914, these two modes of thought pulled together towards the same conclusion, and it would be very hard to say whether at any particular point Grey fell back upon one rather than the other.

REFLECTIONS

The pursuit of explanations for the outbreak of war in 1914 has led a long way. It has also spread out in different directions, some of which involve not so much discussion of the events of 1914 as interpretations of the nature of the past as a whole, and of our understanding of it. It was the refrain at the close of an article by Joachim Remak that 'We have complicated things too much'.[14] Can we not, even in so complex a subject, simplify them a little? Where do we stand?

The problem has always had two parts: the elucidation of events and the finding of a framework of interpretation. The first remains a matter for detailed research, and it is only the second which can be pursued here. The long historical debate has left us with two main problems: how we strike the balance between the idea of guilt (or responsibility) for the war and that of understanding its causes, and what relative importance we attach to underlying forces and immediate events.

The concept of war guilt in 1914 has had a long run, and seems still to have life left in it. It has always involved very difficult questions. What does it mean? What is there to be guilty of? No state or government can be thought of as bearing guilt simply for going to war, because war has been a part of human history. More specifically, during the half-century before 1914 all the major belligerent powers had been engaged in war: Prussia and the Habsburg empire in 1866; Prussia and France in 1870–1; Britain against the Boer republics, 1899–1902; Russia against Japan in 1904–5; Italy against Turkey in 1911–12. Most powers had fought colonial wars. Even that arch-neutral and isolationist power, the United States, was fighting a campaign in Mexico at the very time that war began in Europe. Before 1914 all governments accepted Clausewitz's dictum that war was the continuation of policy by other means. All were prepared for war, and all recognized that in certain circumstances (involving honour, security or ambition) it was necessary and proper to go to war. Of what, then, could any state be guilty in 1914, when all the powers shared the same view of war?

The answer, of course, involves hindsight. The conflict that took place between 1914 and 1918 was not just a war; it was a catastrophe.

The scale, intensity and cost of the fighting were greater than anything known before. The former rules ceased to apply, and the idea of war as an instrument of policy became unacceptable in many eyes. For any state to have deliberately launched such a European disaster was indeed a responsibility, and guilt became a natural description. But to make such an assumption involves a shift in perspective which is in itself scarcely historical. In 1914, no government believed that it was embarking on a war which would last for over four years. It was the almost universal conviction that the conflict would be severe, and would involve vast armies, but would be short – 'over by Christmas' was a common saying. This means that we must look in the first instance for origins commensurate with the idea of a brief, though probably intense, conflict. What causes were sufficient for governments to begin, to accept, or to risk a war of a limited, late nineteenth-century type – *not* the Great War with which our memory is obsessed?

This affects our view of the other balance which has to be struck, that between long-term forces and immediate decisions. It has naturally been believed that anything so tremendous as the war of 1914–18 must have had deep-rooted and powerful causes. As the search has widened to include the causes of war itself, the conduct of whole groups, or the roots of human conduct, this belief has taken a greater hold. But if we are seeking the causes, not of such vast events, but of what might have been a third Balkan war, or a wider version of the Franco-Prussian War, must such explanations be invoked?

The answer is probably not. An exception at once springs to mind: the tension between nationalism and the multinational Habsburg empire, which remains crucial. Other long-term explanations relying on underlying forces moving towards war have all tended to break down at the actual point of contact with the events of 1914. The argument, much used in socialist circles in the 1920s and 1930s, that the war was the result of capitalist and imperialist conflicts over raw materials, markets and fields for investment was weakened by detailed research which showed that disputes over territory in Africa or Asia had often crossed the lines of alliances within Europe. Moreover, the most serious of such conflicts outside Europe had been between Britain and France on the one hand, and Britain and Russia on the other; but these disputes had been resolved peacefully, and the former rivals had fought on the same side in 1914. Again, there was much close cooperation between German and French bankers and industrialists in the complex of coal, iron ore and steel industries which spanned the boundaries between their two countries. In the actual crisis of 1914, some German industrialists were in favour of war, but others were dismayed at the prospect of disruption and loss which war would bring. The study of the underlying forces of economics and imperialism produces as much evidence of international cooperation and opposition to war as it does of pressure towards conflict.

Even the apparently powerful explanations in terms of arms races appear much less clear-cut under close examination. True, the German and French armies were built up in competition with one another. So were the German and British fleets. But the war of 1914 did not emerge directly out of Franco-German conflict, but from conflict between Austria-Hungary and Russia, which had not been engaged in an arms race; and the Anglo-German conflict also came late in the actual crisis of 1914. What did contribute directly to the course of events in July and August was not the general issue of arms races, but the detailed strategic planning for the use of those armaments, especially on land. The role of the Schlieffen Plan, by which if Germany were involved in war with Russia it would *have* to attack France first, was crucial. As soon as the state of an 'imminent danger of war' was declared in Germany, then the plans for mobilization moved with a momentum which could not be stopped; and the German plan for mobilization was also a plan for operations. The one ran directly into the other.

Much the same is true of the long-term explanation from the alliance system. It is true that this system was likely to turn a local dispute into a general war; but the case of Italy also shows that it was possible for a country to ignore its alliance commitments in favour of a calculation of its immediate interests. The alliances worked when they continued to represent vital interests: for example, France and Russia dared not risk isolation, while Germany could not afford to see Austria-Hungary disintegrate; but they did not impose predetermined answers in 1914.

We must return to the exception to this line of argument. The underlying force which exerted a direct and decisive influence on decision-makers in 1914 was the conflict between Balkan nationalism and the multinational Austro-Hungarian empire. Balkan nationalism was a force which had been at work since at least the beginning of the nineteenth century. Gradually, the hold of the Ottoman empire in Europe had been prised loose and one Balkan state after another had attained independence. Then, in a last effort in 1912–13, the Turks had been driven back to a small enclave round Constantinople and the straits, and Austria-Hungary remained as the sole target of Balkan nationalism. In 1914 this nationalism was primarily embodied in Serbia, which had emerged from the Balkan Wars of 1912–13 with substantial gains in territory, and with aspirations to create a Greater

Serbia, or perhaps a new South Slav state. In either case, the Serbs
looked north, towards the populations of Serbs, Croats and Slovenes
within the borders of the Austro-Hungarian empire. Here indeed was
a tide which had been rising for almost a century; and the Austro-
Hungarian empire was looking unhappily like a sandbank. What were
its rulers to do? In 1908 they had contemplated a plan to attack Serbia,
but had in fact stopped short at the annexation of Bosnia-Herzegovina.
In 1912–13 they had simply watched while the Balkan Wars were
fought and Serbian power was increased. The result was that in 1914 a
sense of desperation had developed, and there was a strong impulse to
take action – almost any action – to remove the threat from Serbia. It
was seen as a matter of self-preservation.

This is not to say that the long-term, underlying forces had no weight
– far from it. Though they did not, in most cases, predetermine the
choices made by governments in 1914, they did ensure that war, when
it broke out, could not be limited. The smouldering fire of Anglo-
German naval rivalry, the intense need for security which lay behind
the alliances, and the unappeasable hunger of nationalism all became
concentrated in the struggle once it had begun. The war which began in
Europe in the summer of 1914 was bound to be more than the sum of
immediate events and specific decisions. It would be a concentration of
deep and long-standing antagonisms, not easily to be resolved.

In the light of this review of underlying causes, it is time to look again
at the immediate decisions of July and August 1914. The places to start
must be Vienna and Belgrade. After all, the first declaration of war was
by Austria-Hungary on Serbia, on 28 July. The government in Vienna,
as we have seen, believed that it was acting in self-preservation. It
deliberately forced war on Serbia by delivering an ultimatum which
was designed to be rejected. The Austrian government chose a Balkan
war, and risked something worse, almost certainly in the belief that it
had no alternative. The Serbian government, too, played its part at this
stage, partly by conniving at the nationalist terrorism which produced
the assassination of the archduke, and partly by choosing to take up the
Austrian challenge. If Austria-Hungary sought self-preservation, Serbia sought self-aggrandisement, and believed that with Russian help it
could win a renewed Balkan war.

This takes us to Russia. The methods of Russian decision-making
were confused and its aims uncertain. But it was clear by the middle of
July that Russia would support Serbia, if necessary by war; and Sazonov, the Russian foreign minister, indicated this plainly to the German
and Austrian ambassadors on 18 July. Why was this? Strategic and
economic interests in the straits can be adduced: the importance of

controlling the entrance to the Black Sea, and of securing free passage for Russian exports by the same route. But the prime reasons were surely sentiment and prestige. The restricted circles which made up public opinion in Russia were Pan-Slav in sentiment, and demanded support for Serbia; and Russian prestige – its standing as a great power, capable of backing up its protégé – was at stake.

Again, such motives were amply sufficient for a confrontation, and even a war, on a Balkan issue. Yet the risk of a wider conflict was clearly present; and at this point we must turn to Germany. Germany held the central position in the wider European crisis – central in terms of geography, diplomacy and military action. Geographically, German intervention would turn a Balkan war into a European one. Diplomatically, German support for Austria was bound to stiffen Austria's resolution, which otherwise might have wavered. Militarily, German war plans entailed an immediate attack on France, not Russia. We know what Germany did. It gave complete support to Austria, accepting the near-certainty of a Balkan war and risking a European conflict. The German government also followed the course set out in its military planning to its final conclusion in the invasion of Belgium and France, which changed the whole scale and character of events. The successive waves of historical writing have confirmed this record of German actions, and it is not surprising that debate has concentrated heavily upon the motives which lay behind them. The motives can be easily summed up, but the balance between them is almost impossible to strike. The most straightforward of them and the most readily avowed, were to maintain the Austrian alliance, without which Germany would be alone in a hostile continent, and to score a spectacular diplomatic (or, if necessary, military) success to break free from the encirclement which the Germans genuinely feared and re-sented. Less clear-cut were the further motives stressed by Fischer: the drive to make Germany a world power, and the bid for unity at home to pre-empt the socialist danger. It is with these latter reasons that we move away from motivation commensurate with a limited war, and move to that more appropriate to something wider and more drastic.

This survey has left France and Britain to the last. In so far as France played an active part in the crisis of July 1914, which does not appear to have been very far, it was by supporting Russia, for the well-established reason that she could not afford to lose the Russian alliance and face Germany in isolation. But France's main role was passive, and the French government never had to take the decision whether or not to go to war in support of Russia. The Germans first presented an ultimatum demanding the occupation of French fortresses to ensure French neutrality, and then simply invaded the country through Belgium. In these circumstances the French government had very little to decide. As for Britain, its actions in 1914 had only marginal influence on the course of events. Grey tried to check the move towards war by twice proposing a conference; but such a conference would have put Germany in a minority, and his proposals made no headway. The European war had begun by 2 August, and the question was whether (or perhaps only when) Britain would join it. From the point of view of the origins of the war, this was not a vital question.

It was as the scope of the crisis widened, and a likely Balkan confrontation became a certain European war, with some world-wide aspects, that the long-term, underlying causes of friction came into their own. Imperial rivalries, the arms races, and the alliance system provided the framework within which the crisis of July 1914 took place. They also meant that war, when it came, rapidly involved wider issues than those which were at first at stake. The alliance system represented fundamental security for Germany, France and Russia. Imperial rivalry and the naval race between Britain and Germany meant that, once war had begun, their empires and fleets were at stake; which, for the Britain of that day, meant the very fundamentals of its existence. Thus the underlying forces, which appear to have had little effect on decision-making during the war crisis itself, greatly affected the war which actually came about.

The tragedy was that the war of 1914 became the war of 1914–18 – the Great War. It might not have been so. After all, by the time the Schlieffen Plan ground to a halt, the advance guards of the German armies could see the Eiffel Tower. They were no more than twenty miles from the outskirts of Paris. At that stage, the exhaustion which had overcome marching men, and the French concentration of a new army, brought about the battle of the Marne. The war in the west was not to be decided in six weeks, as the Germans had hoped. By that time, who in western Europe cared what was happening in Serbia? The war had started with a Balkan crisis, but it had rapidly become something much greater. And it is that greater event which historians have been trying to explain for the past seventy-five years.

NOTES

1 Winston S. Churchill, *The Second World War*, vol. 3 (London, 1950), p. 381.

2 L. Albertini, *The Origins of the War of 1914*, 3 vols (Oxford,

1952–7); Italian original published in 1942–3. Vols 2 and 3 deal with the crisis of July 1914.

3 There are valuable chronologies of events in V. R. Berghahn, *Germany and the Approach of War in 1914* (London, 1973), and Z. S. Steiner, *Britain and the Origins of the First World War* (London, 1977).

4 Solid arguments for Germany's primary, though not exclusive, responsibility may be found in Pierre Renouvin, *La Crise européenne et la grande guerre*, 2 vols (Paris, 1934), and B. E. Schmitt, *The Coming of the War*, 2 vols (New York, 1934). Both books have stood the test of time remarkably well.

5 M. Montgelas, *The Case for the Central Powers* (London, 1925); German original published in 1923. E. Brandenburg, *From Bismarck to the World War* (London, 1933); German original published in 1924.

6 G. P. Gooch, *Recent Revelations of European Diplomacy* (London, 1927). Gooch had outlined his ideas in a lecture to the British Institute of International Affairs in Dec. 1922.

7 L. Dickinson, *The International Anarchy* (London, 1926). Dickinson's book was primarily an argument in support of the League of Nations as the solution for the ills of pre-1914 international relations.

8 W. L. Langer, *The Diplomacy of Imperialism*, 2 vols (Cambridge, Mass., 1935); E. L. Woodward, *Great Britain and the German Navy* (Oxford, 1935).

9 F. Fischer, *Germany's Aims in the First World War* (London, 1967).

10 See Mayer's outline presentation of his argument in 'Internal causes and purposes of war in Europe, 1870–1956: a research assignment', *Journal of Modern History*, 41 (1969); and also A. J. Mayer, 'Domestic causes of the First World War', in L. Krieger and F. Stern (eds), *The Responsibility of Power: Historical Essays in Honor of Hajo Holborn* (New York, 1967). For the full development of his ideas, see A. J. Mayer, *The Persistence of the Old Regime: Europe to the Great War* (New York, 1981).

11 For this section see above all J. Joll, *The Origins of the First World War* (London, 1984), ch. 5, pp. 92–119. Joll's conclusion, after discussing the various belligerent powers, is that 'no single explanatory model is applicable to all of them' (p. 119). For a close examination of the British case, see D. Lammers, 'Arno Mayer and the British decision for war, 1914', *Journal of British Studies*, 12 (1973).

12 Steiner, op. cit.; J. Keiger, *France and the Origins of the First World War* (London, 1983).
13 J. Joll, '1914: The Unspoken Assumptions', Inaugural lecture at the London School of Economics (Apr. 1968), reprinted in H. W. Koch (ed.), *The Origins of the First World War: Great Power Rivalry and War Aims* (London, 1972); quotation on p. 309.
14 J. Remak, '1914 – the third Balkan war: origins reconsidered', *Journal of Modern History*, 43 (1971); see esp. pp. 363–4.

FURTHER READING

An excellent review of the whole problem may be found in J. Joll, *The Origins of the First World War* (London, 1984; a second edition is being prepared). Other general discussions are in L. Lafore, *The Long Fuse: An Interpretation of the Origins of World War I*, (London, 1966), which concentrates on Balkan issues; J. Remak, *The Origins of World War I* (New York, 1967), which is brisk and straightforward on a complicated subject; and L. C. F. Turner, *Origins of the First World War* (London, 1967). H. W. Koch (ed.), *The Origins of the First World War; Great Power Rivalry and War Aims* (London, 1972), is a collection of scholarly essays. B. Tuchman, *The Guns of August: August 1914* (London 1972), is a vivid and highly readable narrative. I. Geiss (ed.), *July 1914: Selected Documents* (London, 1972), presents key documents on the war crisis, with an illuminating and combative introduction.

Among older books, S. B. Fay, *The Origins of the World War*, 2 vols (New York, 1928), B. E. Schmitt, *The Coming of the War, 1914*, 2 vols (New York, 1928), and G. P. Gooch, *Before the War: Studies in Diplomacy and Statecraft*, 2 vols (London, 1936 and 1938), remain well worth reading, and illustrate aspects of the historiographical debate between the wars. L. Albertini, *The Origins of the War of 1914*, 3 vols (1952–7), is a historical landmark and repays close study; vols 2 and 3 treat events between the assassination of the archduke and the declarations of war in immense detail. A. J. P. Taylor, *The Struggle for Mastery in Europe, 1848–1918*, puts the events of 1914 in a long historical perspective.

On individual countries, the following may serve as starting-points. **Austria-Hungary**: F. R. Bridge, *From Sadowa to Sarajevo: The Foreign Policy of Austria-Hungary, 1866–1914* (London, 1972). **France**: J. F. Keiger, *France and the Origins of the First World War* (London, 1983). **Germany**: V. R. Berghahn, *Germany and the Approach of the War in 1914* (London, 1973). F. Fischer, *Germany's Aims in the First World War* (London, 1967), and *War of Illusions* (London, 1975), command a special place in the historiography of the subject. They are discussed in J. A. Moses, *The Politics of Illusion: The Fischer Controversy in German Historiography* (London, 1975). **Great Britain**: Z. S. Steiner, *Britain and the Origins of the First World War* (London, 1977); F. H. Hinsley (ed.), *The Foreign Policy of Sir Edward Grey* (Cambridge, 1977). **Italy**: R. Bosworth, *Italy and the Approach of the First World War* (London, 1983). **Russia**: D. Lieven, *Russia and the Origins of the First World War* (London, 1983). **Serbia**: V. Dedijer, *The Road to Sarajevo* (London, 1967).

Strategic issues and military competition are discussed in a collection of essays edited by P. M. Kennedy, *The War Plans of the Great Powers, 1880–1914* (London, 1979). On armies and military plans: G. Ritter, *The Schlieffen Plan* (London, 1958); D. Porch, *The March to the Marne: The French Army 1871–1914* (Cambridge, 1981); J. Gooch, *The Plans of War: The General Staff and British Military Strategy, 1900–1916* (London, 1974); S. R. Williamson, *The Politics of Grand Strategy: Britain and France Prepare for War* (Cambridge, Mass., 1969). On navies and the naval race between Britain and Germany: A. J. Marder, *From the Dreadnought to Scapa Flow*, vol. 1: *The Road to War, 1904–1914* (London, 1961); J. Steinberg, *Yesterday's Deterrent: Tirpitz and the Birth of the German Battle Fleet* (London, 1965).

On imperial and economic rivalries, see D. K. Fieldhouse, *Economics and Empire, 1830–1914;* C. M. Andrew and A. S. Kanya-Forstner, *France Overseas: The Great War and the Climax of French Imperial Expansion* (London, 1981); M. Beloff, *Imperial Sunset*, vol. 1: *Britain's Liberal Empire, 1897–1921* (London, 1969).

6   The Great War and its impact

Philip Bell

The origins of the First World War have remained an obsession because we have failed to understand them. The war itself has remained an obsession because we appear to understand it only too well, and even after so many years we are still appalled and shaken by what we see. The Great War means, above all, the trenches and mud of the western front; Verdun, the Somme and Passchendaele; casualty lists, war memorials and the Last Post. It appears too as a vast symbol of futility, a conflict in which immense effort and sacrifice were misdirected and wasted, achieving nothing. The picture is clear and stark, but how far should we accept it? There are surely questions which need to be examined. On the military side, why did the conflict on the western front take the shape that it did, and are we right to allow that battle zone to fill our horizon to the extent that it does? Next, what were the politics of the war, and why was there no compromise peace despite the immense length and cost of the military conflict? Finally, how true is it that nothing was achieved?

We must start with military events. The outbreak of war in 1914 meant that the fate of Europe was to be decided by force, and we must concentrate first on how that force was used. In the military pattern of events, it is natural to look first at the western front. It was in the west that the length of the war was largely decided. In this process, the first three or four months of the conflict were crucial. It was the German objective, set out in the Schlieffen Plan, to knock France out in six weeks by a great offensive, swinging in a wide arc through Belgium and ultimately hooking round behind Paris. By the beginning of September 1914 this plan had attained immense successes, and yet had failed in its essential purpose. The successes were plain on the map as a virtually unbroken advance to within a few miles of Paris. The failure was that the offensive came to a halt without the French army being destroyed or the government forced to surrender. For this failure there were several reasons. Not the least was sheer exhaustion: the highly efficient German railways took the troops to their starting-points, but then they had to march. After some five weeks they were very weary, and were outrunning their supplies. Then there was a change of plan by the German High Command. In response to Russian pressure in east Prussia, two corps were transferred from the western front to the eastern, thus weakening the all-important German right wing as it swung towards Paris. On the Allied side, Joffre, the French Commander-in-Chief, kept his nerve, formed a new army, and counter-attacked successfully in the battle of the Marne (5–11 September), forcing the Germans to retreat.

The Schlieffen Plan had failed. But so had the French plan for an offensive to recover Alsace and Lorraine and to invade Germany across the Rhine. In this battle the French were defeated with losses amounting to some 300,000 within a month. There was to be no quick victory for either the Germans or the French. By November 1914 the battle lines had settled down along a front which stretched from the Swiss frontier to the Channel coast, and the static nature of the war in the west began to take shape. The armies learned to dig in, gradually creating the trench systems which have become in Britain the symbol of the whole war. Trenches and dug-outs, with reserve lines sometimes extending three or four miles to the rear; barbed-wire entanglements; rifles, machine-guns, and a whole range of other weapons – all combined to give the defence an immense superiority over the attack. A large local advantage in terms of numbers and artillery would secure a small advance, but no more – and even that was at heavy cost. In the next four years, no wholly satisfactory way out of this impasse was found, though many were tried. Massed artillery was used to try to blow a gap through the fortifications; but this was of limited effect, because in 1915 and 1916 most of the artillery ammunition was shrapnel, not high explosive, and in any case there were usually more trenches to the rear. Poison gas was tried, with only partial and temporary success. Tanks, first used by the British in September 1916, promised much, and achieved a dramatic success at Cambrai in November 1917; but alone they could produce only limited results. In the spring of 1918 the Germans achieved striking victories with tactics of surprise and infiltration, but again without achieving the decisive breach which they sought. Victory was eventually won in the west; but for nearly four years stalemate prevailed.

This stalemate left the Germans in control of a large part of northeastern France and almost the whole of Belgium, which they had conquered in 1914. Here lay the key to the strategy of the war in the west. For the French above all, and to a lesser extent for the British too, it was essential to drive the Germans out of these territories; so they had to attack. The Allied offensives on the western front are often described as 'senseless', and indeed they involved grievous casualties for little gain. But the fundamental point behind them was that the Germans simply had to be expelled from their conquests – otherwise they had won. That was why the basic pattern of the war in the west was a series of Allied offensives, beginning in 1915 and going on to the battle of the Somme (July–November 1916 – a new concept in the length of a battle), the French offensive under General Nivelle (April 1917), and the British at the third battle of Ypres (June to November 1917) – which has left its mark on the English language with the name of Passchendaele. The Germans, on the other hand, were mainly content to stand on the defensive, and chose to attack only twice: at Verdun in 1916, when General Falkenhayn set out to destroy the French will to fight by bleeding their army to death, and in the spring of 1918, when it had become vital to win a final victory before the Americans made it impossible.

This strategic impasse, together with what was basically a political imperative for the Allies to persist in their offensives, created the appalling nature of the war on the western front. The life of the trenches and the devastation of the great battles have been caught, not so much by the work of those few who have become known as the 'war poets' – who at the time were highly untypical – but by the everyday letters, diaries and memories of thousands of ordinary soldiers.[1] It was not entirely a new kind of war – the American Civil War and the Russo-Japanese War in Manchuria had produced something like it – but it was experienced by far more men than ever before. It was on the western front that France suffered the vast majority of her 1,327,000 killed, and the United Kingdom most of its 723,000.[2] It was here that the consciousness of the French and British peoples was permanently marked by the war. It was also finally the place where Germany was defeated and the outcome of war decided. This is worth some emphasis, because the disasters of the Somme and Passchendaele have been remembered, while the victories of Amiens, Bapaume and St Mihiel have been forgotten.

So the western front was in many ways decisive; but it was far from representing the whole war. The eastern front involved enormous numbers of troops. It was also much more flexible and fast-moving than the campaigns in the west. Vast distances gave little scope for impregnable trench lines. Great offensives captured large tracts of territory rather than a few muddy square miles. The Russian army for a long time fought well, and with more success than is often remembered. The struggle swayed to and fro. In 1914 the Russians advanced into east Prussia and brought crucial relief to the French, as the Germans moved forces to the east. Then Hindenburg and Ludendorff won brilliant victories at the battles of Tannenberg and the Masurian Lakes; but before the end of the year the Russians had stabilized the position. To the south, in a campaign against Austria-Hungary in late August and early September 1914, the Russians won a great victory. They advanced some 150 miles, occupied most of the province of Galicia, and inflicted at least 350,000 casualties in killed, wounded and prisoners.[3] It was a blow from which the Austrian army never fully recovered.

In 1915 the Germans made their principal effort on the eastern front, with devastating success. In a five-month campaign from May to September, the German army drove the Russians out of large areas of Lithuania, Poland and Galicia. In the centre they advanced about a hundred miles, and captured Warsaw. The Russians lost, in five months, about two million casualties, nearly half of them prisoners.[4] Such a mass of prisoners was a sign of a disintegrating army; yet in 1916 the Russians were able to resume the offensive against Austria. Their armies, under General Brusilov, entered Galicia and Bukovina, capturing in their turn nearly 380,000 prisoners. Encouraged by these successes, Romania seized the opportunity to enter the war on the Allied side, only to be overwhelmed by the German army in one rapid, improvised campaign in December 1916. After two and a half years of war on two fronts, the German military machine was still remarkably effective.

In 1914–16 the Russians thus won great victories against Austria-Hungary, but sustained heavier and more damaging defeats against the Germans. By the end of 1916 Russian casualties were about 3,600,000 dead, wounded, and seriously ill, and about 2,100,000 taken prisoner.[5] These losses included most of the officers and non-commissioned officers of 1914, who had been the backbone of the army. The Russian army stood on the verge of dissolution, and the state on the brink of revolution. The eastern front left a mark upon history at least as great as that in the west.

Western and eastern Europe formed the two main fronts in the military struggle; but there were many others. In May 1915 Italy joined in the war on the Allied side, opening a new front against the Austrians in the difficult terrain of the Alps and the River Isonzo. Here the Italians fought a tenacious campaign, in depressing imitation of the western front, and in harsher geographical and climatic conditions, with no fewer than eleven battles along the Isonzo between 1915 and 1917. They gained no more than a dozen miles, and lost nearly a million casualties.

Another set of fronts was brought into being by the intervention of Turkey, which entered the war on the side of the Central Powers at the end of October 1914. The most famous of the Turkish campaigns was that named after Gallipoli: the Allied attempt to force the straits to the Black Sea, and so bring direct assistance to Russia. It is impossible to say whether this would have brought long-term advantage, even if the military operation had succeeded; was there enough shipping available? were there enough supplies to help the Russians? and could the Russians have made good use of them? But in any case the landing forces (British, French, Australian and New Zealand) which went ashore in April 1915 made little headway, and had to be withdrawn in January 1916 after sustaining appalling hardships and heavy casualties. The only success of the operation was a smooth and bloodless evacuation. Elsewhere, campaigns were fought against the Turks by the Russians in the Caucasus, and by the British in Palestine and Mesopotamia (modern Iraq) – the last being a sign of the importance of oilfields in twentieth-century strategy.

Finally, there was also some fighting in large parts of Africa, in China, New Guinea and the Pacific, mostly to reduce German colonies. It must be doubted whether these campaigns outside Europe really merit the designation of the conflict as a 'world war' – Europe was always the true centre; but they were more than 'side-shows'. Large forces were involved, and the results were often far-reaching. All Germany's colonies were seized by her enemies. The Ottoman empire was broken up and had to be replaced; and in its replacement the forces of Arab nationalism and Zionism emerged in shapes which are recognizable to us today.

One other great zone of operations was the sea. In principle, the two great forces of surface ships, the British Grand Fleet and the German High Seas Fleet, dominated the scene. It was technically possible, in Churchill's phrase, for Jellicoe, the British commander, to lose the war in an afternoon by having his fleet destroyed. But this did not happen. The battle of Jutland (31 May 1916) was for the British a costly and disappointing draw – they had expected another Trafalgar. But they retained command of the sea, with all that was implied in that wide-ranging phrase. It meant control of the oceanic supply routes, along which men and material reached Britain and France from all parts of the world, especially from North America. It also meant the power to curtail drastically the overseas commerce of the central powers. The blockade, which was in effect a slowly developing system of commercial control, could never be complete, because Germany's neutral neighbours, especially the Netherlands and Denmark, offered significant loopholes, and the Germans were able to secure new resources by conquests in eastern Europe. So the Allied grip was never total, but its effects were cumulative and severe.

Germany, too, could apply the weapon of blockade, by the use of submarine warfare. Britain was particularly vulnerable, since at the beginning of the war it imported about two-thirds of its food and large quantities of raw materials for industry. The Germans made two attempts at blockading the British Isles by submarine. In February 1915 the first declaration of a 'war zone' in the approaches to the British Isles was premature in terms of the number of U-boats available. To begin with, there were only 24, of which only one-third could be on station at any given time; and at no point during 1915 were there more than 45 available in all. But in February 1917, when a new phase of unrestricted submarine warfare was declared, the German navy possessed about 120 ocean-going U-boats, of which some could operate right across the Atlantic. Again, it was unusual for more than about one-third of these to be on station, but the losses they inflicted were enormous. In February 1917 British merchant ships sunk by submarines totalled 313,486 tons. In April the tonnage lost reached 545,282 for Britain, and 881,027 for all shipping. The total losses between February and June 1917 were some 3,300,000 tons, of which 2,000,000 tons were British. During April only two U-boats were sunk.[6] Reserves of food supplies fell dangerously, and Britain faced the grim possibility of being starved into surrender. The situation was saved by the entry into the war of the United States, with the deployment of American warships, and above all by the slow and difficult introduction of the convoy system. Losses remained high, but were brought down to manageable levels; and U-boat casualties were pushed up, so that in September more U-boats were lost than launched. But it was a close-run thing.

Land and sea battles had long been the staples of war. In 1914–18, for the first time on any scale, war took to the air. As early as 1915 there were bombing attacks by both the Germans and British on cities in the other country, as well as direct military action over the battle zones. It was the beginning of what was to become strategic air warfare, which made significant strides before the end of the war, with the creation of a separate British air force, including a large long-range bombing force.

Behind all these campaigns on land and sea and in the air lay the crucial war of resources. When the war began, all the belligerents expected it to be short. Industrial production was allowed to run down as men were called into the armies, and general staffs reckoned that they could fight the war on existing stocks of arms and ammunition. This development was particularly drastic in France, where mobilization of men of military age affected a large proportion of the population, depriving both industry and agriculture of manpower in a brutal and arbitrary manner.[7] But by the autumn of 1914 it was becoming clear that the war would not be short, though no one foresaw its actual length; even the far-sighted Kitchener's prediction of three years proved too short. It was to become a war of resources – manpower, industrial production, food supplies and shipping; and also a war of organization, for even the most massive resources could be squandered, while smaller ones could be husbanded.

In terms of resources, the advantage lay with the Allies as against the Central Powers. A calculation of manufacturing production in 1913 showed Germany and Austria-Hungary together as having 19.2 per cent of total world production, while France, Russia and Britain together had 27.9 per cent.[8] Counting of divisions at the front gives uncertain results, because the strength of a division varied in numerical terms from one army to another, and at different times in the war. But it is worth noting that in August 1914 France, Russia and Britain put 202 divisions into the field, Germany and Austria-Hungary 143. In August 1916 the Allies (including Italy and various other states) mustered 405 divisions, the Central Powers (including Turkey and Bulgaria) 369. In broad terms, the Allies held the numerical advantage from the beginning of the war until December 1917, when Russia concluded an armistace; then, with the build-up of American forces, they restored that advantage by the time the war ended in November 1918.[9] That Germany was able to secure repeated military successes and hold out for so long against the industrial and numerical odds, was due to two main factors: its central position, which enabled it to move forces rapidly from one front to another; and the efficiency of its use of resources. German manpower was used to much better effect than Russian.

Still, in the long run Allied superiority in resources told and its superiority developed in a way which was highly significant for the future of Europe. By the end of 1915, France had used up its reserves of manpower, and had no scope to increase its armies. In military terms, therefore, France became increasingly dependent upon Britain, whose forces were still increasing. In economic terms, too, France became dependent on others. The German occupation of north-eastern France deprived the French of much of their industry and many coalmines; and though they worked wonders in the production of arms, ammunition and military equipment, they were only able to do so by importing large quantities of coal, raw materials and industrial machinery from Britain and the United States. The role of Britain thus became rapidly more significant. From being only a minor land power, sending only seven divisions in the original British expeditionary force in 1914, Britain and the empire had seventy divisions on the western front in the spring of 1916. Behind them lay a British armaments industry which in 1916 produced 4,314 guns (as against 91 in 1914), 33,500 machine-guns (300 in 1914), and 6,100 aircraft (200 in 1914).[10] Yet, at the same time, both France and Britain were increasingly dependent upon the United States, partly for munitions, but much more for supplies of food, raw materials and machine tools. They were also heavily dependent on the loans which, from 1915 onwards, were necessary to finance these purchases in the United States. The war of resources was thus producing a new structure of power in western Europe and the Atlantic, with France relying increasingly on Britain, and both on the United States.

To exploit resources efficiently required organization, and above all decisions on priorities. What was the best use for manpower – in the armed forces, in industry, or in agriculture? To take specific examples, was one man more useful as a shepherd, or another on a factory production line, than either would be as an infantryman? Were supplies of nitrates more profitably put into the manufacture of explosives or into fertilizers for agriculture? Who was to decide? The only answer could be the state; and the war saw the rapid extension of government control in all aspects of life. In France, the price of bread – considered to be the key to morale – was fixed shortly after the outbreak of war, and there gradually developed from that action an attempt to control the whole chain which ran back from the baker through the miller to the farmer. This was not a simple task, because when the price of wheat was fixed, farmers showed a natural but distressing tendency to grow barley or some other cereal, so that the machinery of control had to be steadily extended. The French government also intervened to try to increase food production – for example, by releasing agricultural workers from the army, and by requisitioning disused land – but with only limited success.

In Germany, the main effort was put into military and industrial purposes. The Germans kept an enormous army in the field – 94 divisions in August 1914, and 234 in March 1918; and over 13,000,000 men were mobilized in the course of the war.[11] After a fall in industrial production in the few months following the outbreak of war, German industry was rapidly reorganized to produce vast quantities of armaments and military equipment. The Hindenburg Programme, begun in August 1916, introduced wide-ranging controls over manpower and economic resources, and set prodigious new targets for arms and munitions. To meet them, over a million men had to be released from the army late in 1916, and nearly two million in 1917. Agriculture, on the other hand, fell back during the war, and was starved of resources in men, animals and fertilizers. Wheat production fell from 5,094,000 metric tons in 1913 to 2,484,000 in 1917; rye from 12,222,000 tons in 1913 to 7,003,000 in 1917; and potatoes from 54,121,000 tons to 34,882,000 over the same period.[12]

In Britain, which entered the war under a Liberal government temperamentally opposed to state control over the economy, the early slogan was 'business as usual', but this proved impossible to maintain. Almost at once the government had to intervene to provide an insurance scheme for shipping which was an apparently narrow and technical matter, but was of vital importance for a country heavily reliant on seaborne trade. A scheme for the requisition of shipping was introduced in November 1915, and a Shipping Control Committee in January 1916. In the face of a vast, and largely unforeseen, demand for shells, a Ministry of Munitions was set up under Lloyd George in May 1915. Conscription for the armed forces was introduced for unmarried men in January 1916, and for all men within a certain age range in May. This was a drastic departure for the British, who had long prided themselves that they were not as the continental powers, which all had conscript armies. It was at first hotly debated, but then generally accepted, largely because it was seen to be both fairer and more efficient than the voluntary system of recruitment which had raised the Kitchener armies. The formation of the Lloyd George coalition government in December 1916 saw a marked change in the British conduct of the war. Lloyd George introduced a small War Cabinet, with a secretariat to make sure that its business got done; created a number of new ministries to direct the war effort; and transformed the system of Cabinet committees. Of the new committees which were called into existence, two bore names which summed up the wartime situation: the Tonnage Priority Committee and the War Priorities Committee.[13] Under the impact of the German U-boat campaign a serious effort was made to produce more food, though this only produced results in the harvest of 1918, when, as it turned out, the war was almost over. Food rationing was also introduced early in 1918, though only for a limited number of items (including meat, butter, margarine and sugar).

Russia proved a telling example of the need for organization, as distinct from simple productive capacity and resources. Russia achieved striking increases in the production of armaments and munitions, and steel output held up well until 1916; but neither the transport system nor the administration was capable of dealing with the problems of distribution, so that production never achieved its full effect. The system of financing the war was also quite inadequate, producing rampant inflation: the retail price index (for what it was worth) stood at 700 in June 1917, as against 100 in June 1914.[14]

All across Europe the role and powers of the state increased, reaching into areas previously unknown in even the most authoritarian regimes. Yet there were always limits to state power, which were probably more clearly recognized at the time than later. In all countries there was a profound need for unity, and for active support for the war. Governments sought to foster morale by propaganda and censorship, building up national heroes, condemning the enemy's barbarity, and concealing some items of bad news as long as possible. The effects of these efforts were uncertain. There is evidence that people developed a healthy scepticism about official communiqués; and word of mouth, from the wounded or men on leave, spread news from the front readily to those who wished to hear it. Neither propaganda nor censorship had a clear field.

Unity was the watchword; and governments recognized that unity would have to be paid for as well as invoked. On the eve of war the French government decided to make no use of the 'Carnet B', the list of socialist and syndicalist militants who were thought likely to oppose mobilization and disrupt the war effort. This was matched by similar gestures towards the Right: closures of Catholic schools and monasteries ceased, and the anti-clerical Republic sought reconciliation with the Church. The 'sacred union' in France did not just appear; it was sought, on both Left and Right. In Germany, too, a list of socialists to be arrested in the event of war remained unused. In both France and Germany these gestures were successful. Notably, the left-wing parties, despite their earlier anti-militarist sentiments, rallied to the defence of their country. Socialists voted for the war budgets, and in France there were socialist ministers in the government before August was out.

This unity was broadly maintained during the first two and a half years of war. In France and Germany, splits within the socialist parties began to develop during 1915 and grew more serious during 1916. In

Britain the Independent Labour Party and the Union of Democratic Control questioned both the motivation for the war and the need to continue it. In Austria-Hungary the problems posed by the nationalities became more acute. But movements of dissent and opposition to the war did not attain serious dimensions until 1917.

To explain why this was so we must turn to the politics of the war, and above all to the question of war aims, or what the war was believed to be about. In terms of public opinion it was, of course, wise not to discuss war aims in any detail, because the simple unity which could be maintained in the face of enemy attack was likely to be fractured when questions of detail were raised. But as the war went on, the casualties piled up, and the efforts demanded of the people increased, some purposes had to be declared in order to make such sacrifices worthwhile. What were these purposes? They could mainly be expressed in terms of security or predominance (two sides of the same coin) on the one hand, and of a sort of morality on the other. In public, governments naturally tended to stress security and morality, but some territorial issues could command wide public support.

In Germany the Chancellor, Bethmann-Hollweg, drew up in September 1914 – when victory seemed in sight – a programme which would establish German domination of Europe. France and Russia must be so weakened that they would never again be a danger to Germany. In the west, Germany must control Belgium and annex a small part of French territory. In the east, Russia must be pushed out of Europe, and must give up lands which would be formed into states dependent on Germany. Most of Europe, including Scandinavia, would be formed into a great customs union under German management, so that (for example) France would not be able to erect tariff barriers against German exports. This was called 'Mitteleuropa', though it looked uncommonly like *all* of Europe. To this was to be added 'Mittelafrika', to be formed by uniting German, French, Belgian and British colonies in a wide band across central Africa. The historian Fritz Fischer, who attached great importance to Bethmann's September memorandum, also demonstrated that the German government (whether under Bethmann or, later, under Hindenburg and Ludendorff) adhered to these aims as long as there was any chance of victory. In the east they were actually achieved, at the Treaty of Brest-Litovsk in March 1918.

France and Russia were equally determined that Germany must be completely crushed. France wanted to recover (as it was always put) Alsace and Lorraine, which was a limited aim. But in March 1917 the French government also reached an agreement with the new Russian

Provisional Government (formed after the fall of the tsar) by which the Saar and territory west of the Rhine would be detached from Germany. From December 1914 the French government was also set on heavy indemnities; and so the French terms, taken together, became very severe. The same was true of Russian objectives. The Russian government aimed at territorial gains in east Prussia, Posen and Galicia. Sazonov even talked to the French Ambassador about restoring Hanover as a separate state, and restoring Schleswig to Denmark.

British aims were less drastic in terms of territory. Germany must clearly lose all her colonies, mostly to Britain; but in Europe the only stated British objective was the complete restoration of Belgian independence and territory. But here we must move to the other type of war aim, represented as being in some way 'moral'. During the first few months of the war, the French and British premiers, Viviani and Asquith, both spoke of breaking Prussian militarism and destroying the military domination of Prussia. 'Crushing Prussian militarism' came to be a widely accepted war aim; but how could it be achieved? How could one crush Prussian militarism without completely defeating the German army and then dismantling it? Moreover, militarism was a frame of mind and a form of society; did the Allies intend to reconstruct the German state and its mentality? At least to some extent, they did. French socialists were already talking in 1914 of 'liberating' Germany, and bringing to the German people the benefits of the revolution which they had never contrived to carry out themselves.

Viviani was a Radical, Asquith a Liberal; yet they could produce war aims which were as drastic in their own way as those devised by the German Chancellor and Generals Hindenburg and Ludendorff. If these aims were taken seriously – and they were – there was no room for compromise. This was true of all kinds of war aims. In terms of territory, power and morality, no government wanted to restore a balance but wanted to defeat the enemy completely. Raymond Aron has called the twentieth century 'the century of total war', and that is what the Great War became: not a war for a limited aim, but for total victory. This would have to be won in battle. As John Grenville has written, 'No one "stumbled" into war. Nor would any power stumble out of it. The end would be brought about by military imperatives.'[15]

This proved ultimately to be the case. But at the end of 1916, and for much of 1917, it seemed possible that events would turn out differently. The year 1917 was the hardest for all the belligerents – it was the year of doubt and difficulty, of peace moves, mutiny and even revolution. It was then that in Russia the will to continue the war collapsed completely. In March 1917 the tsar, faced with revolution, abdicated and was replaced by the Provisional Government. The promise of peace was one of the great appeals of the Bolsheviks, who seized power in November 1917 in the second revolution of that year. On 15 December 1917 an armistice was signed on the eastern front, confirming what had been the fact for some time: Russia was out of the war. In France, the army was shaken by an outbreak of mutinies which began in April 1917 and continued sporadically for several months, affecting 49 divisions to a more or less serious degree.[16] In most cases the troops limited their action to a refusal to attack, while being willing to hold their lines; but even so it was a grave crisis, casting doubt on the ability of France to continue the war. In Germany the Reichstag met in July 1917, and the Catholic Centre Party and Socialists, who together made up a majority, declared their willingness to discuss a peace based on a return to the position of 1914. On 19 July the Reichstag passed a 'peace resolution', desiring a peace of reconciliation and disavowing territorial conquest to alleviate severe economic conditions. In Britain, Lord Lansdowne, a former Foreign Secretary and Conservative leader in the House of Lords, published in the *Daily Telegraph* (29 November 1917) a letter appealing in powerful language for a compromise peace. In Britain, France, Italy and Germany 1917 was a year of strikes, mainly economic in nature but often arising from opposition to the war.

There were, therefore, many signs that the will to continue the war was crumbling; and one great power dropped out of the conflict altogether. 1917 was also a year of peace moves by governments. President Wilson of the United States attempted mediation in December 1916, and in January 1917 he spoke of 'peace without victory.' Between March and May 1917 the new emperor of Austria-Hungary, Charles, tried to negotiate a compromise settlement. Austria had entered the war in the belief that it was the only way to secure her survival; now, after nearly three years of war, it appeared that the only way for the empire to survive was to make peace. But the plan was far-fetched, because it involved Germany making concessions in Alsace-Lorraine, of which there was no chance; and it led nowhere. In August 1917 Pope Benedict XV published an appeal for peace, with a return to the territorial status quo of 1914 and a renunciation of all financial indemnities. This was not far removed from the peace appeal launched by Lenin after the Bolshevik revolution, using the slogan of 'peace without annexations or indemnities'. When the Pope, Lenin and Lord Lansdowne were saying much the same thing at more or less the same time, it was surely time for governments and peoples to listen. Was not the war costing more in human suffering, economic exhaustion and social dislocation than could ever be recouped even from victory?

Yet the war went on. If not even victory could recover the costs of the war, it was equally true that only victory could justify the sacrifices which had been incurred. And even in 1917 victory still seemed possible for either side, because of two crucial events during that year: the collapse of Russia, and the entry of the United States into the war. We have already seen that Russian fighting power crumbled during the year, and an armistice was concluded in December. This offered Germany the opportunity to concentrate her forces in the west and make one last bid for victory. For Germany, one war in the east had been won, and there was a good chance of victory in the west as well. But in the west, on 6 April 1917, the United States declared war upon Germany. The effects of this could not be immediate, because the USA was not yet a military power and had only a small army. But it had immense industrial capacity. It could build ships at a rate which could, in the long run, outstrip U-boat sinkings, and it was able to supply almost unlimited quantities of food. Moreover, when the Americans mobilized their manpower for military purposes, they could provide a growing army for the western front. In October 1917 there were 3 American divisions in France; in March 1918, 5; in July 25; in October 32; and in November 1918, 42.[17] Every American division was double the strength of a British or French division; and though the troops were not experienced, they were fresh. American intervention meant certain defeat for Germany, if the western allies could hold on long enough.

This they were both determined and able to do. In Britain, Lloyd George became Prime Minister in December 1916 with a programme of organizing the government and the country for a more efficient prosecution of the war, and he was supported in that task by a coalition including Conservative, Liberal and Labour members. In France, General Pétain did much to meet the deep-seated problems which had caused the mutinies, and restored the French army to health. He also had the good sense to indulge in no more great offensives, but to wait for the Americans and the tanks. In November 1917 Clemenceau became premier, on a programme of waging war to the end; and the National Assembly sustained him in that purpose. During the same year Germany became in effect a military dictatorship, under leaders determined to try for final victory. In August 1916 Hindenburg and Ludendorff had taken over the High Command; and in July 1917, after a long period of friction, they succeeded in securing the resignation of Bethmann-Hollweg as Chancellor, and thereafter exercised supreme control. It is worth emphasizing that in Britain and France the rise of Lloyd George and Clemenceau meant the imposition of civilian control on the generals, while in Germany Hindenburg and Ludendorff imposed military control on the civilians. But in both cases the new leadership meant war, which was waged as sternly by the democracies of the *Entente* as by the German militarists.

The entry of the United States thus helped to ensure that the war was continued. It also brought another change in its character, emphasizing still further the 'moral' or abstract element in Allied war aims. President Wilson spoke freely and sincerely of war for democracy, for the rights and liberties of small nations, and for the self-determination of peoples. But what did this mean for the Central Powers? For Austria-Hungary self-determination, if followed to its logical conclusion, meant dissolution. For Germany democracy meant the abandonment of its existing form of government, which would be contrary to both the wishes and the interests of the ruling groups and the Kaiser. Once again the stakes were raised, and the Central Powers were given a further incentive to try once more for victory.

The crisis of 1917 thus passed without the various moves for a compromise peace coming to anything. Only Russia dropped out of the war, reaching in March 1918 the Treaty of Brest-Litovsk, which was in no sense a compromise, but instead simply registered Russian defeat and dissolution. Russia lost Finland, the Baltic provinces, Poland, and the Ukraine, which became for a brief period an independent state. This settlement freed German forces (though large numbers, usually assessed at about a million, had to be left as armies of occupation), and large quantities of artillery and ammunition, for a last offensive in the west. Between 21 March and mid-July 1918 the German army launched a series of offensives, first in Flanders towards the Channel ports, then on the River Aisne towards Paris. They achieved remarkable successes, gaining forty miles in the north and thirty-five miles towards Paris – advances unknown on the western front since 1914. Moreover, they almost broke the Allied front and Franco-British unity, which was saved by the British accepting for the first time in the war an allied supreme commander, Marshal Foch, to coordinate all operations. In the end, the Germans could not maintain the momentum of their advance. Ludendorff's gamble failed, and he was left with a longer line to hold than before the offensives began.

There followed a series of Allied offensives which drove the Germans from most of their conquests in France, though not from the greater part of Belgium, which they still held at the armistice on 11 November 1918. At the end, the collapse of the Central Powers came quickly and all at once. The Turks were defeated in Palestine and Syria. An Allied army broke out of its trenches round Salonika and compelled the surrender of Bulgaria. The Italians destroyed an Austrian army at Vittorio Veneto. But Germany did not collapse because its allies were being knocked away; she had sustained them, not the other way about.

It was Germany which suffered the crucial defeat in 1918, but in examining that defeat it is still difficult to strike the right balance of explanation. The army was losing its fighting power, as the numbers of prisoners made plain; but it did not break. After the war, the generals and later the Nazis made much of the story of the 'stab in the back', that socialists and revolution at home had let down an undefeated army. Yet at the end of September it was Ludendorff who insisted that the government ask for an armistice, not the other way about. On at least one occasion Ludendorff lost his nerve, but for the most part he operated on the calculation that Germany must end the war before the army disintegrated. In this he succeeded, and the war that had begun, at least in part, through the plans of the German High Command came to an end in the same way.

Much later on, when Germany had launched another war in Europe, there was much criticism of the Allied governments of 1918 for not carrying the attack into German territory before granting an armistice. It would have been better, it was argued, to show the German people that they had been defeated, and make them feel the scourge of fighting on their own soil. This course was considered at the time; it was urged, for example, by the French president Poincaré, but he was overruled by Clemenceau and Foch, neither of whom can be regarded as soft or squeamish in their attitudes towards the Germans. Clemenceau was particularly sharp: he would have no more casualties when Germany had admitted defeat. The future peace could be made quite severe enough to convince the Germans of their defeat; meanwhile, to prolong the fighting might encourage the spread of Bolshevism and revolution in Europe, and add to the already great American influence in international affairs. To prolong the war for the sake of fighting on German soil might have seemed the best course twenty or twenty-five years later, but not in November 1918.

The war was over. What were its results, and who – if anyone – had won? And how true is it to say that nothing had been achieved?

One great effect of the war was easier for contemporaries to appreciate than for us. Germany was defeated, and the German army was expelled from Belgium and north-east France. This was no small matter for the countries and peoples concerned. The Allied victory in the west was in itself a major achievement. Yet though they had won, the cost to the whole continent of Europe was enormous. In 1913 it was prosperous, stable and civilized; in 1919 it lay in ruins. In places this was a literal truth; the line of the western front lay like a great scar across northern France and Belgium. But more generally the term was figurative; Europe faced economic ruin, political confusion and psychological uncertainty. The age of progress was at an end.

A large part of the economic loss – as well as the human tragedy of the war – lay in the casualties. In the European belligerent states the dead amounted to about 8,260,000. To these must be added the severely wounded, and also the victims of the influenza pandemic of 1918–19 which struck a population weakened by the effects of war.[18] The physical destruction in the battle zones was accompanied by the cumulative wear and tear of the war years. All across Europe, industry, agriculture and transport had worked at high pressure and without adequate maintenance. Railways and rolling-stock were particularly affected, and the end of the war saw a dislocation of transport all over central and eastern Europe. There were serious shortages of coal and food, caused partly by a fall in production, partly by problems of distribution, and partly by the continuing Allied blockade. Financial and monetary problems were less immediately visible, but in the long run more damaging. Britain and France had been forced to sell large quantities of their foreign investments in the course of the war; Germany had lost much of its own by confiscation. All the European belligerents ended the war with a very heavy burden of internal debt, because much war expenditure had been met by borrowing rather than by taxation. The most insidious and far-reaching effects were those of inflation. In every country (including the neutrals) prices had risen and the value of money had fallen. In France, the wholesale price index rose by a factor of three and a half between 1913 and 1919; in Germany by a factor of four; in neutral Denmark and the Netherlands by a factor of about three.[19]

Against this, states outside Europe had prospered during the war. Japan had been able to export manufactured goods all over east Asia, especially in India, China and Russia, and ended the war with improved export markets and a favourable balance of trade. The greatest benefits were reaped by the United States, which added prodigiously to its already remarkable economic development. Its production of steel doubled between 1913 and 1918; it developed an ocean-going merchant fleet where virtually none had existed before; and above all, it became a creditor instead of a debtor nation. The centre of economic and financial power had crossed the Atlantic.

The political confusion resulting from the war was far-reaching. East of the Rhine and north of the Alps, three great belligerent states had collapsed or even disintegrated. Austria-Hungary had simply disappeared, with its former territories divided between its neighbours or the new, smaller states which replaced it. Russia had suffered defeat, revolution and disintegration. In 1919 the new Bolshevik regime controlled only a diminished and uncertain proportion of the former tsarist territory; Finland, Ukraine and the Caucasian republics had declared their independence. Germany was to a large degree intact, but the ancient Hohenzollern dynasty had fallen, and there were revolutions of a sort in Berlin and Munich. All governments had been shaken, and in some parts of eastern Europe there was no effective government at all. This was not what the rulers of Europe had had in mind when they went to war in 1914.

The fall of the old empires was accompanied by the triumph of nationalism. During the war, each side had promoted nationalist aspirations in order to damage the other. Britain and France, for example, had offered encouragement to the Czechs. The Germans had supported nationalist movements in Poland and the Ukraine in eastern Europe, and in Belgium and Ireland in the west. Across the continent, nationalist expectations had been quickened; but it was impossible that they should all be satisfied. The result was the emergence of a number of new states, based supposedly on the principle of nationality, but all facing problems of national minorities either within or outside their borders. In the establishment of these new states, the decisive element was frequently the use of force: the frontiers arrived at between Poland, Lithuania and Russia between 1919 and 1921 are a case in point. In western Europe, both governments and peoples were gloomily counting the costs of war; but in the east, fighting was paying dividends.

In the new Europe there were few political certainties. It was true that autocratic empires had collapsed, and the democracies in France, Great Britain and the United States had emerged as the victors. But even in the democracies the liberalism and individualism of the nineteenth century had given ground to state control and government initiative. Yet at the same time the loyalty of individuals to their own state and country had been shaken. Wartime propaganda, never as effective as its practitioners hoped, had brought a revulsion of distrust and disbelief. The victors were disillusioned with the fruits of victory, because far too much had been promised. The losers grappled with the grim consequences of defeat, which in Germany were particularly hard to bear because for so long victory had seemed secure. In most countries the great divide between front and rear, between fighting soldier and civilian, continued to leave its mark in peacetime. In these circumstances, men sometimes turned away from their existing forms of government and politics towards an emerging fascism on the one side, or Bolshevism on the other.

This was a time of revolution. The Bolshevik revolution in Russia in November 1917 had lit a beacon in the east which was not to go out for a long time. Bolshevik revolutions followed in Bavaria in January 1919, and in Hungary between March and August; they were short-lived, but were encouraging or alarming according to one's point of view. From Moscow, Lenin looked westward and saw signs of the wider revolution which he so desperately needed; from Paris, the peacemakers looked eastward and saw the flames of Bolshevism licking across the continent. Either way, the possibility of revolution pervaded men's minds. The rise of Bolshevism had another surprising and long-lived effect. The Great War had dealt a tremendous blow to the idea of progress. The age of the Enlightenment should have ended between 1914 and 1918. But deep-seated attitudes of mind are hard to shake; and instead, by a form of displacement, belief in progress was transferred to the Bolsheviks, and the word 'progressive' was to mean, for the next twenty or thirty years, sympathy for Soviet Russia.

The war had proved a disaster for Europe, though nationalists and progressives could find some hope in its effects. What could the victorious powers do to produce a peace settlement which would rescue something from the wreckage and begin to rebuild the shattered continent? The peacemakers of 1919 have been severely criticized by their contemporaries, by their successors, and by historians. Yet we should remember that they attempted, and went far towards achieving, three great objects.

First, they imposed upon Germany a treaty which embodied the major war aims of France and Britain. In terms of territory, France received Alsace and Lorraine; Germany was diminished by losses to Poland, Denmark and Belgium, and lost all its colonies. German militarism, if not crushed, was struck a heavy blow. The army was reduced to 100,000 men; the General Staff, the heart and mind of the German military establishment, was dissolved; there was to be no military air force, and only a truncated fleet. Germany's responsibility for the outbreak of the war was proclaimed, and initially, if in the end uselessly, provision was made for the trial of war criminals, including the Kaiser, Bethmann-Hollweg, Hindenburg and Ludendorff. In these ways, what the victors (politicians and the man in the street alike) had believed the war was about was achieved.

Second, the peace treaties registered and regularized – they could usually do little more – the results achieved by nationalist movements in central and eastern Europe. The new states had to have frontiers; the peace-makers helped to provide them, and the treaties gave them a sort of legitimacy. On the whole, what is striking about the next twenty years is not that there were problems and disputes in eastern Europe, but that the settlement achieved in 1919 proved as stable as it did.

Third, the idealistic aspirations which had flourished during the war in Great Britain and the United States resulted in an attempt to change the whole basis of the international system. Mainly through the influence of President Wilson, but with much of the detailed work being done by Lord Robert Cecil in the British delegation, the League of Nations was brought into existence. It was an organization which could not possibly fulfil the hopes placed upon it in the aftermath of the war; and like the Bolshevik regime it was a new repository of what should have been a defunct faith in progress. But it was a real tribute to those who hoped that the war of 1914–18 had been the war to end war.

These were serious achievements, though they did not last. The peacemakers had not solved the German problem; they had not struck a true balance between the competing claims of many nationalities; they had not replaced power politics by a new form of international conduct. How could they? The Great War had left behind disasters and difficulties which were beyond men's grasp. It still leaves us uncertain and uncomprehending. How was it that the civilized, prosperous and stable states of Europe could fight such a war through to a conclusion, despite the mounting toll of death, destruction and social strain? Do we really know? Many years ago, in his narrative of the Great War, Churchill wrote that 1915 marked the last (and lost) opportunity to confine the conflagration within limits. 'Thereafter the fire roared on till it burnt itself out. Thereafter events passed very largely outside the scope of conscious choice.' In a recent account of the international politics of the war, David Stevenson has written that the conflict was 'a man-made catastrophe not a natural one . . . The war took the course it did because of deliberate decisions.'[20] Which of these judgements is nearer to the truth?

NOTES

1 To put the war poets (meaning nowadays Owen and Sassoon) in perspective, see J. M. Bourne, *Britain and the Great War* (London, 1989), pp. 225–7; cf. 244–5 for some other experiences.

2 Casualty figures taken from J. M. Winter, *The Great War and the British People* (London, 1986), p. 74. All casualty figures, including British ones, are approximate.

3 C. R. M. F. Cruttwell, *A History of the Great War, 1914–1918* (Oxford, 1934), pp. 51–4. Cf. N. Stone, *The Eastern Front 1914–1917* (London, 1975), p. 91, where the Austrian casualties are put at 400,000.

4 Cruttwell, op. cit., p. 185. Russian casualty figures are even more approximate than most; see Stone, op. cit., p. 215, where he describes the complete confusion of the record-keeping system.

5 P. Kennedy, *The Rise and Fall of the Great Powers* (London: Fontana, 1989), p. 341.

6 For different estimates of U-boat strength, see Cruttwell, op. cit., p. 382; for shipping losses, Bourne, op. cit., p. 68, and E. L. Woodward, *Great Britain and the War of 1914–18* (London, 1967), pp. 338–9.

7 3,704,000 men were called up in the first fortnight; see A. Fontaine, *French Industry during the War* (London, 1926), p. 26.

8 Table in Kennedy, op. cit., p. 333.

9 Table in M. Ferro, *The Great War 1914–1918* (London, 1979), p. 129.

10 Table in Kennedy, op. cit., p. 345.

11 Figures in Ferro, op. cit., p. 129, and Kennedy, op. cit., p. 347.

12 Figures in Kennedy, op. cit., p. 349, and B. R. Mitchell, *European Historical Statistics 1750–1970*, abridged edn (London, 1978), p. 113.

13 For the reorganization of government in Britain, see J. Ehrman, *Cabinet Government and War, 1890–1940* (Cambridge, 1958), ch. 3.

14 Price index figures in Kennedy, op. cit., p. 340.

15 R. Aron, *The Century of Total War* (London, 1954); J. A. S. Grenville, *A World History of the Twentieth Century*, vol. 1: *1900–1945* (London: Fontana, 1980), p. 192.

16 G. Pedroncini, *Les Mutineries de 1917* (Paris, 1967), p. 63.

17 Table in Ferro, op. cit., p. 129.

18 Figures in Winter, op. cit., p. 75.

19 Mitchell, op. cit., pp. 390–1.

20 Winston S. Churchill, *The World Crisis: 1915* (London, 1923),

p. 17; D. Stevenson, *The First World War and International Politics* (Oxford, 1988), p. v.

FURTHER READING

The notes on this chapter deal mainly with statistics and quotations used within it. For guidance on reading, the following note refers to a few of the most valuable books in English; I have tried to keep it to little more than two dozen.

Among a mass of material on the Great War, it is best to start with two chapter-length introductions in B. Bond, *War and Society in Europe, 1870–1970* (London, 1984), and J. Gooch, *Armies in Europe* (London, 1980). C. R. M. F. Cruttwell, *A History of the Great War, 1914–1919* (Oxford, 1934; reissued 1964), is still valuable; more recent and briefer discussions are in M. Ferro, *The Great War, 1914–1918* (London, 1973), and K. Robbins, *The First World War* (Oxford, 1984).

Among many military studies, J. Terraine, *The Western Front, 1914–1918* (London, 1964), and the same author's *Douglas Haig: The Educated Soldier* (London, 1963; reissued 1990), are part of a long attempt to change ingrained views on the conduct of the war in the west; for another view, see e.g. L. Wolff, *In Flanders Fields* (London, 1959). For a short, balanced and comprehensive study of the British military effort and its background, see J. M. Bourne, *Britain and the Great War, 1914–1918* (London, 1989). On high command, see C. Barnett, *The Sword-bearers: Studies in Supreme Command in the First World War* (Harmondsworth, 1966); at the other end of the spectrum, the experience of the men at the front is movingly caught in M. Middlebrook's *The First Day on the Somme* (London, 1971). On trench warfare, T. Travers, *The Killing Ground: The British Army, the Western Front and the Emergence of Modern Warfare, 1900–1918* (London, 1987), is excellent.

On the home fronts, F. P. Chambers, *The War Behind the War* (London, 1939), and J. Williams, *The Home Fronts: Britain, France and Germany 1914–1919* (London, 1972), remain useful. On Great Britain, there are excellent discussions in A. Marwick, *The Deluge: British Society and the First World War* (London, 1965); J. M. Winter, *The Great War and the British People* (London, 1986); and K. Burk (ed.), *War and the State: The Transformation of British Government, 1914–1919*. On France, see J. J. Becker, *The Great War and the French People* (Leamington Spa, 1985); on Germany, G. Feldman, *Army, Industry and Labour in Germany, 1914–1918* (Princeton, 1966), and

M. Kitchen, *The Silent Dictatorship: The Politics of the German High Command under Hindenburg and Ludendorff, 1916–1918* (London, 1978).

On war aims and the politics of war, see the excellent all-round treatment in D. Stevenson, *The First World War and International Politics* (London, 1969); also B. Hunt (ed.), *War and Strategic Policy in the Great War* (London, 1977). On Germany, F. Fischer, *Germany's Aims in the First World War* (London, 1967); on Britain, V. H. Rothwell, *British War Aims and Peace Diplomacy, 1914–1918* (Oxford, 1971). As introductions to the peace settlement, see H. Elcock, *Portrait of a Decision: The Council of Four and the Treaty of Versailles* (London, 1972), and S. Marks, *The Illusion of Peace: International Relations in Europe, 1918–1933* (London, 1976).

7 State and society under Lenin and Stalin

Edward Acton

'Spare me from living in interesting times.' The generation which experienced the age of Lenin and Stalin had better cause to invoke the old Chinese prayer than any in modern European history. Not only did the country pass through a bloody civil war (1918–20), three devastating famines (1921–2, 1932–3, and 1946–7), and the catastrophe of the Great Patriotic War (1941–5), but its political, cultural, social and economic life was turned upside down. During the revolution and civil war period, divine-right monarchy sanctioned by Russian Orthodoxy gave way to one-party communist rule sanctioned by Marxism-Leninism. The traditional social structure was demolished as the nobility and industrial bourgeoisie were expropriated. In the period of the First, Second and (truncated) Third Five-Year Plans (1928–32, 1933–7, 1938–41), the pace of change accelerated again. The collectivization of the land saw the proportion of the population classified as members of individual peasant households, operating the age-old strip-farming system, plummet from 75 per cent to less than 3 per cent. In the same period the urban population leapt by thirty million and the number of workers rose from one-eighth to one-third of the population, in the course of a massive shift from agriculture to industry. Huge new coalmines and steelworks were opened, more than quadrupling total production in these key sectors. The output of oil almost trebled, while that of electrical energy rose almost tenfold. Whole new industrial complexes, towns and major cities recast the landscape.

In their different approaches to the period, Soviet and Western historians have performed a strange *pas de deux*. Until the mid-1980s, the orthodox Soviet view presented it above all as a triumph of popular creativity. In 1917 the overwhelming majority of the population had thrown their weight behind Lenin and the Bolshevik party and created the world's first socialist government. The Soviet people under the leadership of the party then proceeded, despite the devastation of war and civil war, international isolation and the opposition of an embittered minority, to construct a new society free from unemployment and exploitation. It was a society in whose defence the people would make any sacrifice, and for which some twenty-seven million people paid the ultimate price in the heroic struggle against the brutal Nazi war machine.[1]

In the West, by contrast, the long-dominant 'totalitarian' view of developments under Lenin and Stalin offered a virtual mirror image of this account. In 1917, skilfully exploiting the chaos reigning in war-torn Russia, Lenin and his small group of conspirators launched a successful *coup d'état*. They consolidated their power by brute force and the suppression of all civil liberties. At the end of the 1920s, Lenin's successor, Stalin, imposed a ruthless programme of collectivization and forced-pace industrialization which was accompanied by appalling deprivation, the creation of a multi-million slave-labour camp system, and the death of millions by starvation and execution. Society was transformed through the application of mass terror by a doctrinaire one-party dictatorship. The Soviet people repelled the Nazi onslaught despite, rather than because of, the trauma they had been put through.[2]

Since Gorbachev's accession to power in 1985, discussion of the period among Soviet historians has been transformed. For many, it has become the most urgent social duty to break away from the triumphalist stereotypes of the old orthodoxy. The social, economic and military achievements of the 1930s and 1940s, the mass literacy drive, the welfare provision, the creation of a mighty industrial base, the defeat of fascism, so Soviet historians now tend to argue, have been celebrated long enough. The 'blank pages' of Soviet history must now be written and the spotlight turned upon the dark stains in the record. Many of the problems which beset the contemporary Soviet Union are to be found in the crimes committed in this period against human rights and democracy, and in the economic irrationalities and monstrous waste of the 'command economy'. Until all the horrors of the period are brought to light, the ghost of the past cannot be exorcized.

By the late 1980s, revisionist Soviet historians were vying with each other in the frankness with which they denounced the Stalinist system. Those who, in the pre-Gorbachev era, had been silenced for voicing criticisms of collectivization and terror, now find themselves overtaken by more radical voices. To admit of anything positive in the Stalinist record is to invite attack as an apologist. When more cautious voices suggest that wholesale denunciation amounts to vulgar anti-Stalinism, the champions of the new line reply that this is equivalent to speaking of 'vulgar anti-banditry'.[3] The victims of the show trials of the late thirties have now been rehabilitated, and where once currents of opposition to the party line under Stalin were dismissed as peripheral and essentially counter-revolutionary, they are now hailed for having saved the honour of the party. Equally, where once western analyses were scorned as vicious bourgeois distortions, the notion of Stalinism as 'totalitarianism' is rapidly gaining currency.[4]

The drastic reappraisal by Soviet historians now getting under way, however, comes at a critical juncture in the development of western study of the period. Among western specialists, the last two decades have seen the gradual discrediting of the 'totalitarian' model. It has been faulted for presenting a schematic and bogus picture of continuity between the revolution of 1917 and Stalinist coercion, for over-simplifying the process which led to the creation of the Stalinist state, and for misconstruing the manner in which that state operated.[5] A number of western 'revisionists' have taken matters further, moved the focus away from high politics, and concentrated instead upon more detailed analysis of the workings of the party and administrative apparatus, of the experience and aspirations of workers, of shifts in the social structure, and of the cultural upheaval of the period.

The revisionists have not gone unchallenged in the West. Critics have warned that their work tends to sanitize Stalinism and reduce the historically unique scale of state intervention to the small change of interest-group bargaining.[6] The charge that social historians tend to write history with the politics left out is not a new one. But even those sympathetic to the goal of examining the 'social dynamics' of Stalinism have insisted that it is a particularly grave charge in this instance. Whatever its deficiencies, the totalitarian model rightly placed the nature and role of the Stalinist state at the centre of attention. The agenda now before western and Soviet historians alike, therefore, is to 'theorise the state-society relationship';[7] to develop a framework for understanding the origins and dynamics of Stalinism which makes full allowance for the power and pretensions the Soviet state developed, yet acknowledges the extent to which the will of the Kremlin was supported by some elements within society, evaded by others, and frustrated by its own servants.

The point of departure must be the revolution itself. For in the course of 1917 the state, a defining characteristic of which is the capacity to exercise coercive authority, virtually ceased to exist. It was this process which rendered the Provisional Government helpless in the face of the Bolshevik-led uprising in October. From the moment when the tsar was forced to abdicate and the Provisional Government took office, the coercive force available to it had been minimal. The army remained intact, but traditional military discipline collapsed. Soldiers elected committees to represent them, and made clear that they would accept the authority of their officers and of the new government only conditionally, and would repudiate orders with whose purpose they disagreed. The discredited tsarist police force disappeared, and the new government proved unable to establish control over the armed militia organized by workers. This opened the way to the dispersal of power among an array of popular institutions – factory committees, trade unions, soviets and peasant committees – rapidly created by workers and peasants.

The effect of these developments was to render the liberal-dominated Provisional Government incapable of enforcing its will, and to make it dependent instead upon society's voluntary acceptance of its policies. But those policies proved increasingly unpopular. After introducing the full panoply of civil liberties, and setting in train the democratization of local government during its first weeks in power, the Provisional Government wished to concentrate national energies on pursuing the war until a general peace had been won. It therefore sought to postpone resolution of other major issues until a Constituent Assembly had been elected, and to proceed without undue haste towards such an election. This flew in the face of popular aspirations. Among workers, frustration with declining living standards and threats to employment, and anxiety to see government intervention on their behalf, became intense. In the countryside, peasant impatience for radical land reform and the distribution of noble estates became ever more evident. Among several of the national minorities, demands for autonomy rapidly gathered momentum. Anti-war feeling among rank-and-file soldiers, fuelled by the government's attempt to launch a new offensive in June, became increasingly widespread. Popular defiance of the government's authority became endemic as workers challenged management, peasants seized land, soldiers ignored officers, and minority nationalists repudiated Petrograd. The Mensheviks and Socialist Revolutionaries (SRs), having joined the cabinet and failed to steer government policy in a more radical direction, forfeited much of the enormous popularity and prestige they had initially enjoyed. Workers, peasants and soldiers sought representatives more responsive to their demands.

It was in this context that support mounted for radical socialists – Left SRs, Internationalist Mensheviks, anarchists, and above all Bolsheviks. In terms of organization the Bolsheviks had the edge over the other extremist groups on the Left, but during 1917 they were far from being the highly centralized and disciplined body once envisaged by Lenin. The party was 'internally relatively democratic, tolerant and decentralized'. Differences over policy were fiercely debated at every level of the party, the disciplinary sanctions at the leadership's disposal were minimal, and Lenin's authority was repeatedly flouted.[8] What underlay the Bolsheviks' increasing influence was the appeal of their policies. Urged on by Lenin from above and by militant rank-and-file members from below, they took a line of outright opposition to the Provisional Government. They committed themselves to a programme of immediate peace, confiscation of noble estates, drastic reform of industrial relations and intervention to prevent economic collapse, and the principle of national self-determination. They called for the downfall of the Provisional Government and the transfer of 'all power to the soviets'. These policies attracted an influx of workers and soldiers into the party, and membership soared from 10,000 or so in February to some 300,000 by October.[9] In the late summer the party made sweeping advances in elections to soviets in most urban areas, and won a large following in the army. By October the Bolsheviks had become a mass party supported by the great majority of urban workers and a substantial proportion of the soldiery. The Constituent Assembly elections held in November 1917 demonstrated that among the peasantry and therefore the country as a whole, the SRs were dominant. But the party had established itself as the most effective vehicle for achieving popular goals. So widespread was popular support for its call for the transfer of 'all power to the soviets' that when the party, operating through the apparatus of the Petrograd Soviet, launched the armed rising of 24–5 October, Kerensky and his colleagues were unable to offer effective resistance.

The 'state' that the Bolsheviks took over was an extremely fragile affair. The support of armed bands of workers, soldiers and sailors was sufficient to crush immediate political threats to the new government, notably that posed by the Right SR-dominated Constituent Assembly, which was forcibly dispersed after its first meeting in January 1918. And popular action expropriated the property and undermined the institutions of the traditional élites in city and countryside. But Bolshevik organization in the rapidly disintegrating army was patchy and fragmented, while the structure of the workers' militia and Red Guards was too irregular and decentralized to provide a disciplined force at Lenin's beck and call. In any case, the government initially abided by the long-standing Bolshevik goal of dispensing with both a standing army and a regular police force, relying instead upon 'the universal arming of the whole people', upon voluntary, democratic and locally organized workers' militia.[10]

On taking office, therefore, the Bolshevik government was under powerful compulsion to tailor its policies to popular wishes. Indeed, during its first months it was arguably more responsive to mass pressure than any government in Russian history. Despite the wish of many in the party leadership to reject Germany's Carthaginian terms and launch a 'revolutionary war', pressure from the soldiers ensured that an armistice was rapidly signed, and formal peace was concluded at the Treaty of Brest-Litovsk in March 1918. Despite the leadership's preference for immediate steps towards collective farming, the new government gave legal sanction to the peasantry as they parcelled out the private land through the agency of the traditional village commune. Even in the factories, where Bolshevik influence was most deeply rooted, the assertion of direct control by workers, and widespread demands for the nationalization of enterprises threatened with closure, went far beyond anything the party leadership considered compatible with economic recovery. And, despite Bolshevik conviction that it would be a retrograde step for the minority nations to break away from Russia now that it was in truly revolutionary hands, the new government had little choice but to proclaim their right to do so.

In the course of 1918, however, the Bolshevik government acquired in full measure the coercive power of a state. From mid-1918, initial reliance upon local voluntary efforts at policing began to give way to the creation of a regular and centrally controlled police organization. At the same time, the Red Army was rapidly transformed into a centralized body based on conscription and traditional military discipline. From the spring, the 'All-Russian Extraordinary Commission for Combating Counter-Revolution and Sabotage' (the Cheka), set up shortly after the revolution on a temporary basis to deal with overtly counter-revolutionary activity, swiftly expanded and developed into a nationwide political police force numbering some 40,000 by the end of the year.[11]

In the eyes of the Bolshevik leadership these developments were made necessary by the threat of counter-revolution from a dispossessed minority. But their effect was to make it possible for the government to pursue policies which placed it at loggerheads with most peasants and many workers. That it did so was the result of the catastrophic economic breakdown which followed October and the manner in which the government chose to react. The trade nexus between town and countryside, which had been steadily eroded as peasants withdrew from the market for want of industrial goods to buy, broke down altogether. Both grain and raw materials all but ceased to reach the cities. In desperation, *ad hoc* detachments of workers, soldiers, and officials went into the countryside to requisition supplies. From the middle of 1918 the government's Food Commissariat, backed by the Cheka and the Red Army, began to take requisitioning into its own hands. The government sought to win support from 'poor peasants' and to extract grain only from 'rich peasants', but in many areas its actions amounted to little less than an assault upon the peasantry as a whole.

There was a parallel, if less direct, confrontation between the government and industrial workers. The dislocation resulting from the collapse of trade between city and countryside was compounded by the precipitate military and economic demobilization which followed the armistice signed with Germany. By mid-1918 no less than 60 per cent of Petrograd's workforce were unemployed, as the abrupt cessation of military orders brought much of industry to a halt.[12] With bread rations falling below subsistence levels, industry was further undermined by absenteeism and demoralization. Lenin's early confidence in workers' initiative gave way to alarm, and in the spring of 1918 the leadership began to urge the need for strict industrial discipline under firm one-man management. Many factory committees themselves endorsed the call for discipline, an end to strikes, and the introduction of work-books, bonus incentives, piece-rates and the threat of dismissal. With factory committees gradually being incorporated into the trade unions and subjected to centralized control from above, rank-and-file workers found their voice ignored.

Menshevik, Right SR and anarchist activists who aspired to articulate the resentment of peasants and workers were subjected to growing harassment by the Cheka, and their press was severely circumscribed. Even the newly-established Left SR party, which had briefly formed a coalition government with the Bolsheviks before resigning in disgust at the Treaty of Brest-Litovsk, was subjected to ever-tighter restrictions. Rival parties were driven from effective representation in the soviets, elections to which became less and less frequent and meaningful. Soviet executive committees, dominated by Bolsheviks, ceased to be responsive to democratic pressure, and the same process ran right through the Soviet pyramid. At the apex, the Supreme Congress of Soviets and its Central Executive Committee lost control over Lenin's cabinet, the Council of People's Commissars. The soviets, for all the sovereignty entrusted to them by the constitution adopted in 1918, became subordinate in practice to the Bolshevik party.

Moreover, during 1918 the Bolshevik party itself became increasingly unresponsive to pressure from below. As economic crisis was compounded by full-scale civil war in the summer, the party underwent a rapid process of centralization. From above, Lenin and his colleagues became impatient with democratic niceties; from below, rank-and-file members urged greater control from the centre in order to maximize the use of limited personnel and resources against the party's enemies. The sheer growth in the administrative burdens placed upon party members reduced the time and energy available for democratic political consultation. Party cells met less often and were ever more dominated by local committees. The local committee itself was increasingly subordinate to its secretary, who in turn owed his office more and more often to appointment from above rather than to election from below. Thus, as the party's priorities shifted from political and ideological struggle to administrative and military activity, it became more a pliant instrument at the command of the leadership than a medium through which popular aspirations could be expressed.

Why did workers and peasants fail to prevent this erosion of their influence over government policy? In the first place, economic catastrophe generated bitter divisions among them. The desperate struggle for jobs, for fuel and above all for grain pitted workers against workers, peasants against peasants, city against countryside, and one national group against another. In this situation, with some groups and some regions standing to benefit from government intervention, the creation of a united front against the Bolsheviks proved impossible. Second, many of the workers who had shown the greatest political initiative in 1917 were themselves drawn into the apparatus of the state: the Soviet bureaucracy, the Cheka and the Red Army. Those workers who remained at the factory bench tended to be less skilled, less educated, and less well equipped to organize resistance. Third, and most important, was the impact of the civil war. It was this which, ironically enough, enabled the Bolsheviks to consolidate their hold on power. In one sense, the war intensified the friction between the government and its erstwhile popular base, as the need to feed and supply the Red Army accentuated the burden on workers and peasants alike. But at the same time the emergence of White armies, threatening to reverse the upheaval in property relations which workers and peasants had secured during 1917, made the new government the rallying-point for popular resistance to counter-revolution. However much peasants resented the impositions of the Reds, they tended to detest the Whites even more. Among workers, the determination to defend the gains of the revolution was fierce, and it was they who provided the core of the victorious Red Army.

Although the erosion of soviet democracy destroyed popular participation in the making of government policy, it did not remove all constraints upon the state. Once the civil war was over, the attempt to maintain the policies of 'war communism', to continue grain requisitioning, to intensify measures against black-market trading, and to impose military-style discipline upon workers in the drive to restore the country's devastated industry and transport system, provoked massive opposition. Widespread peasant disturbances, a rash of industrial strikes, and open revolt at the naval base of Kronstadt in 1921 compelled Lenin and his colleagues to make an abrupt U-turn. The New Economic Policy (NEP), adopted at the Tenth Party Congress in March 1921, saw the Bolsheviks come to terms with the mixed economy. Requisitioning was ended and private trade legalized. The semi-militarization of labour was abandoned, and the trade unions, though still headed by party members selected by the party leadership, provided a measure of protection for the working class. In the cultural sphere, too, the reins of control were slackened. Despite party censorship, uncommitted artists and writers enjoyed a limited degree of independence, and in history and the social sciences non-Marxist specialists gained considerable scope for research and publication.

However, during the 1920s neither peasants nor workers, still less petty traders (NEP-men) and non-party intellectuals, consolidated their influence over state policy. The remnants of the Menshevik and SR parties were suppressed, and the Soviet Union became a one-party state. Likewise, within the Bolshevik party itself, expressions of dissent and criticism of the leadership became increasingly difficult. The same Congress which saw the introduction of the NEP also imposed a 'temporary' ban on the formation of 'factions' within the party. Moreover, despite lamentation from all the leading Bolsheviks, the processes which had eroded internal party democracy during the civil war were not reversed after its conclusion. The system whereby important posts were filled by appointment from above rather than by election from below became entrenched. And that system concentrated power at the top, specifically in the hands of Stalin, whose position as General Secretary gave him a wide measure of control over key appointments. The influence which rank-and-file members were able to exercise over the leadership was very limited. The 200,000 workers recruited to the party in 1924 to strengthen its links with the proletariat played little part in policy formation.[13] The fraction of the membership living in the villages played virtually none.

Control over policy, therefore, was restricted to the upper echelons of the Bolshevik party. This did not predetermine the course that would be taken during the 1920s. True, all the leading Bolsheviks were committed to the acceleration of economic recovery and the development of the country's industrial base. Industrial expansion would underpin the socialist state's security in a hostile capitalist world, increase the 'socialist' sector of the economy and the size of the proletariat, and provide the productive power for the mass prosperity that was socialism's promise. But they were deeply divided over how to accumulate the resources for investment that were necessary to achieve the goal. On this the Bolshevik heritage was ambiguous.

Bukharin, who emerged as the champion of the NEP and warned against placing an excessive burden on the peasantry, had as good Bolshevik credentials as any, and defended his relatively gradualist position with copious references to Lenin. Trotsky and the 'Left Opposition', who pressed for a more active investment programme and for heavy taxation of kulaks and NEP-men, were equally insistent that it was they who represented true Leninism. That the party committed itself to the massive investment programme of the First Five-Year Plan is to be explained by mounting anxiety about the Soviet Union's international vulnerability, and by a rising tide of optimism within the upper echelons of the party that such a programme could be implemented without disrupting the NEP. Gosplan, the State Planning Commission, drew up a draft Five-Year Plan in 1927. It presented a tantalizing vision in which increases in productivity and agricultural output would make it possible to combine a massive investment in heavy industry with a rise in living standards. As General Secretary, Stalin was in a pivotal position, free to moderate or inflate this optimism. During the mid-1920s his attitude had been ambiguous. While he broadly supported Bukharin and denounced the 'adventurism' of the Left Opposition, he insisted on the possibility of building 'socialism in one country'. Once he had used his control over appointments within the party to outmanoeuvre Trotsky and his allies, he threw his own weight behind a programme of investment which exceeded anything they had advocated. Rival groups of planners were encouraged to vie with each other in advancing ever more ambitious targets, and in an atmosphere of mounting euphoria the optimists of 1927 were left behind. Targets were constantly revised upwards, and in March 1929 the Politburo enthusiastically endorsed a fantastic 'optimum' variant of the Plan.

The optimism was quickly confounded. While investment soared, increases in productivity were a fraction of those planned, and agricultural output actually declined. If the investment programme was to be sustained, peasants and workers would have to bear a heavy burden. The constraints which they would try to impose upon the state would have to be broken. As the measure of coercion that this would involve became apparent, a minority in the party, headed by Bukharin, protested and urged a slowing of investment tempos. But this so-called 'Right Opposition' was overridden. The majority of the leadership, headed by Stalin, was prepared to take the gamble that the state was now strong enough to overcome any resistance that society could offer.

Although such resistance was widespread and bitter, Stalin won his gamble. When peasants reacted to lower grain prices by withdrawing from the market, forced requisitioning was instituted. When even these 'extraordinary measures' yielded disappointing results, the state resorted to a more drastic solution: the forcible collectivization of agriculture. Peasants offering the most active resistance were denounced as 'kulaks', and were isolated and deported *en masse* to remote regions in the east and north. The bulk of the land and farm machinery was taken out of peasant hands and subordinated to state control. The state gained an unshakeable grip on the grain harvest. Equally, the state remained immovable in the face of workers' protests against the burdens of the industrialization drive, the pressure to raise work norms and tighten discipline, the sharp fall in real wages, the gross overcrowding, and the chronic shortages. Those union leaders, headed by Bukharin's ally in the Politburo, Tomsky, who sought to give voice to workers' resentment were purged and replaced by more compliant men. During the 1930s the trade unions became adjuncts of the state apparatus, supporting economic officials, enterprise managers and technical specialists in the campaign to increase productivity with minimal concern for welfare and wages. Similarly, the cautious notes of criticism struck by non-party intellectuals were silenced by a wholesale purge of 'bourgeois' elements in every academic, professional and educational field.

Unlike in 1920–1, then, society proved unable to deflect the government from its chosen course, from the hectic, forced-pace drive for industrialization. The state burst asunder the constraints upon it. That it was able to do so can be explained in part by the extent to which its apparatus had been strengthened during the 1920s. The Red Army, rapidly run down after 1920, was gradually built up. The network of the Ogpu, successor to the Cheka, was extended. The bureaucracy was rationalized and significantly expanded, especially in the provinces.[14] But the fact that the state prevailed is to be explained, too, by the support it received from groups within society. A variety of motives lay behind this support: ideological commitment, patriotism, and personal ambition. The NEP had frustrated the idealism of party members old and new, especially among the rapidly growing Communist Youth Organization (Komsomol). Among workers generally, there was little love for the NEP with its high rate of urban unemployment, painfully slow improvement in working-class wages and conditions, and widening differentials favouring managers and specialists. For some, the rhetoric of class warfare in terms of which the Plan was implemented struck a responsive chord. It promised a return to the heroic tradition of October and the Civil War, and an attack on bourgeois deformities, on NEP-men, kulaks and privileged members of the intelligentsia.

Activists lent support 'from below' on various different 'fronts' of the First Five-Year Plan. In the 'battle for grain' and the implementation of collectivization, for example, alongside the party and state officials and police and military units who were involved, an important role was played by industrial workers. Tens of thousands took part. Most prominent were the so-called 25,000ers, an elite group of volunteers hastily trained in the winter of 1929–30. They were despatched to the countryside to assist both in cajoling the peasantry into collective farms, and in establishing the farms once they had been created.

In the cultural sphere, the attack upon 'bourgeois' fellow-travellers was pressed not only by the state and party leadership from above, but also by radical groups within society. Theorists who had despised the compromises of the NEP period seized the opportunity to press for their visionary ideas. In each academic discipline – from history and literature to philosophy, in the sciences, even in mathematics and town planning, and certainly in education and law – militant enthusiasts denounced bourgeois deformities and undertook a frantic search for truly 'proletarian' approaches. Marx's dream was coming true; socialism was taking form, and the market was giving way to planned distribution. The end was in sight for all that was bourgeois – from the state to religion and the family.

In industry, during the First Five-Year Plan period there was a surge of enthusiasm among a minority of activist workers. They vied with each other to increase productivity, and urged fellow workers in workshops and whole factories to engage in 'socialist competition', to speed production and to exceed planned targets. Groups of a dozen or so young workers, initially with little encouragement from management, trade unions or the party, formed 'shock brigades' to raise output and efficiency by experimenting with new methods and by rationalizing production, and to act as a model of responsibility and self-discipline. From the beginning of 1929 both the 'shock worker' movement and the movement for socialist competition were taken up by the party and the planning agencies, and turned into a national campaign.

Of longer-term significance was the enthusiasm with which a minority of workers seized the new opportunities for education and training which the industrialization drive afforded. In the First Five-Year Plan period enrolments in higher education almost trebled, approaching half a million, and the proportion of working-class students soared from 25 to 50 per cent. Between 1928 and 1932 over 100,000 adult workers (*vydvizhentsy*) were enrolled in crash courses in higher education, while many more rapidly acquired new skills on the job.[15] While it was on the initiative of the state, then, that collectivization, forced-pace industrialization and the momentous social and cultural transformation of the 1930s were launched, they were implemented with the support of a small but significant minority within society.

Yet the frenzied support 'from below' in 1929 and 1930 soon began to abate. On the one hand, disillusionment spread among activists. The 25,000ers sent to assist in collectivization found the task of establishing viable farms and gaining the cooperation of peasants extremely difficult. The enthusiasm of the early shock brigades was diluted to vanishing-point as millions of workers enrolled as shock workers for form's sake and for the rewards membership would bring, rather than out of genuine commitment. On the other hand, the political authorities became dismayed by the disruption that the upsurge of support from below had caused. The removal of skilled workers, be it to the countryside or into white-collar positions, was severely exacerbating industry's desperate shortage of skilled labour. In October 1930 a two-year halt to all such promotions was called, and in December 1931 it was announced that the 25,000ers were to be released from duty and, should they wish, they could return to their factories. Likewise, the visionary experiments of the cultural revolution were reined in. Traditional structures were restored in education and the legal system; earlier attacks on the family gave way to an emphasis on parental responsibility and authority; and the more extreme anti-religious activities of the Komsomol were toned down.

The effect of the upheaval of 1928–31, however, was radically to redraw the boundary between state and society. Many of the activists of 1928–30 crossed the notional line between the two, and were absorbed into the state. Workers involved in collectivization who remained in the countryside took up positions in the local party and state hierarchies; enthusiasts of the cultural revolution were set to work to enforce the increasingly centralized control of scholarship, art and education; and shock workers and *vydvizhentsy* were appointed to specialist and managerial posts. They blazed a trail followed by hundreds of thousands of upwardly mobile children of workers and peasants who, in the course of the 1930s, took office in the vastly expanded administrative, economic and coercive apparatus. In doing so they extended the reach of the state deep into every facet of social life.

Virtually every citizen became an employee of the state. Private commerce and independent artisan production were suppressed, and although collective farms notionally belonged to their members, in practice management was taken out of their hands, and they too became state employees. Thus, to impose its will, the state combined the sanctions available to it as employer, and as the source of welfare benefits in housing, education, and health care, with direct legal sanctions. The 1930s saw a stream of increasingly stringent decrees designed to regulate in minute detail the conditions in which its employees worked, from wage norms to the length of the working day and the provision of holidays. In 1932 a system of internal passports was introduced, to tighten control over migration; every worker was compelled to carry a labour book containing a detailed record of his labour performance; draconian legislation in 1940 made absenteeism – defined to include arriving twenty minutes late for work – a criminal and imprisonable offence; and special permission was required to change from one job to another.

Outside the workplace the state's omnipresence was no less evident. Virtually all institutions were subordinated to the state and run by party appointees. The press, the radio and publishing were under direct party supervision. The content of the school curriculum was laid down from above, and contained a large dose of ideological instruction. In every cultural field, firm central control was established. Not only was Marxism-Leninism treated as the guide to all knowledge, but the party leadership's views – and specifically those of Stalin – were to be taken as the key to that guide. A narrow and restrictive orthodoxy was laid down in every discipline, from art and literature to pure science and psychology. In history, for example, the *Short Course in the History of the Communist Party of the Soviet Union*, published in 1938, imposed a crude and rigid interpretative framework on discussion of the past and became the basic text from school to professorial level.

Moreover, not only did the law seek to regulate ever wider areas of private life, but the apparatus for its enforcement was vastly expanded.

In the course of the 1930s the state security police, or NKVD (successor to the Cheka and the Ogpu), became intimately involved in every sphere of social activity – in the supervision of collective farms, industrial enterprises, education, welfare, and organized leisure pursuits – and developed a seemingly ubiquitous network of informers. Nor did conformity with the law, praise for Stalin, or support for the party bring a guarantee of immunity; no individual, from Politburo member to humblest peasant, was secure. An integral feature of the NKVD's power was its seemingly indiscriminate exercise of power and the acute insecurity it bred. It carried away not only members of social groups defined as enemies of the people, such as 'kulaks', and public figures identified with dissent from one or another aspect of party policy, but countless individuals who could think of nothing they had done to attract the attention of the police and the nocturnal knock on the door.

Nevertheless, there were limits to the state's ability to control the lives, let alone the ideas and loyalties, of its citizens. Two such limitations merit particular emphasis. The first concerns the collectivization of peasant agriculture. In the face of the peasantry's bitter hostility to the new order, the state was compelled to grant one major concession. Each household was permitted to retain a plot of somewhat less than an acre for its own use, together with a small amount of livestock, and to sell its surplus produce. And, contrary to the whole ethos of collectivization, the peasantry devoted an entirely disproportionate amount of their time and effort to these small plots. Every device used to motivate and discipline peasant labour on collective land, on the other hand, proved dismally unsuccessful. Monetary incentives were minimal, limited as they were to the size of the surplus left after both the state's insatiable appetite and the farm's running costs had been met. In this situation even the most diligent of farm managers found the problem intractable. Intervention by local party and state authorities into the detailed running of the farms did little to improve matters. Based as it often was on minimal knowledge of agriculture in general and local conditions in particular, it served only to alienate the peasantry further. Peasant apathy, neglect and petty insubordination amounted to a form of passive resistance which all the seemingly unlimited power of the state could not overcome.

An analogous situation limited the state's control over industrial workers. True, collective protest was kept to a minimum. The trade union leadership was firmly in the hands of party appointees. Deep fissures within the working class – between established cadres and the influx of rural migrants, and between young and old, skilled and unskilled – which had been further exacerbated from 1931 by widening pay differentials, militated against the creation of new, independent organizations. In any case, attempts at coordinated opposition and intermittent strike action were rapidly dealt with by the NKVD. Yet the state proved unable even to approximate the degree of control over the individual worker to which it aspired. What prevented it from doing so was the fact that, despite their lack of independent collective organizations, workers retained a rudimentary amount of autonomy and bargaining power. This was guaranteed by the enormous demand for labour entailed in the ambitious targets of successive Five-Year Plans. The effect was to compel managers to compete with each other in order to secure and retain labour, thereby limiting their ability to discipline their workers. If the management of one factory was too heavy-handed, a worker could move on and sign up in another where the demands made upon him were less exacting, wages were higher or conditions were better. As a result, no matter how furiously the state hurled down decrees against the high turnover rate of labour, or against absenteeism, slipshod work, defiance of management and damage to machinery, managers were severely inhibited about implementing them. As on the collective farm, what happened on the factory floor was in large measure beyond the control of the state.

Moreover, there was a chronic leakage of power within the apparatus of the state itself. On the face of it, that apparatus was supremely centralized, a 'bureaucratic leviathan' in which Stalin and his colleagues at the centre presided over a rigidly hierarchical structure. Officials belonging to every arm of the state – an industry and agriculture, the party, and the commissariats, the soviets, education and the welfare services, the police and the military – defied orders at peril not only of their jobs, but of their liberty and possibly their lives. Besides being supervised by their immediate superiors, every branch of the apparatus was monitored by a party hierarchy bound by the strict principles of 'democratic centralism'. As if that were not enough to guarantee the scrupulous implementation of the centre's will, party officials themselves were closely watched by a police apparatus armed with virtually limitless disciplinary authority. Yet closer analysis suggests that the leadership was constantly frustrated by its own servants.

In part this arose from the sheer size of each hierarchy, the hectic speed with which they expanded, and the explosion of paperwork to which the state-driven industrialization programme gave rise; from poor communications across a vast country embracing a hundred different nationalities; from the low level of education of many officials; and from the ill-defined and overlapping responsibilities entrusted to each agency. But these problems only exacerbated more deeply rooted contradictions. A critical area of conflict between the centre and its officials revolved around the implementation of the chronically overambitious targets set by successive plans. There was permanent tension between, on the one hand, the desire of industrial and agricultural managers and officials to secure low, or at least feasible targets, and to exaggerate their achievements, and, on the other, suspicion at the centre that they were underrating capacity when production quotas were being set and exaggerating production when results were reported. Moreover, regional party officials charged with monitoring the implementation of Moscow's orders became enmeshed in the same net. In seeking to achieve their targets, to ensure that their commissariat, their region, their city or their enterprise secured scarce labour and raw materials, officials in party, state bureaucracy, and economy alike were drawn into semi-official and often corrupt networks lubricated by patronage and bribery. What to local officials seemed to be the legitimate fruits of office, of skilful flexibility, and of forceful organization, all too easily appeared in Moscow's eyes as embezzlement, contravention of socialist legality, or deliberate wrecking and treason.

The apparent recalcitrance of its officials posed the centre with massive problems. When not only workers and peasants, but the state's own officials, failed to implement orders and deliberately fed back misleading information, rational planning became all but impossible. The 1930s were marked by successive crises, rooted in poor coordination between interdependent sectors of the economy, and in the monstrous waste caused by enterprises devoting all their energy to achieving gross output targets, regardless of quality. Fierce disputes arose within the Politburo over how the centre was to impose its will, and a variety of strategies were adopted. One method was to appoint plenipotentiaries to break through what appeared from Moscow to be deliberate obstruction. Part of the purpose in despatching the 25,000ers to the countryside in 1930, for example, was to enable Moscow to reassert control of local officials who showed either excessive or inadequate zeal in the drive for collectivization. Another strategy was to invite pressure from below: to encourage workers to denounce instances of inefficiency, corruption and wrecking by state officials and industrial managers. One important motive behind the official support for the Stakhanovite movement in the mid-1930s was to compel management to adopt new production methods, by combining pressure from above with demands by model workers from below. To tighten control over members of the party itself, there were repeated attempts to 'cleanse' the party, to verify the credentials of members, and to expel those who from incompetence, inertia or opposition failed to observe instructions and party norms.

Most drastically, the centre resorted to the arrest and in many cases execution of suspect officials. The precedent was set in the Shakhty affair of 1928, when fifty specialists in the coal industry in the Donbass were charged and found guilty of using their position deliberately to sabotage economic planning. In 1930 and 1931, fabricated cases against the 'Toiling Peasant Party', the 'Industrial Party', and the Mensheviks' 'Union Bureau' took a heavy toll of economists, agrarian and industrial specialists, and other officials involved in the state planning agencies. In the course of the First Five-Year Plan period there was a massive purge, both of rural state and party officials and of trade union officials. An even more extensive and far bloodier attack on officialdom formed an integral part of the Great Terror of 1936–8. Stalin unleashed the NKVD not only against the one-time lieutenants of Lenin whom he mistrusted or resented, but against countless loyal Stalinists as well. The hierarchy of every branch of the state – the trade unions, industrial management, the commissariats, the judiciary, education, the army, and above all the party itself – was ravaged as hundreds of thousands of officials were dismissed, arrested, and in many cases executed. At the end of 1938 Stalin began to take alarm at the havoc caused, and the terror abated. But the 'problem' remained. The decimation of the country's skilled and experienced specialists and administrators proved a poor remedy for inefficiency, corruption, and endemic tension between centre and periphery.

During this period, then, the relationship between state and society passed through a series of fundamental changes. The state which the Bolsheviks seized in October 1917 was hardly a state at all. It was during the civil war that the new government assembled centralized coercive power. As it did so, control over policy became concentrated within the upper echelons of a Bolshevik party increasingly insusceptible to popular pressure. Until the late 1920s, the semi-independent institutions of workers and the economic weight of the peasantry continued to impose constraints on the state. But in the 'great turn' of the First Five-Year Plan, the state forcibly broke free of those constraints, with a measure of support from a minority of activists within society. From the early 1930s, many of these activists were incorporated into the state and became part of a sprawling apparatus, which continued to expand throughout the 1930s and acquired a historically unprecedented capacity to intervene in the daily life of the citizen.

Drastic though that intervention was, however, it fell far short of the systematic control to which the government aspired. Peasants and workers developed residual defence mechanisms, and the apparatus itself was marked by a level of abuse, waste, confusion, incompetence and insubordination, both unwitting and deliberate, which constantly frustrated official policy. By 1941 the power of the Stalinist state was prodigious. But it was power of the most crude, clumsy and counterproductive kind.

NOTES

1 See e.g. M. P. Kim *et al.*, *History of the USSR: The Era of Socialism* (Moscow, 1982).
2 For a classic definition of a totalitarian system, see C. Friedrich and Z. Brzezinski, *Totalitarian Dictatorship and Autocracy* (Cambridge, Mass., 1956), pp. 9–10.
3 I. V. Bestushev-Lada, *Istoriia SSSR*, 5 (1989), pp. 60–91.
4 For a sparkling guide to the upheaval in Soviet historiography, see R. W. Davies, *Soviet History in the Gorbachev Revolution* (London, 1989).
5 For a detailed critique see S. Cohen, *Rethinking the Soviet Experience* (Oxford, 1985).
6 P. Kenez, 'Stalinism as humdrum politics', *Russian Review*, 45 (1986), pp. 395–400.
7 G. Eley, 'History with the politics left out – again?' *Russian Review*, 45 (1986), p. 394.
8 A. Rabinowitch, *The Bolsheviks Come to Power: The Revolution of 1917 in Petrograd* (New York, 1976), p. 311.
9 See V. I. Miller, 'K voprosy o sravnitel'noi chislennosti partii bol'shevikov i men'shevikov v 1917g.', '*Voprosy istorii KPSS*, 12 (1988), pp. 109–18.
10 For Lenin's attitude in the first six months after October, see N. Harding, *Lenin's Political Thought*, vol. 2 (London, 1981), pp. 168–200.
11 G. Leggett, *The Cheka: Lenin's Political Police* (Oxford, 1981), p. 100.
12 W. G. Rosenberg, 'Russian labor and Bolshevik power after October', *Slavic Review*, 44 (1985) pp. 222–3.
13 T. H. Rigby, *Communist Party Membership in the USSR, 1917–1967* (Princeton, NJ, 1968), pp. 116–17.

14 See S. Sternheimer, 'Administration for development: the emerging bureaucratic élite, 1920–1930', in W. M. Pintner and D. K. Rowney (eds), *Russian Officialdom: The Bureaucratization of Russian Society from the Seventeenth to the Twentieth Century* (London, 1980), pp. 316–54.
15 S. Fitzpatrick, *Education and Social Mobility in the Soviet Union, 1921–1934* (Cambridge, 1979), pp. 187–8.

FURTHER READING

A valuable general treatment is G. Hosking, *A History of the Soviet Union*, rev. edn (London, 1990). M. Lewin, *The Making of the Soviet System: Essays in the Social History of Inter-war Russia* (London, 1985), brings together several brilliant essays, including the best brief treatment of the First Five-Year Plan period. The relevant sections in J. F. Hough and M. Fainsod, *How Russia is Governed* (Cambridge, Mass., 1979), are full of useful insights. On the economy, A. Nove, *An Economic History of the USSR*, rev. edn (London, 1982), is a most lucid guide.

An introduction to the revolution in terms of the controversy surrounding it is E. Acton, *Rethinking the Russian Revolution* (London, 1990). The key work on the October revolution is A. Rabinowitch, *The Bolsheviks Come to Power: The Revolution of 1917 in Petrograd* (New York, 1976). D. H. Kaiser (ed.), *The Workers' Revolution in Russia, 1917: The View from Below* (Cambridge, 1987), includes essays by the authors of some of the most valuable recent monographs on the events of 1917.

E. H. Carr, *The Russian Revolution: From Lenin to Stalin* (London, 1979), provides an admirably concise summary of his great 14-volume history of the first decade after the revolution. The best volume on the civil war is E. Mawdsley, *The Russian Civil War* (London, 1987). On the early development of the Bolshevik state, see T. F. Remington, *Building Socialism in Bolshevik Russia: Ideology and Industrial Organization, 1917–1921* (Pittsburgh, 1984); G. Leggett, *The Cheka: Lenin's Political Police* (Oxford, 1981); F. Benvenuti, *The Bolsheviks and the Red Army, 1918–1922* (Cambridge, 1988). For the transformation of the Bolshevik party, see R. Service, *The Bolshevik Party in Revolution: A Study in Organizational Change 1917–1923* (London, 1979). O. Figes, *Peasant Russia, Civil War: The Volga Countryside in Revolution (1917–1921)* (Oxford, 1989), is a brilliant study of the peasantry in the period.

For the political struggles and economic debates of the 1920s, see S. Cohen, *Bukharin and the Bolshevik Revolution: A Political Biography, 1888–1938* (Princeton, NJ, 1974). On the experience of the working class, see C. Ward, *Russia's Cotton Workers and the New Economic Policy* (Cambridge, 1990), and W. J. Chase, *Workers, Society and the Soviet State: Labor and Life in Moscow, 1918–1929* (Chicago, 1987).

For the major western treatment of collectivization, see two volumes by R. W. Davies: *The Socialist Offensive: The Collectivization of Soviet Agriculture, 1929–1930* (London, 1980) and *The Soviet Collective Farm, 1929–1930* (London, 1980). L. Viola, *The Best Sons of the Fatherland: Workers in the Vanguard of Soviet Collectivization* (Oxford, 1987), examines sympathetically the role of the 25,000ers in collectivization. Four recent monographs dealing with the working class during the first Five-Year Plans are V. Andrle, *Workers in Stalin's Russia: Industrialization and Social Change in a Planned Economy* (Hemel Hempstead, 1988); D. Filtzer, *Soviet Workers and Stalinist Industrialization: The Formation of Modern Soviet Production Relations, 1928–1941* (London, 1986); H. Kuromiya, *Stalin's Industrial Revolution: Politics and Workers, 1928–1932* (Cambridge, 1988); and L. H. Siegelbaum, *Stakhanovism and the Politics of Productivity in the USSR, 1935–1941* (Cambridge, 1988).

The process of upward social mobility is examined in S. Fitzpatrick, *Education and Social Mobility in the Soviet Union, 1921–1934* (Cambridge, 1979). The experience of white-collar specialists and managers is treated in N. Lampert, *The Technical Intelligentsia and the Soviet State: A Study of Soviet Managers and Technicians 1928–1935* (London, 1979), and K. E. Bailes, *Technology and Society under Lenin and Stalin: Origins of the Soviet Technical Intelligentsia 1917–1941* (Princeton, 1978). For a fascinating collection of essays on the 'cultural revolution', see S. Fitzpatrick (ed.), *Cultural Revolution in Russia, 1928–31* (Bloomington, 1978).

The best treatment of the terror of the 1930s is R. Medvedev, *Let History Judge: The Origins and Consequences of Stalinism*, rev. edn (New York, 1988); it is the work of the leading Soviet dissident historian of the Brezhnev years. The best known western account is R. Conquest, *The Great Terror: Stalin's Purges of the Thirties*, rev. edn (London, 1990). A recent, highly controversial contribution which removes Stalin from centre-stage is J. A. Getty, *Origins of the Great Purges: The Soviet Communist Party Reconsidered, 1933–1938* (Cambridge, 1985). A broader analysis is G. Gill, *The Origins of the Stalinist Political System* (Cambridge, 1990). For a wide-ranging commentary on new Soviet discussion and documentation of the Stalin era, see W. Laqueur, *Stalin. The Glasnost Revelations* (London, 1990). D. Volkogonov, *Stalin. Triumph and Tragedy* (London, 1991) is a shortened version of the most important Soviet biography to appear during the Gorbachev years.

8   The triumph of Caesarism: Fascism and Nazism

Paul Hayes

When it is so hard to reach agreement about the nature of Fascism and Nazism,[1] it is obviously difficult to make comparisons between the movements. This is further complicated by the fact that among political scientists and historians there is serious disagreement about the extent to which the history of pre-1914 Italy and Germany is relevant to the evolution of Fascism and Nazism. While all are agreed that both international and domestic factors are relevant, it is the question of relative importance which is crucial. Some commentators have emphasized the significance of the international situation, in particular the rapid social and economic development throughout the Western world in the late nineteenth and early twentieth centuries. As Organski put it, 'three related societal changes are important in the study of fascism: political mobilization, social mobilization, and economic development. All three are increasing rapidly in the period preceding a fascist episode.'[2] Others have stressed the importance of the uniqueness of Fascist movements in particular countries, viewing them primarily as unrelated to each other, and certainly not linked with other totalitarian movements. In Germany this debate has become entangled with that of *Sonderweg* (the unique form of the evolution of Germany),[3] thus making interpretations still more hazardous.

Another important, and related, question is the extent to which the rise of these movements could have been predicted. Friedrich, for example, argued that 'in the general studies concerned with man and society, totalitarianism is the most perplexing problem of our time. It has burst upon mankind more or less unexpected and unannounced.'[4] These views were buttressed by an earlier generation of liberal-minded historians, notably Fisher, with his emphasis on 'the play of the contingent and the unforeseen'.[5] The opinions of Friedrich and Arendt[6] were moulded by their own experiences and, perhaps, by a feeling that their generation had missed, or even betrayed, opportunities to establish democratic and pluralistic systems more widely. There was thus a need to explain Fascism and Nazism (and, later, communism too) in terms of uniqueness - awful, but non-recurring; this explanation was made all the more convincing by the belief that the apparent irrationality of the Fascist movements rendered their rise quite unpredictable. While there is much to be said for this viewpoint, it should not be forgotten that the rise of Fascism was not entirely unpredicted. In 1918 Spengler had argued that 'the Caesarism that is to succeed approaches with quiet, firm step'.[7] As it turned out, his emphasis upon force and power as the characteristics of the coming political system was prescient. But could the rise of Hitler have been predicted from Mussolini's success? Are, in fact, the cases of Italian Fascism and German Nazism at all comparable except at a superficial level? It is to these questions that we now turn.

The situations of Italy and Germany, victor and vanquished, were both similar and different. For all the trappings of victory, Italy had gained little from participation in the war. During 1915–18 Italy had fought a series of bloody battles, never penetrating Austrian territory very far; and after the disaster at Caporetto in October 1917, most fighting was within Italy's pre-1914 borders. By the end of the war Italy had lost over 600,000 dead and nearly a million wounded – half of these being seriously disabled. At the conference of 1919 Italy made some modest territorial gains in Istria, Trentino and the Alto Adige, together with a job lot of overseas concessions of dubious value. The prize of Fiume and a large area of Dalmatia completely eluded Sonnino. Many Italians, especially those on the left, had doubted the wisdom of involvement in the war. After the very modest gains of 1919 the nationalist Right was extremely dissatisfied, especially with the lofty moralizing of Wilson and with what was seen as the treachery of Clemenceau and Lloyd George. D'Annunzio spoke for not only the Right, but for much of the Centre and Left, when he referred to 'the mutilation of Victory'.[8] Italy had paid a fearful price for victory, not only in manpower but also in resources. The most severe price of all – the destruction of an already enfeebled political system – was yet to be paid, and was closely linked to the fact that many Italians regarded the war as a defeat, not a victory.

By contrast, Germany had lost the war in 1918. The territorial concessions made in 1919 – the loss of Alsace-Lorraine, Eupen, Malmédy, West Prussia and parts of Silesia, part of Schleswig-Holstein, the Memelland, and all the colonies – ought alone to have convinced

German opinion that the war had indeed been lost. Reinforcing this point were the vast reparation payments agreed, the renunciation of the gains of Brest-Litovsk, the exclusion of Germany from the League of Nations, the war guilt clause, and the loss of control in the Saar to the League, and in the Rhineland to Allied forces of occupation. If further evidence were needed, it could be found in the change of government from empire to republic, and the enormous losses of men during the war. During just over four years of conflict Germany lost over 1,800,000 dead and more than 4,200,000 injured; in addition, others were lost and never accounted for. Yet many Germans remained unconvinced that the war had indeed been lost, except in the sense that sheer perfidy by a corrupt gang of politicians had stabbed Germany in the back. Apart from a short period in 1914 there had been no fighting on German soil; expectations of victory had remained high until almost the end, and German armies did not seem obviously defeated in 1918 – as had apparently been recognized by the Allies' agreeing to an armistice. While Germans knew that the war had not been victorious, many of them saw it not as a defeat but as a setback which, with suitable leaders and policies, could be overcome. Thus even the period of occupation, foolishly believed to be a guarantee of security to France and Belgium, acted as an irritant, perpetually reminding Germans that important work – the destruction of the *Diktat* – remained to be done.

The potential for political instability in Italy and Germany was thus considerable. It was exacerbated by disappointed hopes, economic difficulties, the weakness of post-1918 governments in both countries, the continued existence of powerful groups of veterans, and poor leadership. It was in Italy that the combination of problems first became acute. As Mack Smith observed, 'postwar problems were everywhere difficult, but in Italy the ruling classes were so bewildered that they lost both control over events and confidence in themselves.'[9] The old political system of management, transformism, was swept away in the aftermath of the election of 1919, when the Catholic Popolari won 100 seats and the Socialists 156. Old leaders such as Nitti, Giolitti, Salandra, Bonomi and Facta remained important because of factionalism and lack of leadership in the two large parties. Practising old politics in a new situation was, however, quite inadequate. Shortly before the elections of 1919 a severe shock was administered to Nitti and his government when, in September, a motley force mainly composed of veterans marched under the leadership of D'Annunzio and seized the city of Fiume. The state of public opinion in Italy was such that this action was widely supported, both openly and covertly.

Although both the new regime in Fiume and the government's mis-handling of the episode were more suited to Feydeau farce than serious politics, the consequences for Italy were grave. An already weak government was further discredited at home and abroad, while those who favoured direct action, rather than the pursuit of goals through a representative system, were greatly encouraged. The refusal of Nitti to eject D'Annunzio, coupled with threats against Yugoslavia when its government wished to resume control of the city, showed that resent-ment against the 1919 settlement was prevalent even among the lib-eral, educated classes.

In this atmosphere it is hardly surprising that demands for direct action to solve problems spilled over into domestic politics. As in so many other European states, the post-war economic situation was bleak. Demobilization had been followed by mass unemployment. The decline of war-related industries added to this problem, while the waste of resources during the war had severely reduced the availability of capital to reconstruct peacetime industries. The pre-war taxation systems had been unfair and inefficient, and many burdens had been added in attempts to increase revenue during the war. Inflation, al-ready high, rose sharply after 1918, exacerbating social tensions. Two of the worst-affected groups – landless peasants and poorly paid fac-tory workers – soon resorted to the seizure of land or to strikes and factory occupations. The owners of property were terrified by this militancy and resentful at the government's apparent toleration of illegality. By 1920 fears of an Italian version of the events of 1917 in Russia were widespread among the upper and middle classes.

It was in this situation that Fascism found its voice. Its leader was Mussolini, who had so recently been decisively rejected by the elector-ate.[10] The strikes and civil unrest of 1920 and early 1921 gave this former socialist agitator an opportunity to reconstruct a political career. As editor and owner of *Popolo d'Italia* he had available the means to spread his ideas of how to set Italy back on its feet and, in due course, to ensure Italian domination of the Mediterranean. Much of what Mussolini wrote was imprecise and even self-contradictory; this enabled him to acquire support from very different sections of the population.

> He continued to campaign for nationalisation of the land, workers' participation in the running of factories and partial expropriation of capital; but he took care to confuse the issue by stressing that inside his movement there was room for all political beliefs or none at all,

wrote Mack Smith.[11] Mussolini's prospects gradually improved in the months following the 1919 election, as governments under Nitti and then Giolitti conspicuously failed to solve Italy's problems. In September 1920, following the failure of wage negotiations, a wave of occupations and lockouts struck the industrial centres of the north. The situation was widely seen as revolutionary, though there was little evidence of coordination and still less of deeper and more sinister motives. But Giolitti's reluctance to intervene alarmed the middle classes, who feared anarchy. Landowners and industrialists formed their own organizations and recruited private armies, mainly from the ranks of the unemployed war veterans. Increasing disorder lent credibility to Mussolini's vehement attacks on the lack of government authority, and made him more attractive to the aristocracy and the bourgeoisie.

Giolitti, in common with many others, exaggerated the danger from the Left. By early 1921 he had so far lost his nerve that he was willing to bring the Fascists into a national bloc, hoping thus to contain socialism. At a local level there had already been official collusion in Fascist attacks on socialists and communists for several months. Counter-attacks by enraged socialists and trade-unionists had served only to increase Mussolini's prestige among those with influence and authority. In these chaotic conditions the premier decided to call an election in May 1921. The Fascists were admitted to the national bloc and were thus afforded protection by the police, the army and the administration. The election campaign was characterized by much violence and intimidation, and some fraud. Squads of Fascists broke up meetings, attacked party offices and newspapers, and were active in beating and killing political opponents. Their experience in protecting property interests, initially in the countryside and later in many urban areas, served them well in a campaign of violence unprecedented in Italian politics. The election result was a great disappointment to Giolitti, who soon found himself replaced by Bonomi. Mussolini secured over 7 per cent of the vote and 35 seats in the Chamber; it was not a good result, but a great improvement on 1919. Once Giolitti's usefulness was over, Mussolini promptly abandoned him and the national bloc, and joined the opposition in the task of rendering government impossible.

At this point Mussolini seems to have realized that continued public disorder, coupled with the discrediting of parliamentary institutions, offered him some prospect of power as a strong man to save Italy from disintegration. He proclaimed the virtues of dictatorship, attacked republicanism, democracy and the parliamentary system, and made a strong bid for the support of extreme nationalists by his bitter tirades against the powers who had created and supported the Versailles system. Inside the Chamber he intrigued ceaselessly to destabilize governments, and was inadvertently aided in this process by the mutual jealousies of the leading politicians, antipathy between various Leftist factions, and the failure of the Popolari and the Socialists to reach an accord. While these tactics enjoyed some success, they also caused problems. Mussolini's changes of tack, and his apparently elastic political principles, caused difficulties for him inside his party. During the period from August to November 1921 he had to struggle to establish his claim to lead the Fascists, and it was only at the third Fascist congress in November that he asserted his primacy. At grassroots level, however, the Fascists were increasing in number and in confidence. This arose principally from the activities of the Fascist squads, headed by the energetic and ruthless Balbo. Opponents of Fascism were not safe whatever their position, and in September a socialist deputy was killed. Capitalizing upon the support of the veterans, the *squadristi* adopted the black shirts, songs and salutes of the *arditi*. Paramilitary power and a reign of terror on the streets became the hallmarks of Fascism. The fact that the Fascists provided 'order' of a kind comforted and attracted many property owners driven to despair by the feebleness of government.

The replacement of Bonomi by Facta in February 1922 opened the last phase of democratic government in post-war Italy. Mussolini's response was to launch a reoccupation of Fiume and, when that proved successful, to start a campaign of terror in a number of important cities. Collusion in Fascist attacks on the persons and property of socialists and trade-unionists was widespread among the administration and the police. The army did nothing to restrain Fascist illegality. In Rome Mussolini continued to intrigue, and in the provinces his able and unscrupulous deputies, Balbo, Farinacci and Grandi, made local deals and arrangements with whichever political groups best served the tactical needs of the moment. The socialists at last responded with the futile gesture of a general strike. Mussolini's reply was an ultimatum stating that if the government did not stop the strike, then the Fascists would. In early August the Fascists seized control in a number of key cities, the most important of which was Milan, while the government looked on. Their reward was increased finance and political support from the powerful federation of industrialists.

During the last weeks of democratic government Mussolini pursued a two-pronged policy. He continued to negotiate with parliamentary leaders, making numerous contradictory promises and thus ensuring the impossibility of a coalition against him. In most cases he spoke of partnership, suggesting that the Fascists would make an effective junior partner in a reconstituted government. Even experienced politicians succumbed to this offensive, and support from the press, especially the *Corriere della Sera*, persuaded much of the political nation that even a government headed by Mussolini could be safely controlled. At a different political level, contacts were opened or strengthened with leading figures in the Court, the army and the Church. It was essential to avoid opposition from the king and the armed forces if power were to be seized. Meanwhile, the mobilization of Fascist forces continued, and on 16 October at a secret meeting the leadership of the party agreed on a *coup d'état*. Eight days later Mussolini spoke openly of a march on Rome, and two days after that the Fascists began to mobilize. The events of 27–8 October were confused by the resignation of Facta, the refusal of Mussolini to participate in a coalition, the demand of General Badoglio to be given full powers to crush the Fascists, the continuation of Facta in office on a temporary basis, and finally, early on 28 October, Facta's decision to impose martial law. When, however, he went to secure the consent of the king, it was refused. A last-minute attempt to construct a government under Salandra failed, and he advised the king to appoint Mussolini. On 29 October Mussolini was made prime minister, and by the next day he had assembled a cabinet. The march on Rome now became a mere symbol of a triumph of political intrigue, though in order to satisfy both the *squadristi* and the need for a myth, it was depicted as a real and important event involving the violent seizure of power.

What conclusions can be drawn from these events about the nature of Fascism and its support? The most obvious point is that perhaps not even Mussolini himself knew what Fascism stood for. Fascist rhetoric emphasized power, violence, nationalism, revolutionary change, the need for leadership and the inadequacy of other political ideas. There was no intellectual consistency in Fascist doctrine or policy; indeed Mussolini frequently, and possibly correctly, gave the impression that he made up policy as he went along. There were revolutionary elements, both social and economic, in Fascist propaganda throughout 1919–22, but from 1920 onwards Mussolini was plainly ready to adapt his beliefs to the needs of the situation. This is clearly shown in his revised attitudes towards the monarchy, the Church, industry, trade unions, land seizures and property rights. There was, however, consistency in his contempt for democracy and the parliamentary process, his hatred of socialism and communism, and his readiness to use direct, often brutal, means to achieve his objectives. Fascism played upon a common weakness in democratic societies: the readiness of many to accept the elements of a political programme which attracted them, while simultaneously ignoring or downgrading those elements which they disliked. Fascism thus drew strength, rather than weakness, from its incoherence and inconsistency. This would not have been possible in a society less strained and tense, or in a country better led and governed. Fascism was not, of course, all things to all men, but it was something of importance to many.

The fact that the Fascists came to power as a result of political intrigue and a breakdown in government is in itself an important piece of evidence concerning the nature of Fascist support. At the very least it shows that there was widespread tolerance of Fascism among the ruling political and economic élites.[12] This conclusion is further supported by evidence from before Mussolini's advent to power of sympathy and collusion among central and local government officials, the police and the army. Additionally, the Fascists were the recipients of large subsidies from industrialists and landowners. All of this suggests that the social, economic and political establishments accepted Mussolini and his movement as a means of defending their interests. Some dissented from this view, but the behaviour of De Bono, Federzoni and Volpi was more typical. However, it should not be assumed that the Fascists were without support among other sections of society. Many middle-class Italians saw Mussolini as a more effective bastion against the Left than the weak and disunited governments of 1918–22, and while they did not vote in large numbers for his party in 1921 they were probably, even then, willing to tolerate his methods. By the autumn of 1922 toleration had been converted into enthusiasm among many who were hitherto cautious. Nor was Fascism unsupported among the poor. In urban centres, with the aid of finance from industrialists, the Fascists were often able to ensure employment for their followers; in agrarian areas it was not uncommon to find support for Fascism among smallholders, leaseholders and sharecroppers.[13] Fascism benefited from the failure of the Popolari and the Socialists to represent effectively the interests of those who voted for them in 1919 and 1921. For those who were desperate or frightened, rule by a strong man, a man of the people who stood outside the ruling classes, did not seem so dreadful a fate. If those who positively supported Mussolini in 1922 were not that numerous, there were many who were willing to let him try his hand, and few who were ready and able to oppose him.

The rise of Nazism in Germany was, of course, related to general circumstances which bore some relationship to those which facilitated the triumph of Italian Fascism. But the history of the rise of Hitler to power is significantly different from that of Mussolini, and sufficiently different to make it hard to see how it could have been imagined that Hitler would readily act as a puppet. Hitler and his party, the NSDAP, were much less of an unknown quantity in 1933 than were Mussolini and the Fascists in 1922. By 1933 the NSDAP had been in existence for thirteen years, having been founded out of the wreck of the DAP, a small party which Hitler had joined in September 1919. Whereas the Italian electorate had only two opportunities to judge the policies of the Fascists, the German electorate had far more information at its disposal. Quite apart from presidential elections, there were six general elections in this period in which the NSDAP participated. These took place in May 1924 (6.5 per cent), December 1924 (3 per cent), May 1928 (2.6 per cent), September 1930 (18.3 per cent), July 1932 (37.3 per cent) and November 1932 (33.1 per cent).[14] Furthermore, there were fewer ambiguities about Hitler and his policies – inevitably so, given his exposure to free public debate since 1920, and the particular attention he won after the stunning electoral advances of September 1930 and July 1932. Additionally, he had published his own account of his beliefs and intentions in the two volumes of *Mein Kampf* in 1925 and 1926. While there were inconsistencies in the text and a considerable amount of invective and polemic, it can hardly be denied that Hitler made his general intentions clear. As Nicholls accurately observed, 'Generally speaking the book mirrored Hitler's character and fundamental attitudes faithfully enough.'[15] Furthermore, the principal modification of the views expressed by Hitler in the mid-1920s was to place greater emphasis on the role of the leader; this in itself ought to have demonstrated the inherent implausibility of regarding him as a potential puppet for other forces.

The lack of success of Nazism in the decade 1920–30 is, perhaps, less a testimony to the strength of the Weimar Republic and its system of government than it is evidence for the lack of distinctive appeal of the NSDAP. For those who wanted revenge for Versailles, a strong foreign policy, Germany for the Germans, anti-Marxism, or anti-capitalism, there were plenty of other parties in the field offering variations on these themes. The most obviously distinctive theme of Nazism in this period was anti-Semitism, and this alone was not enough to rescue the NSDAP from marginality. In fact, anti-Semitism was comfortably catered for in more orthodox political groupings, for hostility to the Jews was quite widespread in German society, and even more deeply rooted in Austria.[16] Hitler and his party also suffered from identification with the abortive Beer Hall putsch of 8–9 November 1923. Many who sympathized with Hitler's views preferred to work through the existing establishment to achieve their objectives, and frowned upon overt illegality. If there were to be a revolution, then, they felt, it would be best achieved by stealth and manoeuvre rather than by challenges in the street. Furthermore, the socialist and revolutionary rhetoric of Hitler did not altogether seem readily compatible with their views of a highly structured and regimented society. At the same time, his emphasis on nationalism and his hostility towards democratic values repelled many on the Left who subscribed, in part at least, to his more radical views about society and capitalism.

During most of the 1920s, therefore, Nazism proved quite unable to take advantage of widespread hostility to the Versailles system, of indifference to the republican form of government, and of a succession of weak, disunited and vacillating administrations. Clearly, the gradual, if slow, recovery of the economy from the trough of 1923, the reduction of reparations, the withdrawal of Allied forces, the diplomatic triumphs of Stresemann, and the ascendancy of conservative forces – especially after the election of Hindenburg as president in 1925 – did nothing to help Hitler. Yet by the autumn of 1930 the NSDAP was a force with which to be reckoned, having won 107 seats in the Reichstag as compared with the 12 of 1928; only the Socialists, with 143 seats, had a larger parliamentary representation. How can this be explained?

The general conditions which permitted this dramatic advance are many. They can be roughly divided into two categories: the problems faced by all industrial countries after 1929, and the particular difficulties which existed in Germany. The impact of the crash of 1929 and the depression which followed was severe on all industralized countries. In Germany the worst effects were not felt until 1931–2, but by the summer of 1930 it was quite evident that the economic advances of the post-1923 period were fast disappearing. As a major trading nation Germany was bound to suffer severely from any decline in international trade, and duly did so. A crisis could hardly have been avoided. Other countries with longer-established political systems also endured great difficulties and, in due course, underwent political metamorphoses. Britain acquired a National Government in the summer of 1931; in the autumn of 1932 the advocates of a New Deal were triumphant in the United States. But in both cases the existing political systems were sufficiently strong to contain change within democratic structures.

The problems faced by Germany were, however, unique. Ever since 1919 Germany had been heavily dependent on American loans and capital investment. After 1929 these sources virtually dried up. The issue of reparations acted as a focal point for national resentment, even though in practice they were a negligible financial matter. The fierce debate in 1929 over the Young Plan showed how this question could activate crude nationalism and stoke the fires of resentment against the Allies. Even in an age of undistinguished political leadership, Germany was very poorly off. Stresemann died on 3 October 1929, and Hindenburg was old and feeble. The principal figures in the democratic parties found it hard to comprehend the seriousness of the problems which now surrounded them, and hence failed to see the need to work positively together. The system of proportional representation had compelled the creation of delicately balanced coalitions; now it inadvertently encouraged parties to identify strongly with the protection of interest groups at the expense of compromise. Behind the scenes, powerful forces in the army, the judiciary and the bureaucracy were hostile to republican government and democratic values. Many ordinary Germans had only a tepid belief in the Weimar Republic, as it was commonly identified with defeat and humiliation. This made it easy to blame social and economic disaster on the democratic system, thus encouraging extremist parties in their rhetoric and violence. These were characteristics of German political life which politicians in other countries were fortunate enough, on the whole, to find absent from their own political cultures.

These were also the conditions of which Hitler was able to take advantage. He was greatly aided by disunity among his opponents. The bitter rivalry between the parties to the Left, which was foolishly encouraged by Stalin, meant that no possibility of a Popular Front existed. Additionally, the Socialists were quite unable to agree with the moderate parties of the Centre and the Centre-Right on how to tackle German problems. The issues of unemployment and the provision of benefit to the unemployed proved particularly difficult to treat, and led directly to the fall of Müller's government at the end of March 1930.[17] From this time onwards the Socialists declined to participate in government, disastrously reducing the capacity of the democratic parties to find a solution to Germany's problems. The effect of this was to put Brüning into power, in the absence of a secure majority in the Reichstag, until he in turn was ejected from office in late May 1932. During a period lasting well over two years, despite mounting evidence of social and political instability, the leaders of German democracy proved unwilling and unable to make the compromises which might have enabled it to survive.

Unlike many other politicians, Hitler realized that the chaotic state of affairs gave him and his party a real chance of power. His emphasis on the need for leadership struck a chord that was greatly attractive to the increasingly desperate masses; his unequalled talent for demagogy provided him with the means to communicate.[18] As Bullock put it, 'Hitler, with an almost inexhaustible fund of resentment in his own character to draw from, offered them [the Germans] a series of objects on which to lavish all the blame for their misfortunes.'[19] Hitler was greatly aided in his propaganda offensive by the able Goebbels and by the generally sympathetic, if often somewhat patronizing, attitude of much of the nationalist press. The party organs, the *Völkischer Beobachter* and *Der Stürmer*, were probably useful in maintaining morale among party members, but can have played little part in making converts to Nazism. To maintain a prolonged campaign, in effect from early 1930 to January 1933, was very expensive. Hitler, like Mussolini before him, needed substantial financial support. In part the party was an effective raiser of funds itself, through both legitimate political activity and protection rackets. However, the scale of operations demanded much more substantial sums than these activities could provide. Hitler's violent nationalism and anti-Marxism was the key to the coffers of the wealthy, particularly those of industrial magnates, property tycoons and the owners of great landed estates. The veneer of respectability given to the NSDAP by leading members such as Göring, Schwarz and Amann – all of whom were involved in fund-raising – was plainly important. Yet, with one significant exception, it was not until 1932, following Hitler's speech at the Düsseldorf Industry Club on 27 January, that there was a major breakthrough in obtaining finance from a substantial number of the wealthy. Before 1932 the NSDAP largely depended on subventions from Thyssen, who controlled the United Steel Works, and to a lesser extent from Kirdorf the coal magnate. Their support was crucial in enabling the campaign of 1930 to succeed, for by the close of polling the NSDAP was financially in very deep water.[20]

The party depended heavily upon the enthusiasm and organization of its activists. As the slump deepened, so membership rose quickly. In summer 1929 the NSDAP had 120,000 members, increasing to 178,000 by the end of the year; in December 1930 membership had risen to 389,000 and it stood at more than 800,000 a year later.[21] The various departments of the party were well organized, though serious problems were caused by rivalry between Goebbels and the Strasser brothers. In June 1930 Otto Strasser was driven from the party, but Gregor Strasser remained an influential figure until December 1932, when disagreements with Hitler about relations with the chancellor, Schleicher, caused his fall. Quite apart from the normal proselytizing and fund-raising, many party members were enrolled in the Sturmabteilung (SA), founded in 1921, or the Schutzstaffel (SS), which had its origins in Hitler's own personal bodyguard but was first properly organized in 1925. Holding the leadership of both bodies created problems for Hitler, but these seemed to be solved when in October 1930 Röhm was appointed to lead the SA; in January 1929 Himmler had been given charge of the SS, which in the autumn of 1930 became in effect a separate organization. Members of these groups played a major part in street-fighting, intimidation of opponents and political violence of all kinds, including attacks upon Jews and their property, on a scale far in excess of that of the Fascist *squadristi*.

An important factor in demoralizing the democratic parties and filling the ranks of the NSDAP and its paramilitary groups was the growth of unemployment. In January 1930 the registered unemployed numbered 3.2 million, a year later almost 4.9 million; during the whole of the last year of the Weimar Republic's existence, unemployment never fell below 6 million. It is generally believed that the real figure, including those who did not register, was 10 per cent higher than this. Only about two-thirds of the traditional workforce were in employment, and about 20 per cent of these were on short-time. Many of the unemployed abandoned the traditional parties and looked instead to Nazism or communism for some answer to their problems. The NSDAP was by far the greater beneficiary, as it was able to call for a distinctively German solution and did not seem to be controlled from outside. Nazism also made many converts in rural areas, long the bastion of traditional conservatism. Many farmers, especially in the east, were inefficient, but even in the areas where farming was more prosperous incomes fell dramatically. Hitler and his colleagues made a deliberate attempt to capture the farming vote, and as early as March 1930 produced an agrarian programme much to the liking of the peasantry. In the elections of 1930 the NSDAP made major gains in rural areas, though mainly in predominantly Protestant areas; rural Catholics tended to stick to the Centre Party.

The other section of the German electorate which swung heavily towards Nazism between 1928 and 1932 was the lower middle-classes: white-collar workers, small businessmen, shopkeepers, and those on fixed incomes. As Bullock pointed out,

What Hitler offered them was their own lower middle-class brand of extremism – radical, anti-Semitic, against the trusts and the big capitalists, but at the same time (unlike the Communists and the Social Democrats) socially respectable, nationalist, pan-German, against Versailles and reparations, without looking back all the time (as the Nationalists did) to the lost glories and social prestige of the past and the old Imperial Germany.[22]

While it is true that the lower middle-classes in many areas abandoned the bourgeois parties in favour of the NSDAP, what is not true is the assertion that it 'never numbered more than a relatively small proportion of workers among its members and voters'.[23] The appeal of Hitler transcended the natural divisions of the electorate – Protestant and Catholic, old and young, urban and rural, union and non-union labour, working and middle-classes, and so on. Hitler's support was strong in many areas of Germany and in many different parts of society. In July 1932, when nationally the NSDAP polled 37.3 per cent of the vote, it exceeded this level in no fewer than fourteen of Germany's thirty largest cities; in only one, Dortmund, did the level sink as low as 20 per cent. It seems very likely that among the young working-class unemployed the NSDAP had a large and vociferous following; many, after all, joined the SA. Hitler was skilful in being able to hold together this coalition of improbable associates.

Unlike Mussolini, therefore, Hitler came to power partly because of his known appeal to the electorate. He also had to reach agreement, as did Mussolini, with influential people and their interests. Although compromises had to be made throughout the period 1932–4, in the end Hitler's concessions were relatively unimportant to him. He was, of course, gravely underestimated by those with whom he dealt. Papen, who played a key part in helping Hitler become chancellor in January 1933, later admitted, 'My own fundamental error was to underrate the dynamic power which had awakened the national and social instincts of the masses ... we believed Hitler when he assured us that once he was in a position of power and responsibility he would steer his movement into more ordered channels.'[24] Hitler's belief in himself played a significant part in the events of 1932. It was a bold decision to run against Hindenburg, the national hero, on a ticket which was substantially nationalist in character. In the presidential elections of March and April Hitler won 30 per cent and 36.8 per cent of the vote respectively. The political landscape had changed decisively. Hindenburg, candidate of the Right in 1925, was elected essentially by votes from the SPD, from the predominantly Catholic Centre Party, and from ultra-conservative Protestants. Voters from the old bourgeois parties seem to have deserted to Hitler in large numbers, confirming Goebbels' taunt in the debates of 23–6 February in the Reichstag: 'Hindenburg is praised by the gutter journals of Berlin and lauded by the party of deserters.'[25] Even after the election reverse of November 1932, Hitler still stuck to his campaigning, believing that the establishment would have to give way to public pressure to give his party office.

As previously mentioned, however, Hitler did not neglect his parallel route to power. Contacts were maintained and strengthened with key figures in the establishment, and he was greatly aided by the infighting between Brüning, Papen and Schleicher. If he had ever had doubts about the need to preserve these links, they were resolved by the events of 14 April 1932. During the presidential election campaigns the SA, and to a lesser extent the SS, had appeared almost out of control. Röhm had talked openly of a coup and had mobilized his forces on 13 March, the day of the first election. Subsequent investigations by the police discovered a good deal of evidence damaging to the NSDAP, and on 14 April a decree dissolving the SA, the SS and all affiliated organizations was promulgated. Hitler accepted this ruling, at least to the extent of removing the uniforms of his followers, and realized that Röhm's tactics were dangerous to his plans – a realization which in the longer term was to contribute to his willingness to remove Röhm in June 1934. Meanwhile, Hitler and his close circle redoubled their efforts to obtain the agreement of the establishment not to obstruct the rise of the NSDAP to power. Negotiations with Schleicher expedited the fall of Groener, the Minister of the Interior, on 13 May, and of Brüning seventeen days later. With Papen installed as chancellor, assured of NSDAP tolerance, the ban on the SA and SS was lifted on 16 June; this greatly assisted Hitler towards his electoral triumph in July.

The summer and autumn of 1932 witnessed ever more complex political intrigues, at the centre of which were placed Hindenburg, Papen, Hugenberg, Schleicher and Hitler. Following the elections Hitler was excluded from power, only to respond by procuring the election of Göring as president of the Reichstag. Papen responded in turn by dissolving the Reichstag after it had sat for less than a day. Up to a point Papen's strategy worked, since in the election of early November the NSDAP lost 2 million votes, 34 seats and 4.2 per cent of the total poll. Following this reverse, however, Hitler played the political game much more cautiously than he had in August. Although he still demanded power, he did so in more measured terms and warned that Papen's policy would lead to the victory of the KPD.

Schleicher now abandoned Papen, who resigned on 17 November. A week of negotiations followed, during which Hitler was unable to form a governmental coalition; Hindenburg refused to allow him to form a minority government and rule by decree. Further wrangles between Papen and Schleicher prolonged the crisis until, on 2 December, Schleicher informed Hindenburg that Papen no longer commanded the confidence of the army. On the same day Schleicher was commissioned to form a government. Hitler again refused to join, despite growing financial difficulties within the NSDAP and evidence of declining electoral support. In early January 1933, however, contact between Papen and Hitler was resumed. A couple of weeks later it became clear that Schleicher's attempts to form a government had failed, and on 28 January he resigned. On 30 January, with the support of Papen and Hugenberg, Hitler became chancellor.

Hitler became chancellor, then, because the political, military and financial establishment believed that he could be controlled and used to serve their ends; in due course, doubtless, he could be discarded. Great faith was put in the belief that with only two minor offices given to the NSDAP in addition to the chancellorship, the new leader could easily be controlled. In this sense Bullock's observation that 'Hitler did not seize power; he was jobbed into office by a backstairs intrigue'[26] is true, but it is not the whole truth. It does not properly deal with the question of what government could be formed if Hitler and the NSDAP continued to stand outside the system. As long as divisions remained between the democratic parties, and as long as the KPD and the NSDAP continued to obtain significant votes – and there were precious few signs of either of these conditions ceasing to exist in early 1933 – a stable government could not be formed. To sum up, then, the verdict of the electorate had made it imperative that Hitler and the NSDAP be brought into government; and the jealousies of parties and politicians, the reassurance of minority status for the NSDAP, and the private guarantees given by Hitler and his entourage to key figures in the establishment, made it seem safe to acknowledge the force of that imperative. Within five weeks Hitler had made nonsense of the arcane calculations of Papen, Hugenberg and their associates, with fatal consequences for the republic and the German people.

It is now necessary to turn to the impact of Fascism and Nazism upon the societies they controlled, and to examine the modes of control employed and the relationships established with powerful interest groups. In peacetime conditions the Fascists were in power in Italy for almost three times as long as their German counterparts: 1922–40, as contrasted with 1933–9. However, the impact of Hitler and his party proved much greater than that of Mussolini and his followers. In part this can be attributed to the different nature of administration in the two countries. While it is possible to over-generalize, it is nevertheless fairly accurate to say that the bureaucracy in Germany was both much more efficient, and more officious, than in Italy. Once in control, then, it was easier for Hitler to assert his will than for Mussolini. This tendency was reinforced by the fact that Germany was a more modernized society, had better communications, and had a citizenry more accustomed to accepting administrative instructions.[27] In addition, Hitler was, in all probability, much more seriously intent on the conversion of his compatriots into the kind of citizens he wanted them to be; he had a much stronger belief in ideology than Mussolini. A further stimulus to action was, simply, the need to reward loyal followers. During the long years of struggle Hitler had acquired many obligations which needed to be discharged to the benefit of party stalwarts. The comparative brevity of Mussolini's campaign left fewer to reward, and less pressure so to do.

In post-1922 Italy and post-1933 Germany it was hazardous to remain a member of another political party or movement. The speed and energy with which other parties were controlled or suppressed was, however, very different in the two states. In Italy Mussolini controlled only a small number of seats until the Acerbo law, passed in late 1923, ensured the Fascists of a majority in the elections of April 1924. In fact, the Fascists secured 65 per cent of the vote, though how much of this was attributable to fraud and intimidation is largely conjectural. However, it is widely agreed that there was a majority vote for the groupings assembled behind Mussolini. The election result effectively rendered the other parties redundant, and it was only upon realizing this fact that liberal, radical and socialist forces set about trying to rectify the situation. It was, of course, far too late. Even the obloquy hurled at Mussolini after the murder of Matteotti scarcely dented the Fascist position. In early 1925 all the other parties were outlawed and those deputies, 123 in number, who had participated in the so-called Aventine secession of June 1924 were deemed to have forfeited their seats. Thereafter the parliament was a cipher, and non-Fascist political activities had to be carried out in clandestine fashion. Punishment for illegal political activities was severe, though much less so than in Hitler's Germany.

The political parties in Germany were eliminated much more quickly. A decree of 28 February, the day after the Reichstag fire, suspended a wide range of individual liberties. Thereafter the KPD ceased to exist as an effective force, most of its leaders having been arrested. On 23 March the Enabling Bill was passed, making the chancellor almost all-powerful. On 26 May the KPD was abolished, to be followed on 22 June by the SPD; their assets were all seized. In the days which followed, other parties in rather curiously obliging fashion announced their voluntary dissolution: the Democrats on 28 June, the People's Party and the Bavarian People's Party on 4 July, and the Centre Party on 5 July. Not at all voluntarily, and despite appeals to Hindenburg, the Nationalists were suppressed on 28 June. On 14 July the NSDAP was legally recognized as the only political party in Germany. Political activity continued, but illicitly and at high risk to those involved.

The authority of local government was similarly attacked. The not inconsiderable power of the *Länder* disappeared as a result of the decree of 28 February and the manipulated elections which followed. Control of the police passed into the hands of the NSDAP. At the same time Hitler began the process of transforming the local organizations of his party into the new administrations of the states. Local elections were abolished and Reich Administrators (almost invariably the local Gauleiters) were appointed to rule in place of the locally elected heads of government. On 30 January 1934 all local assemblies were abolished, and states were made totally subservient to central rule. Thereafter party strength was built up steadily at a local level, and in such a way that the roles of local administration and party organization became almost completely intertwined.

In Italy the reduction of local power was more attritional in character, and also less effective. The most important change was the replacement of the elected mayors by the appointed *podestà*. Most of those chosen were party hacks, often of negligible administrative skills. In consequence, local notables were frequently able to continue to wield some power or influence. A further complicating factor was that whereas in Germany the party was essentially subservient to Hitler, in Italy Mussolini found that party functionaries had their own ideas and policies. A long struggle ensued, until Mussolini achieved mastery over his party; it was probably not until 1928 that his victory was assured.[28] Uncertainty about such matters made it easier to escape fully centralized control, especially in areas remote from Rome, and for some of the old networks of patronage to survive in fairly recognizable form.

Control of the judiciary and the civil service also needed to be wrested from independent bodies. According to constitutional theory the civil administration was supposed to be quite separate from the administration of justice. In fact, in both Germany and Italy there were many links between the various arms of administration, and their existence made politicization easier. Purges of the civil service, extending to the highest levels, replaced opponents with party members or time-servers. The growth of competitive cadres and institutions both politicized and confused the administration. The ability to rule by decree tended either to ruthless efficiency, or to chaos and competition, according to circumstances. The demand by party members for jobs produced in Germany what Speer called 'our system of overbred organization'.[29] The dictators revised existing legal codes and appointed to high office those who showed themselves to be particularly compliant. In the last months of the Reich the proceedings of the People's Court under Freisler revealed the utter debasement of justice in Germany.

The Italian experience was similar. Pressure for places, combined with a perceived need for centralized control and enthusiasm for corporatism, soon led to a vast system of graft and corruption – much worse than in Germany. Efficiency, rational planning and allocation of resources, honest administration and effective direction were all conspicuous by their absence. Justice often became a matter of how much was paid or what pressures were brought to bear. An already rickety structure of administration was further weakened by the post-1926 politicization of the prefects, and vast sums of money were spent on expanding the security services – despite the fact that it was not until 1936 that the regime became generally unpopular. An administration of indifferent quality prior to 1922 became within a decade a byword for delay, corruption and confusion. The Fascists exercised general control, but over a deeply flawed instrument.

The exercise of control over trade unions and industry posed very different problems in the two countries. In Germany the trade unions were reduced to a mere cipher within a few weeks of the electoral victory of 1933. This was important, given the large numbers of well-organized trade-unionists and the close links between them and the SPD. After several weeks of organized attacks on trade union offices, on 2 May the SA and SS seized all trade union property and buildings. Commissioners were appointed to administer affairs, and leading activists such as Grassmann and Leipart were arrested. On the same day, Ley announced the merging of all the non-Christian trade unions into the 'Deutsche Arbeitsfront', under his leadership. Eight weeks later the Christian trade unions were also forcibly incorporated. During the next few months a complicated restructuring of professional and trade bodies took place. Throughout the years which followed there were serious disputes concerning the demarcation of authority between Ley, the ministries of labour and of economics, and the Trustees of Labour.[30] Once war began these problems were exacerbated by competition for labour and skills, and the overall result seriously hampered the war effort.

Whereas links between labour and the SPD or KPD made it both politically and economically necessary to subordinate trade unions to state control, industry, banking, business and agriculture posed different problems. Important vested interests (often with links to Hindenburg and the armed forces) in all these sectors had given significant support to Hitler in his struggle for power. An early attempt to impose control might have proved imprudent. Yet strong forces within the NSDAP demanded radical change. Darré desired a reduction both of interest rates and of the capital value of agricultural debt. Wagener wanted to seize control of the industrial employers' association. Zeleny and Renteln campaigned against chain stores on behalf of middle-class business interests. Feder advocated a strongly anti-capitalist programme certain to attract much opposition from industry, business and the banks. How, then, was Hitler able to adjust to such a complex situation? The answer lay in a mixture of change and caution.

Some pressures led to immediate changes. In March 1933 Renteln's Combat League of Middle-class Traders spearheaded a party drive to boycott Jewish businesses and large-scale trading enterprises. By early May the retail trade and handicraft organizations had been taken under corporatist control, and later that month Renteln and Hilland, despite fierce protests from Hugenberg, captured the organization of local chambers of commerce and industry. But economic realities limited the extent of change. Fear of mass unemployment led to the reduction of chain store business rather than its elimination; and middle-class traders did not even benefit much from this decline, because civilian consumption was limited in the late 1930s by the demands of the construction and armaments industries. Darré was likewise unable to revolutionize agriculture, though it proved easy to seize control of agrarian organizations. Cartelization did take place, though a high bureaucratic planned economy was largely avoided. On 15 July 1933 a formal, corporatist reorganization of agriculture was instituted, to be followed on 13 September by measures for market and price controls. On 29 September a law concerning entailment was also promulgated, though this was to prove even less of a success than the other two pieces of legislation. By 1934 the infighting so common in the Third Reich had overtaken the various offices and levels of control dealing with agriculture, to the general disadvantage of agrarian interests. In due course agriculture, like small businesses, fell under the control of Göring, following the establishment of the Four-Year Plan in 1936. Even in these areas, then, where radical pressures had been strongest in 1933, changes led ultimately to corporatist control, but a control largely devoid of firm economic direction.

The strongest evidence for Hitler's caution can be found in his appointments to key positions dealing with industry, banking and economic management. On 17 March 1933 Schacht resumed office as president of the Reichsbank,[31] and on 27 July 1934 he became Minister of Economics, succeeding Schmitt who had held office for some thirteen months. The real significance of these appointments is that they placed at the head of affairs two men who knew the German system of industry and banking well. Schacht and Schmitt represented a defeat for the radical wing of the NSDAP, and the careers of Wagener and Feder did not recover. Schmitt, who had been managing director of German's largest insurance company, was 'in his business and economic outlook ... a Liberal ... impelled to don the SS uniform very quickly'.[32] Krupp continued as president of the Association of German Industry, and the power of vested interests was demonstrated by the creation in July 1933 of a General Economic Council dominated by representatives of heavy industry and banking. Attempts to extend state control were resisted by Schmitt, and in August 1933 Renteln's career was checked when his Combat League was dissolved. Only after early 1934, when, with Schacht's support, rearmament began, did a widening of state control over the economy become feasible. After Hindenburg's death the partnership between Hitler and the armed forces determined the direction of production, and the economy fell increasingly under the control of the state.[33] Schacht – plenipotentiary for the war economy in addition to his other offices – played a key part in subordinating traditionally powerful interests to Hitler's will. Those who dissented, including ultimately Schacht himself, were removed or prudently fled. The most important sectors of the economy were thus not subjected to restructuring as part of a deliberate ideological process, but rather evolved towards an often inefficient corporatism as a result of the demands of rearmament and construction. Many of those with vested interests found it possible to live within this system, and dissent was largely ritualized until it became clear that the war was being lost.

Mussolini's treatment of trade unions and industry was very different. Industrial interests exercised a very strong influence inside the party and not only put a brake upon any radical tendency to pursue anti-capitalist policies, but even opposed the elimination of competing trade union structures – essentially on the grounds that a divided labour movement posed less of a problem for management. Yet both Mussolini's own political instincts and the strongly corporatist opinions of many Fascists argued against the survival of independent trade unions or other forms of association. As in Germany, there were close links between political parties and trade unions, adding to Mussolini's desire to be rid of both. The most powerful organizations were the CGL (General Confederation of Labour), closely linked to the Socialists, and the Catholic CIL (Italian Confederation of Labour). Without the active cooperation of industry, these institutions were too powerful to be challenged in 1922. Fascist policy was thus to build up Fascist unions, though this then posed the difficulty of what these bodies' attitude would be towards calls for strikes by their members. This problem continued to vex the party for several years after it attained power.

Those who advocated integral syndicalism, based upon a monopolistic system of obligatory unions, believed that they held the answer. Rossini, the head of the CNCS (National Confederation of Trade Union Corporations), and Farinacci both favoured corporatism, though from different perspectives. The growth of industrial unrest in 1924, coupled with governmental failure to cajole the CIL and CGL into greater cooperation, lent urgency to the debate. Even when internal agreement between the party, the government and the corporations had been achieved on 23 January 1925, the Confindustria (Confederation of Industry) continued to resist the development of corporatism. During the summer and early autumn of 1925 a long struggle was waged between employers resisting the pressures for corporatism, and the Fascist bodies. On 2 October 1925 the Palazzo Vidoni agreement recognized the Fascist unions' claim to sole representation, while the industrialists were bought off with practical concessions. The losers were Italian workers, who were henceforward able to strike only in the most exceptional circumstances. A system of arbitration also made collective bargaining superfluous. Free unions thus had no obvious function to discharge, and by early 1927 both the CGL and CIL had admitted their powerlessness. In the meantime state control had been formalized by the creation of a Ministry of Corporations in the early summer of 1926, aptly described as 'a new bureaucratic empire, whose tasks were essentially those of surveillance over the unions'.[34]

Industrial and financial interests were not so easily tamed. Rather, their power grew during the next decade. The protectionist lobby encouraged the adoption of autarkic policies once it had forced the liberal free-trader, De Stefani, from the Ministry of Finance in July 1925. Volpi, his replacement, was both a representative and a tool of big business, and although a planned economy was introduced, its character tended to be formed more by the industrialists than by the government. In 1927 the employers forced through wage cuts, thus destroying any worker support for Fascist corporations. Cartelization and monopolistic practices increased. The extent of the power of vested interests was shown by the response to world depression. In 1933 the government set up the IRI (Institute for Industrial Reconstruction) to save banks and to prop up imperilled industries. Intervention became common, but government control, except in the matter of permits and authorization, was not very effectively exercised until the drive towards a war economy began to take effect. Then, perhaps for the first time, it became clear to industrial and financial interests that their capacity for independent action had been sapped by increasing dependence on the state for the control of labour and the supply of capital. Their decline in influence was illustrated by the inability to oppose effectively either the attack on Abyssinia or participation in the war in 1940, despite widespread opposition to these ventures. Ultimately, therefore, Mussolini won a victory of a kind over big business interests by his decisions in foreign affairs.

In both Germany and Italy the lack of resistance by the armed forces to the dictators played a key role in their assumption and consolidation of power. Although the army had traditionally played a much larger part in German than in Italian politics, it is arguable that the Italian army had a much better, and more legitimate, opportunity of preventing Mussolini's coup than the German army had of excluding Hitler from power. In 1922 Mussolini enjoyed only tenuous electoral support, and the Italian army was not disgraced by overt intervention in domestic politics; in 1933 Hitler enjoyed substantial public backing, and the army had already forfeited much credibility because of its recent involvement in politics. However, this viewpoint does not take sufficient account of the important parts played by the king in Italy, and by the president in Germany; in both cases their influence crucially affected relations between the dictators and the armed forces.

In Italy the army could have opposed Mussolini in 1922, though there was some risk of internal division because of the pro-Fascist views of a group led by De Bono. The fact is that Badoglio was perfectly prepared to enforce martial law, but the king refused to sign the decree. Once this opportunity had passed, there was little further resistance from the army. Mussolini was careful after 1922 to keep its leadership in good humour. He paid respect to the sacrifices of

1915–18, and his belligerent utterances and occasional actions over such issues as Corfu and Albania were, on the whole, well received by the officer class. In general, too, the incomes and status of officers were protected. The upper echelons of the army were thus inevitably drawn into the conspiracy which pretended that Italy had become a first-class military power. Once committed, the army could not easily reverse its stance. As Mack Smith commented on Badoglio as chief of the general staff, he 'had been allowed to hold this post since 1925 precisely because he was ready to go on underwriting Fascist policy even though he knew it was bluff'.[35] Thus, after 1922 the army was little capable of influencing Fascist policy.

In Germany it seems certain that the army would have resisted any attempt by Hitler to seize power, and that Hitler took this into consideration during the period up to January 1933. Hindenburg's decisions to appoint Hitler and then to tolerate NSDAP excesses made it easier for Hitler and the generals to think in terms of an accommodation. The age of the president made this an urgent concern, and in June 1934 the nature of the bargain was in part clarified with the purging of the SA. Two weeks later Hitler acknowledged that the army was the sole bearer of arms within the Reich, and on 2 August he received an oath of loyalty from the leaders of the armed forces in response to his assumption of full powers following Hindenburg's death. In the space of a mere thirty-three days the army, without fully realizing either the fact or the consequences, had become bound to Hitler. As Blomberg was to admit in 1945, 'before 1938–9 the German generals were not opposed to Hitler'[36] – indeed, why should they have been, since they had undertaken actions to strengthen his grip on power? They agreed, after all, with Hitler's policies on rearmament and territorial restoration, though not necessarily with *Lebensraum*. By 1938, at the time of the Czech crisis, the assumption of the military caste that Hitler could easily be removed was no longer valid. In fact, the collapse of the army as a potentially independent source of power can be dated to 4 February 1938, when Blomberg and Fritsch were pressed into resignation and command of the army passed into more obliging hands – those of Brauchitsch and Keitel, both of whom were directly under Hitler's personal control. Indeed 'the Olympian position of the Army as a "State within a State" was shattered for ever. . . . Power the Army had held, and power they had cast away. Now they were to reap the harvest of their errors'.[37]

Religious bodies also posed, in theory, a threat to the dictators' drive to establish absolute control. Hitler's task was easier than that of Mussolini. There were four principal groups of believers in Germany –

Lutherans, Catholics, Calvinists and Jews – of which the first two were large and the other two much smaller in size. Almost needless to say, Hitler did not let Jewish interests stand in his way, and even before the Nuremberg Laws were passed in September 1935, most forms of collective participation in civil life had been denied to Jews. On the night of 9–10 November 1938, *Kristallnacht*, Jews all over the country were subjected to assault, destruction of property, arrest and death. Thereafter Jews were barely suffered to exist and, following the Wannsee Conference of 20 January 1942, the final bureaucratic arrangements for their extinction were made. The churches provided little resistance either to these atrocities or to the extension of Nazi power, though individual churchmen of course did. The collective failure of the churches stemmed not merely from lack of unity but also from their political and social history. All the churches, especially the Protestant ones, had a tradition of submission to state power. The Catholic Church, through the Centre Party, had actively participated in Hitler's final arrival in power and was fatally compromised as a result. Anti-Semitism too was a strong force among many staunch believers, being particularly virulent in predominantly Catholic areas. In addition, Hitler was perceptive enough to emphasize certain traditional values, strongly approved by religious leaders, which enveloped him in a cloak of respectability. His privately expressed contempt for the churches was very strong,[38] and certainly the religious organizations barely restrained his post-1934 actions at all.

Mussolini, on the other hand, had to deal with a powerful Catholic Church sustained by the presence of a Pope established in the heart of Rome. Despite his publicly acknowledged atheism, Mussolini saw the necessity of reaching agreement with the Church. By 1922 some arrangements had already been made, as can be seen from the Church's withdrawal of official support from the Popolari and its refusal to denounce Fascism as hostile to Christian values. In 1929 the Concordat was agreed. The Vatican City was recognized as a sovereign territory and the Church as the state religion, supported by financial aid and tax exemptions. The Church also acquired an increased role in education, control over marriage laws, and received support for discrimination against Protestants. In return the Papacy recognized the state of Italy and therefore by implication, approved Mussolini's government. Despite some conflict in the 1930s, the Church's compromises rendered it incapable of effective institutional resistance. As Mack Smith observed, 'while the Pope boldly protested at Mussolini's more strident heresies no government in Italian history had received anything like so much ecclesiastical approbation'.[39] When persecution of the Jews began in 1938, the Church was more inclined to speak softly than to wield its big stick.

Perhaps the most obvious and immediate danger to the establishment of control lay in a free press, radio and cinema. In both Italy and Germany this danger was quickly dealt with and, on the whole, effectively. In 1922 Mussolini began with a programme of intimidation, including occupation of offices and destruction of whole issues. Some newspapers were bought, and some editors forced out. Mussolini's mouthpiece, the *Popolo d'Italia*, however, was never highly regarded by the Italian public, which preferred the *Corriere della Sera*. Unfortunately, its editor, Albertini, initially viewed Mussolini as the saviour of Italy from Bolshevism, so during the crucial period of 1922–4 this newspaper was not very effective as a critic. When Albertini and some other editors turned against Fascism, the proprietors of the leading newspapers were persuaded to dismiss them and replace them with official nominees. On 20 June 1925 new press laws were passed and press liberty became a thing of the past, especially after the Journalists' Union began to expel members with anti-government views. In the first decade of Fascism radio was not so important, but from 1934 it began to emerge as a significant medium for propaganda, as it was firmly under state control. From 3 April 1926 all cinemas were obliged to show official newsreels, and from 1931 the Public Safety Law promoted an elaborate system of control. By the late 1930s the only significant, and far from consistent, voice of dissent was the *Osservatore Romano*, the official journal of the Vatican. Even this was controlled after 16 May 1940, and its circulation then rapidly declined.

Hitler's exercise of control was even more rapid and effective. Bans on some newspapers, most notably *Vorwärts*, began in February 1933. Laws introduced prohibiting the 'defamation' of the government made it difficult for any newspaper to criticize the regime. Once the process of *Gleichschaltung* (coordination) was under way, the socialist and communist press disappeared immediately, soon followed by the Catholic newspapers. The circulation of the *Völkischer Beobachter* rose sharply; as the official organ of the NSDAP, this is hardly surprising. Traditional newspapers of an independent outlook, such as the *Berliner Tageblatt* and the *Frankfurter Zeitung*, survived, but in such an emasculated form that they posed no threat.[40] The rest of the press was even less independent and accepted government hand-outs and instructions without demur. Minor infractions or inadvertent infelicities were likely to lead to severe punishment; in 1943 the *Frankfurter Zeitung* was closed down because of an insufficiently adulatory obituary of Troost, once Hitler's favourite architect. In March 1933 radio, cinema and theatre were placed under Goebbels' control, through the Ministry of Public Enlightenment and Propaganda – there being a good deal less of the former than of the latter. Radio was seen as a particularly important vehicle of propaganda, and considerable efforts were made to expand its audience.[41] Cinema increasingly suffered from an over-rich diet of propaganda and dismal films showing the pernicious role of the Jew in society, but, nevertheless, gave instant access to a wide audience. In the late 1930s cinema newsreels ensured that millions of Germans heard what the government wished them to hear.

What conclusions concerning the comparability of Fascism and Nazism may be drawn from this brief survey? Perhaps the most obvious is that comparisons are limited by the different political cultures, social structures and economic resources of Italy and Germany. Furthermore, Hitler and Mussolini, though having much in common, were also very different. What they shared was a belief in their roles as men of destiny, as figures towering above ordinary people; they believed that they could shape institutions, alter laws, impose new values and change society. Nothing was immutable save that they deemed it so. These attitudes made it unlikely that they would seek to rule on behalf of others. If other interests were promoted, this was the product of convenience or necessity – and was usually of rather short duration – rather than of desire. Once in power, both dictators found it fairly simple to eliminate or downgrade the influence of interest groups. Greater constraints were placed upon Hitler and Mussolini by lack of economic resources, governmental inefficiency, over-bureaucratization, or intra-party squabbling, than by the press, the armed forces, the Churches, big business or the judiciary.

The most obvious differences were those of will and power. The different reactions of the Fascists and the Nazis to problems of control, and their different levels of success in attaining such control, cannot be obscured by a theoretical similarity of ideology. Whatever the reasons are, it is evident that, in both the long and short term, Fascism affected Italians much less than Nazism affected Germans. This may, perhaps, reflect the extent to which Nazism truly represented a more deeply held set of attitudes in Germany than did Fascism in Italy. In international affairs Hitler's influence was more profound than that of Mussolini, and though it is often convenient to ascribe this largely, though not entirely, to the possession of greater resources, it may also be that the key factor was the much stronger sense of purpose and dynamism of the Nazis. In order to understand this difference fully, it is necessary to look far back into the history of both countries. Thus, often superficial similarities of ideology did not make Nazism interchangeable with Fascism.

NOTES

1 See e.g. P. M. Hayes, in *Modern History Review*, 1 (2) (1989).
2 A. F. K. Organski, in S. J. Woolf (ed.), *The Nature of Fascism* (London: Weidenfeld & Nicholson, 1968), p. 30.
3 See H.-U. Wehler, *Entsorgung der deutschen Vergangenheit?* (Munich: Beck, 1988); R. Augstein *et al.*, *Historiker 'Streit'* (Munich: Piper, 1988); or, for an earlier thematic treatment, A. J. P. Taylor, *The Course of German History* (London: Hamish Hamilton, 1946).
4 C. J Friedrich (ed.), *Totalitarianism* (New York: Harvard University Press, 1964), p. 1.
5 H. A. L. Fisher, *A History of Europe* (London: Edward Arnold, 1949), p. v.
6 H. Arendt, *The Origins of Totalitarianism* (New York: Harcourt Brace, 1951).
7 O. Spengler, *The Decline of the West* (London: Allen & Unwin, 1971), p. 507.
8 A. Rhodes, *The Poet as Superman: D'Annunzio* (London: Weidenfeld & Nicolson, 1959), p. 165.
9 D. Mack Smith, *Italy: A Modern History* (Ann Arbor: Michigan University Press, 1969), p. 321.
10 D. Mack Smith, *Mussolini* (London: Weidenfeld & Nicolson, 1981), pp. 35–7.
11 ibid., p. 40.
12 This point is well developed in Mack Smith's *Mussolini*, pp. 50–7.
13 See A. Lyttelton, *The Seizure of Power: Fascism in Italy 1919–1929* (London: Weidenfeld & Nicolson, 1973), pp. 54–76.
14 R. F. Hamilton, *Who Voted for Hitler?* (Princeton: Princeton University Press, 1982), p. 476.
15 A. J. Nicholls, *Weimar and the Rise of Hitler* (London: Macmillan, 1979), p. 106.
16 See especially G. L. Mosse, *Germans and Jews* (London: Orbach & Chambers, 1971); P. G. J. Pulzer, *The Rise of Political Anti-Semitism in Germany and Austria* (New York: John Wiley, 1964).
17 For a full, although not entirely detached, account see E. Eyck,

A History of the Weimar Republic, vol. 2 (London: Oxford University Press, 1964), pp. 226–52.

18 These skills are acknowledged by almost all biographers and historians of the period. They are very effectively described in A. Speer, *Inside the Third Reich* (London: Weidenfeld & Nicolson, 1970).

19 A. Bullock, *Hitler: A Study in Tyranny* (London: Odhams, 1964), p. 159.

20 There are many accounts of the financing of Hitler, including the memoirs of Thyssen. An interesting, if not entirely convincing, account of the wide-ranging contacts of the NSDAP, and the efforts of some financiers to resist Hitler, can be found in J. Pool and S. Pool, *Who Financed Hitler* (London: Macdonald & Jane's, 1979).

21 Bullock, op. cit., pp. 141, 150, 190.

22 ibid., p. 159.

23 S. Miller and H. Potthoff, *A History of German Social Democracy* (Leamington: Berg, 1986), p. 108. They are far from being alone in their favourable assumptions about the relative immunity of the German working classes to Nazism.

24 F. von Papen, *Memoirs* (London: André Deutsch, 1952), pp. 256–7.

25 Quoted in Eyck, op. cit., p. 356.

26 Bullock, op. cit., p. 253.

27 The German saying 'Befehl ist Befehl', loosely translated as 'Orders are orders', was not just a product of literary imagination.

28 Lyttelton, op. cit., pp. 269–307.

29 Speer, op. cit., p. 213.

30 M. Broszat, *The Hitler State* (Harlow: Longman, 1982), pp. 138–64; K. D. Bracher, *The German Dictatorship* (Harmondsworth: Penguin, 1973), pp. 411–23.

31 For his own account of his dealings with Hitler, see H. Schacht, *My First Seventy-six Years* (London: Allan Wingate, 1955), pp. 300–94.

32 Schacht, op. cit., p. 313.

33 For a fuller account see Bracher, op. cit., pp. 411-23; Broszat, op. cit., pp. 164–82.

34 Lyttelton, op. cit., p. 326.

35 Mack Smith, *Mussolini*, p. 240.

36 J. W. Wheeler-Bennett, *The Nemesis of Power* (London: Macmillan, 1961), p. 383.

37 ibid., p. 374.

38 H. Rauschning, *Hitler Speaks* (London: Thornton Butterworth, 1939), pp. 59–65.

39 Mack Smith, *Italy: A Modern History*, p. 443.

40 The best account of the press is given in O. J. Hale, *The Captive Press in the Third Reich* (Princeton: Princeton University Press, 1964).

41 The best general account of propaganda is given in Z. A. B. Zeman, *Nazi Propaganda* (London: Oxford University Press, 1964).

FURTHER READING

The literature on Fascism, Nazism and inter-war Italy and Germany is enormous. Every year brings forth a flood of additions. The following, however, are likely to be of particular help.

The ideological basis of the movements is covered in A. J. Gregor, *The Ideology of Fascism* (New York, 1969), and *The Fascist Persuasion in Radical Politics* (Princeton, 1974); A. Hamilton, *The Appeal of Fascism* (London, 1971); S. J. Woolf (ed.), *The Nature of Fascism* (London, 1968), and *European Fascism* (London, 1968); P. M. Hayes, *Fascism* (London, 1973), and F. Stern, *The Politics of Cultural Despair* (Berkeley, 1961).

The identity of those who voted for the Fascist parties is covered in S. U. Larsen *et al.* (eds), *Who Were the Fascists?* (Oslo, 1980); R. F. Hamilton, *Who Voted for Hitler?* (Princeton, 1982); G. Salvemini, *The Origins of Fascism in Italy* (New York, 1973). The structure of the political movements, and developments in society and culture before and after the capture of power, are examined in E. Nolte, *Three Faces of Fascism* (London, 1965); A. Lyttelton, *The Seizure of Power: Fascism in Italy 1919–1929* (London, 1973); J. J. Linz *et al.* (eds), *Breakdown and Crisis of Democracies* (Baltimore, 1979); W. Laqueur (ed.), *Fascism: A Reader's Guide* (Berkeley, 1976); A. J. Gregor, *Italian Fascism and Developmental Dictatorship* (Princeton, 1979); E. R. Tannenbaum, *Fascism in Italy: Society and Culture, 1922-45* (London, 1973); F. Neumann, *Behemoth: The Structure and Practice of National Socialism, 1933–1944* (New York, repr. 1966); M. Broszat, *The Hitler State* (London, 1981); K. D. Bracher, *The German Dictatorship* (London, 1973); J. C. Fest, *The Face of the Third Reich* (London, 1970); R. Grunberger, *A Social History of the Third Reich* (London, 1974); I. Kershaw, *The Nazi Dictatorship: Problems and Perspectives of Interpretation* (London, 1985); Z. A. B. Zeman, *Nazi Propaganda* (London, 1964); J. M. Ritchie, *German Literature under National*

Socialism (London, 1983). A useful guide is R. S. Wistrich, *Who's Who in Nazi Germany* (London, 1982). Also valuable is J. Steinberg, *All or Nothing: The Axis and the Holocaust, 1941–43* (London, 1990).

There are also standard biographies of the leading figures involved in the movements, most notably A. Bullock, *Hitler: A Study in Tyranny* (London, 1964); W. Maser, *Hitler* (Munich, 1971); D. Mack Smith, *Mussolini* (London, 1981); C. Hibbert, *Benito Mussolini* (London, 1962); as well as studies of other important leaders, including Hess, Himmler, Goebbels, Göring, Ciano and Farinacci. The memoirs or diaries of Ciano, Speer, Schacht and Papen are very revealing – often inadvertently.

9 Between democracy and autocracy: France, 1918–45

Nicholas Atkin

The history of France between the two world wars has been overshadowed by the defeat of 1940. As a result, many accounts of the Third Republic during this period are written as an explanation of the military catastrophe. For a long time, it was fashionable to blame defeat on the weaknesses of French parliamentary democracy which, it was alleged, had failed to provide stable government and strong leadership. Cabinets came and went with alarming alacrity and rarely produced significant reform. Furthermore, historians have stressed the Republic's economic shortcomings. Hampered by a low birth rate, France remained a peasant society, unable to compete with the leading industrial powers of western Europe. And, finally, the Republic has been seen as unpatriotic, 'a weakling in a society of nations'.[1] Political divisions were so deep-rooted that few French men and women were prepared in 1940 to sacrifice their lives for their country. Small wonder, then, that France was so comprehensively beaten on the battlefield. It had lost the fight even before the war had begun.

To what extent are these criticisms justified? Was France inevitably doomed in 1940? In recent years, the Republic has been more favourably treated by historians. It has been shown that in the 1920s France enjoyed an impressive period of political stability and steady economic growth. Admittedly the 1930s were a more turbulent decade, yet the Republic retained an inner strength which enabled it to fend off internal threats. When defeat came, this was due more to the failings of the French High Command than to the weaknesses of parliamentary democracy. In 1940 the Republic was no nearer to collapse than was Napoleon III's Second Empire in 1870. Ultimately, it was war which destroyed the Republic and gave birth to the authoritarian government of Marshal Pétain.

The Third Republic had been created in 1870 following the defeat of

France by Prussia. At the time, few believed it would survive. However, the Republic surmounted a series of crises and, on each occasion, emerged stronger than before. In 1914 the Republic faced its biggest test yet: that of war. No modern French regime has survived defeat in war, and it is likely that the Republic would have collapsed in 1918 if Germany had not capitulated. Thus the declaration of peace was met with considerable rejoicing in the streets of Paris. But not everyone was so sanguine. Many realized that victory had been won at great cost and created its own difficulties. Broadly speaking, these problems were threefold: the re-establishment of peacetime government; the reconstruction of the economy; and the quest for international security.

Given the magnitude of these problems, it is often argued that what France needed in the post-war world was strong government, something the Republic was unable to provide. Certainly the Republic is renowned for its political instability. Between 1919 and 1940 France had forty-two governments, each of which lasted on average no longer than six months. Nor can it be denied that this rapid turnover of cabinets made reform extremely difficult. When parliamentary majorities could not be found to support tough measures, for example during the depression years of the early 1930s, parliament had little alternative but to allow the government to rule by decree.[2] One possible solution to this uncertainty would have been a strong presidency. Yet the fear of a repetition of Louis Napoléon's *coup d'état* of 1851 ensured that, under the Third Republic, the president enjoyed little more than ceremonial powers.

Even so, the Republic was far more stable politically than is sometimes recognized. It must be remembered that the fall of a ministry did not lead to a general election, but merely to the creation of a new cabinet which largely comprised the same people as before. During the inter-war period up to eighty per cent of one ministry survived into the next. Moreover, considerable agreement existed within French politics. Although ideological battles could be fierce, French politics were not divided into two blocs of Left and Right. As has been remarked, 'A fair degree of consensus existed at the centre, which parliament faithfully represented.'[3] The centre, in turn, was dominated by the Radicals who often formed the basis of any government. Despite their name and their championing of the revolutionary tradition, the Radicals were never very radical, and saw their role as protecting the interests of small shopkeepers and farmers. The real parties of the Left were the Socialists and Communists; both these groups shared doubts about participating in 'bourgeois' politics, yet the Socialists remained committed to parliamentary democracy. Similarly, the Right had largely reconciled itself to the Republic, and only a few traditionalists dreamt of restoring the monarchy.

The inherent stability of this system ensured that France overcame the first problem of the post-war world: the return to peacetime politics. Indeed, stability and unity were the watchwords of the new government elected in 1919. This was largely made up of deputies from the Alliance Démocratique, moderate Republicans who had formed an electoral pact known as the *bloc national*. Thus the elections marked a swing away from the Radical-dominated chamber of 1914 and, overall, it is fair to say that the 1920s belonged to the moderate Right. Although in 1924 the Radicals and Socialists formed an electoral alliance to establish the 'Cartel des Gauches' government of Edouard Herriot, this fell the following year. The Socialists refused posts in Herriot's cabinet, which struggled to cope with a series of financial crises. In 1926 the chamber turned to the former president, Raymond Poincaré, who led a number of right-wing ministries until 1929. The Radicals would have to wait until 1932 before they regained control of parliament.

The 1920s were therefore one of the most stable periods in the political history of the Republic. This stability was further underlined by the failure of political extremists to launch a serious challenge to the regime. The growth of the far Right will be discussed later; in the early 1920s it was the Left which was perceived to pose the most dangerous threat. In 1919 the deputies of the *bloc national*, mindful of events in Russia, were worried about revolution in France. Their fears were heightened in December 1920 when an enthusiastic majority at the Socialist Congress at Tours broke ranks to establish the Parti Communiste Français (PCF). Even so, the Communists struggled to maintain a momentum and lost support to the Socialists, who rejected the notion of violent revolution. In any case, French society was not in the mood for dramatic change. Although a new industrial workforce endeavoured to improve its economic standing, France remained a country of landowning peasants and self-employed members of the middle class who had no interest in redefining the social system.[4] Thus, the majority of the population was content with things as they were, and was not prepared to countenance revolutionary upheaval.

The appeal of political extremism was also limited by the fact that the 1920s were a period of steady economic growth for France. It will be recalled that the second major issue confronting the Republic in 1919 was economic recovery. There were several aspects to this problem. The first was the rebuilding of those areas of northern and eastern

France which had been devastated by war. This task was carried out with impressive speed and efficiency. In turn, reconstruction made a significant contribution to the overall development of French industry. During the 1920s French industrial production rose faster than anywhere else in Europe. This growth was largely due to developments in new industries such as chemicals and motor cars, which benefited from the rationalization of production. Even so, these developments did not fundamentally transform the nature of the French economy. For the most part, industry remained concentrated in small family firms which employed only a handful of people. Moreover, France still depended heavily on agriculture. Although by 1931 the urban population had outgrown that in the countryside, the rural population still represented one-third of the workforce and agriculture provided nearly a quarter of the nation's wealth. Yet agricultural production remained sluggish, hampered by primitive techniques and the Napoleonic inheritance laws which insisted on the equal division of property between heirs – thus ensuring that the size of holdings decreased over the nineteenth century as land was passed down from fathers to sons.

A further problem was that of finance. Before 1914 the franc had been one of the most stable currencies in the world, yet the war had destroyed that stability. Consequently, in the 1920s French politicians were obsessed with the value of the franc and were convinced that its strength determined the overall health of the economy. Many small investors were also concerned about the franc. In the course of the First World War they had lent heavily to the government, which had subsequently built up a huge national debt. It had been hoped that Germany would pay for this by way of reparations. Yet in 1923 Germany defaulted on her repayments. Before long, the value of the franc had dropped and there was a crisis of confidence in government. Successive ministries attempted to raise new loans with little success; financial stability was restored only in 1926 when Poincaré, who enjoyed the support of the business community, returned as premier.

However, even the authority of Poincaré was unable to redress the most deep-rooted economic problem confronting France in the post-war world: the decline in the population. During the pre-war phase of the Republic the French population had been largely static, and in 1914 it stood at around 39.5 million in comparison to the 67 million of the German empire. Four years of war left France with 1.3 million dead, a further 1.1 million badly wounded and a severe fall in the birth rate. The 1919 parliament attempted to compensate for these losses by outlawing abortion, by restricting information on contraception and by launching a propaganda campaign to encourage women to have large families. Governments in the 1920s even welcomed the immigration of foreign workers, which was to create problems in the 1930s when unemployment began to rise. Yet no real financial inducements were offered to families to have more children, and by 1939 the size of the French population was much the same as it had been in 1913.

Demographic strength also had a bearing on France's standing as a great power. This was the remaining issue confronting the Republic in 1919: the quest for international security. It was understood that victory had been achieved only through the support of the allied powers. In future, France could no longer depend on their assistance. Thus security against Germany was paramount.[5] In order to achieve this, between 1919 and 1924 France pursued a hard-line policy towards its former enemy. At the Versailles Conference of 1919 France recovered the lost provinces of Alsace-Lorraine, was given control over the coalmines of the Saar, and was awarded heavy German reparations. The French also hoped to dismember the German state by creating a separate Rhenish Republic. Yet this was not acceptable to the Allies, and France had to settle for a demilitarized Rhineland. At least it could take comfort from American and British treaties guaranteeing French security. But these offers became worthless in 1920 when the United States refused to ratify the Treaty of Versailles. As a result, France looked to the creation of new alliances. Refusing to trust exclusively in the newly-created League of Nations, between 1920 and 1924 France signed military agreements with Belgium, Poland, and the 'Little *Entente*' powers of Czechoslovakia, Yugoslavia and Romania. Meanwhile, the French insisted upon the strict enforcement of the Versailles settlement, in particular the recovery of reparations. As previously mentioned, in 1923 Germany defaulted on the repayments. In an attempt to exact payment by force, French and Belgian troops occupied the industrial area of the Ruhr. This plan backfired, however. Not only did the occupation provoke international condemnation, it also exposed the weaknesses of French public finances. The troops were withdrawn, and in 1924 a commission was established to look into the question of reparations. The Dawes Plan, as it became known, reduced significantly the amount of German repayments, and France was again compelled to reconsider its policy towards Germany.

This task fell to the experienced diplomat Aristide Briand, who was foreign minister between 1925 and 1932. Aware of the failings of a hard-line policy, Briand adopted a more conciliatory approach. In 1925 he supported Germany's entry into the League of Nations, and in the same year he was one of the creators of the Locarno Treaty whereby France, Belgium and Germany agreed to respect the frontiers of 1919. Three years later he secured with Frank Kellogg, the US Secretary of State, a pact which denounced war as an instrument of policy unless used in national defence. Although nearly every country in the world adhered to this declaration, it accomplished little in practice, and France was not confident of its security. Its fears were heightened after 1929 when, in the wake of the Wall Street Crash, Germany again encountered difficulties in meeting reparations. In 1930 the amount of repayments was once more reduced, and in 1932 they were scrapped altogether. Thus, even before Hitler took power in January 1933, French hopes about security had been undermined.

Although France was uncertain about its international position, the 1920s were a successful decade for the Republic. The First World War had not weakened its political institutions, and economically it had made good progress. The 1930s were a more troubled period. The onset of the Depression gave rise to political extremism, and democracy was severely tested. Nonetheless, the Republic stood up to the challenge well.

In 1929 the Wall Street Crash unleashed a world economic crisis, yet it was not until 1931 that France felt the effects of the Depression. By June 1930 French industrial production was still increasing, whereas in the United States and Germany it had declined steeply since June 1929.[6] The reasons for France's relative immunity from the crisis are still not fully understood. One explanation is that since the stabilization of the franc in 1926, France was regarded as a haven for capital.[7] A further explanation is that because French industry and agriculture were largely small, self-financing enterprises, they were less immediately vulnerable to the impact of foreign collapse than were their European counterparts. However, when the Depression finally arrived, it was more protracted than elsewhere. The crisis manifested itself in various ways. The initial consequences were the fall in the volume of overseas trade and a huge balance of payments deficit. A further repercussion was the decline in industrial production. Bankruptcies soon followed. Although big established firms were able to weather the storm, many smaller industries went to the wall.

The effects of the Depression were uneven. It was probably the countryside which was worst affected. Agricultural overproduction and the decrease in demand led to a steep fall in prices and a drop in incomes. Many peasants resorted to rioting; others joined ultra-right political groupings such as Henri Doguères's Défense Paysanne. The Left also sought to mobilize the peasantry; both the Communists and

Socialists established peasant trade unions. By comparison, the urban working class suffered less from the Depression. The fall in prices raised their standard of living, yet this was little consolation to those out of work. Although unemployment was not as severe as in Britain, Germany and the United States, statistics reveal that unemployment in France rose from 54,600 in 1931 to 433,700 in 1936.[8] Those least affected by the Depression were the bourgeoisie and small shop-keepers, who were protected by government policies. Even so, the French middle classes experienced a profound sense of insecurity and looked anxiously to the future.

How did the government respond to the crisis? Between 1929 and 1932 (with a brief interval in 1930) the premiership was in the hands of André Tardieu, a former associate of Clemenceau. He embarked on an ambitious programme of economic planning and social reform. But these policies won him little support in parliament. The Left was worried that Tardieu might undermine its own schemes for reform, whereas members of the Right became concerned about the levels of public spending. Together these concerns led to Tardieu's fall in 1932. In any case, the elections of that year were won by a cartel of Radicals and Socialists; yet they had not learned the lessons of 1924. Once again, Socialists refused to join the cabinet. Even more serious were divisions over economic policy. The Radicals favoured a milder ver-sion of the deflation proposed by the Right; by contrast, the Socialists advocated reflation.[9] The result was ministerial confusion and a rapid turnover of cabinets between 1932 and 1934. However, in 1934 the debates over economic policy were overshadowed by the Stavisky Affair.

This scandal arose from the activities of a petty crook, Serge Sta-visky. In 1933 he had been instrumental in issuing a large number of counterfeit bonds for a Bayonne pawnshop. The press soon discovered Stavisky had been wanted for police questioning since 1927, but had friends in high places who had saved him from prosecution. Taking advantage of the general sense of unease created by the Depression, the extreme Right used these revelations to denounce the corruption of parliamentary democracy. The Radical government of Camille Chautemps tried to hush up the affair, but this proved impossible after Stavisky's suicide in January 1934. Chautemps resigned, and another government was formed on 29 January under the premiership of Edouard Daladier, a Radical from Provence. Daladier attempted to defuse the situation by dismissing Jean Chiappe, the head of the Paris police, who had shown a marked toleration for right-wing demonstrations, but this only made matters worse. On 6 February 1934 right-wing protestors converged on the Chamber of Deputies, apparently bent on storming the Assembly. Rioting broke out; 15 people were killed and a further 1,435 wounded. The following day, Daladier resigned and Gaston Doumergue, a former president, established a government of national union comprising politicians from a wide variety of parties.

With the benefit of hindsight, it may be seen that the events of 6 February 1934 were not a deep-laid plot on the part of the Right to overthrow the Republic;[10] the demonstrators lacked coordination and a sense of purpose. Yet this was not how Republicans viewed the protest at the time. They believed France had been saved from a March on Rome, and were worried about the rise of French Fascism. Historians, however, have been concerned with the broader question of whether there was such a thing as French Fascism. Some have argued that the right-wing organizations of the 1930s were not Fascist, but belonged to an established tradition of extreme nationalism. Although this might have been the case with certain of the leagues, it cannot be denied that France did possess its own Fascists.

The oldest of these organizations was the neo-royalist Action Française (AF). Founded in the 1890s, the AF was anti-parliamentarian, anti-Semitic, and anti-communist. Yet it was not Fascist. Its leader, Charles Maurras, was not a man of action like Mussolini or Hitler, but an ageing intellectual. In any case, by the 1930s the AF was past its peak. Although in 1934 it could claim 60,000 members, younger right-wing militants accused the AF of being stale and lethargic. This had led to the creation of new organizations such as the Jeunesses Patriotes in 1924 and the Faisceau in 1925. Consciously modelling themselves on the Italian Fascists, these movements attracted support among ex-servicemen, yet lost influence after 1926 when the right-wing government of Poincaré took power. More influential was the Solidarité Française, established in 1933. With its distinctive blue shirts, it was organized on Nazi lines and was prominent in the riots of 1934.[11] Yet this league could not match the strength of the Croix de Feu. Founded in 1927, this began life as veterans' association. However, in 1931 it was joined by Colonel de la Rocque and was transformed into a mass movement. By 1934 it boasted 150,000 supporters and was regarded by the Left as the most dangerous of the leagues. Although de la Rocque emulated Mussolini, he denied he was a Fascist, and in 1936 he was forced to dissolve the Croix de Feu and reorganize it as a political party, the Parti Social Français (PSF). Less ambiguity surrounds the overtly Fascist Parti Populaire Français (PPF) created in 1936 by the former communist, Jacques Doriot. A man of action and impressive orator, Doriot was more successful than other

Fascists in winning the support of the working classes, and by 1937 the PPF claimed a membership of 100,000.

Despite the impressive growth of the leagues, their appeal was always limited. Unlike Germany, France had not suffered national humiliation in 1918 and was fortunate in that it possessed a political system which offered some hope to those groups most susceptible to the appeal of Fascism. As has been remarked, 'the interests of the small shopkeeper and peasant proprietor had been effectively represented by the Radical party, which had no equivalent of comparable strength in Germany and Italy.'[12] Even so, the French Left was deeply troubled by the rise of the leagues and was galvanized into action. Before 1934, an alliance of the Left was out of the question. Both the Socialists and the Communists questioned the left-wing credentials of the Radicals, and the Radicals, in turn, feared the Socialists' electoral strength. Yet the real obstacle to an alliance was the Communists. Watched over by Moscow, the PCF had set out to emulate the Bolsheviks. It set little store by winning elections, and preferred to build up a network of cells in factories. Yet, despite this sectarianism, it was the PCF which made the first moves towards establishing left-wing unity. Frightened by the rise of the extreme Right both at home and abroad, the party began to think in terms of constructing a Popular Front against Fascism. Moscow, in turn, encouraged these moves, and in July 1934 a joint Communist-Socialist pact of unity was agreed. Yet this was not enough for the PCF, which now believed it had to win over those members of the middle classes who might be tempted by the lure of Fascism. Thus the PCF began to court the Radical party. At first, the Radicals were suspicious of such overtures, but in October 1935 they too joined the Popular Front. This change of heart arose not only from their frustration with the right-wing governments of Flandin and Laval which had succeeded Doumergue's cabinet of national union, but also from their worries about recent Socialist and Communist victories in municipal elections. Accordingly, the Radicals believed their best chance of fighting the 1936 parliamentary elections lay in a broad alliance of the Left. In the event, the Radicals lost seats, but overall the elections were a resounding triumph for the parties of the Popular Front.

In many ways the victory of the Popular Front augured a strengthening of democracy in France. On a personal level, this was reflected in the figure of Léon Blum, the Socialist leader, who became premier in June 1936. Having spent all of his political life in opposition, this Jewish intellectual had not been caught up in the political game of government, and this distinguished him from other Republican politicians.[13] He was a 'new man' who believed that the Popular Front should set out to promote the regeneration of France. Moreover, the Popular Front was not a hastily contrived electoral alliance which would disintegrate once the moment had passed, but a genuine reform movement with a wide-ranging programme for social legislation.[14] Its electoral manifesto, published on 11 January 1936, promised an extension of civil liberties to trade unions; an end to the deflationary policies of Flandin and Laval; the partial nationalization of the Bank of France; the removal of corruption in parliamentary life; the abolition of the right-wing leagues; and a commitment to world peace and disarmament. All in all, it was a bold programme, which raised the hopes of French workers. The expectation of change soon gave rise to a massive strike movement in French industry. By the end of May, there were some two million sit-down strikers. Each contemporary account of these protests recalls the carnival atmosphere of the strikers as they looked to the new government to resolve their economic difficulties.[15] However, these hopes quickly turned sour as Blum encountered a series of unforeseen difficulties.

Broadly speaking, the problems confronting the Popular Front were fourfold. First, Blum needed to end the occupation of the factories. This he did with particular skill, although, as we shall see, his solution was later to undermine his government's economic standing. On 7 June employers and workers were brought together at the Hôtel Matignon, the premier's residence, to discuss a reform programme. The Matignon agreements, as they became known, established the compulsory right of collective bargaining and pay rises of up to 15 per cent. Further legislation inaugurated a forty-hour week and paid holidays for workers. By the end of June most strikers had returned to work. A second problem was the opposition of the Right. On 18 June the leagues were dissolved without any real difficulties; yet conservative fears about the Popular Front were substantial. Many on the Right believed that France was on the verge of revolution, and were aghast at the Matignon agreements and the extension of government controls over the Bank of France. The right-wing press railed at Blum, chastising him for his Jewishness. This polarization of Left and Right was hardened by a third issue: the Spanish Civil War. The Left called for France to intervene on the side of the Republicans, whereas the Right supported General Franco. Although sympathetic to the Republican cause, Blum kept his country out of the war on the grounds that French intervention might provoke civil conflict on home soil. He was also concerned not to alienate the British government, which was against foreign involvement in Spain. In turn, Blum's policy of

non-intervention embittered the PCF. Preferring to support the Popular Front from the back benches rather than by accepting cabinet posts,
the Communists now became exceedingly critical of the premier. Yet
more serious was a fourth question: the financial and economic crisis.
The introduction of a forty-hour week and wage increases exacerbated
inflation, stifled production and contributed to a steep rise in the cost
of living. In this situation, employers flouted the Matignon agreements
and exported capital abroad; meanwhile, workers resorted to further
strike action. Blum attempted to deal with these problems by devalu-
ing the franc in October 1936, but this had little effect. By June of the
next year the financial situation had not improved, and Blum tendered
his resignation.

Ever since, historians have been divided in their attitude to Blum.
Those on the Left blame him for his timidity, and argue that he should
have used the occasion of the Popular Front to launch a full-scale
revolution; a difficult proposition, given that the Communists never
supported such an idea. Others point to the impossible political situation in which Blum found himself. Neither the Radicals nor the
Communists were reliable allies. In contrast, economic historians have
criticized the cost of his social programme, arguing that the introduction of a forty-hour week should have been delayed and devaluation
carried out earlier. There is certainly something in these arguments,
although, as has been pointed out, they overlook the fact that the
Popular Front 'was committed to doing something for the workers:
they expected it, and it was no more their due after years of government indifference'.[16] It should also be remembered that in order to
fight fascism the Popular Front spent more on rearmament than on
financing its social policies. Yet, whatever the reasons for its demise,
the Popular Front was not a total failure. Although its achievements
fell short of its supporters' expectations, 'its existence at least demonstrated the possibility of socialist government in a largely conservative
society.'[17] Accordingly, it would provide a continuing source of inspiration for the French Left; in 1981, at the time of another Socialist
victory, President Mitterrand would speak of completing the work first
undertaken by the Popular Front.

With the fall of Blum in June 1937, ministerial confusion reigned
until March 1938, when Daladier returned as premier. His government
marks another stage in the political history of the Republic. Breaking
away from the Socialists, Daladier led the Radicals in a rightwards
direction. This was reflected in tough economic measures, a policy of
reconciliation with the Catholic Church, and the Family Code of 1939
which attempted to reverse France's demographic decline by granting

family allowances. For some historians, Daladier's policies foreshadow those of the Vichy regime. But this is not to say that democracy was dead in France; it was merely moving in a different direction. It was the declaration of war that sounded the death-knell of the Republic.

It will be recalled that France had been worried about its international standing long before Hitler's rise to power. Thus, to many French men and women, Hitler was one of a long line of German leaders bent on further aggression, and they were not surprised by his decision in 1933 to pull Germany out of the League of Nations. To provide extra security, France courted the Soviet Union in 1934 and Italy in 1935, but these overtures resulted in little. Then in March 1936 came Hitler's decision to remilitarize the Rhineland. Although this was a flagrant breach of the Locarno Treaty, France did not act. The existing government under Albert Sarraut was a stopgap administration whose job it was to hold the fort until the general election in two months' time. Such a government was unwilling to risk mobilization, especially when French public opinion was against intervention. The High Command also opposed unilateral action and deliberately exaggerated the numbers of German troops. Confronted with these problems, Sarraut looked for guidance from Britain. The British government, in turn, believed that Germany had only occupied her 'own back garden' and discounted any retaliatory measures. Thus the issue blew over and the crisis was contained.

The Rhineland occupation had a significant bearing on French security. If France had been prepared to resist Hitler, then it is likely that she would have been dragged into a war. Yet in 1936 military circumstances were more favourable to France than they were in 1940. Thus an opportunity for victory had been lost. In future, France would think more and more in terms of a defensive strategy based on the Maginot line, a series of underground fortresses situated on the eastern frontier. Furthermore, the Rhineland occupation revealed to the world that France no longer possessed the will to maintain the 1919 settlement. Aware of this weakness, the government regarded an *entente* with Britain as providing the best guarantee of security and came to champion the cause of appeasement. This policy won considerable public support, particularly among members of the bourgeoisie, who had been frightened by the Popular Front and now considered Hitler less of a threat than Blum. Support for appeasement reached its peak in 1938 during the Anschluss and the Munich conference. By this stage, France was no longer prepared to support its eastern European allies; yet it possessed little room for manoeuvre.

After the Munich agreements, the British government resolved to stand up to Hitler, leaving France few options other than to support Britain. Thus in March 1939, following Hitler's seizure of Czechoslovakia, Britain and France promised to guarantee Polish independence. In August Hitler signed the Nazi–Soviet pact, which removed his fear of a war on two fronts; in the following month he invaded Poland. Even at this stage France hesitated about going to war; but given its commitment to Britain, it found itself dragged into a conflict which it had always dreaded and never wanted.

In terms of equipment France was well matched to fight a war with Germany. French rearmament had been proceeding at a rapid pace since 1936. Yet once German forces crossed over into French territory in May 1940, France was defeated in four weeks. Why did defeat come so swiftly? One explanation is that the 'phoney war' of September 1939 to May 1940 undermined national unity. Many believed that the fighting would be confined to the east and carried on their lives regardless. Certainly public morale was not as strong as it had been in 1914; even so, the most convincing explanation of French defeat is a military one. This has two aspects. First, the French High Command pursued a misguided strategy. Expecting the Germans to invade through Belgium and Holland, as they had done in 1914, Gamelin, the Commander-in Chief, moved French and British troops to the north. In the event, the main thrust of German tanks came through the heavily-wooded Ardennes, which had previously been regarded as impenetrable. Unused to the tactics of *Blitzkrieg*, the allied forces were unable to make a successful counter-attack and discovered themselves outflanked by the enemy. Second, the French High Command, wedded to defensive tactics, was profoundly pessimistic. This defeatism was quick to surface. On 21 March 1940 Daladier was replaced as premier by Paul Reynaud, a former minister of finance. Frustrated by the ineptitude of Gamelin, Reynaud appointed Weygand, a veteran of the First World War, as Commander-in-Chief, and on 18 May included in his cabinet Marshal Pétain, another veteran of the Great War. Neither of these old soldiers knew how to save the situation, and each urged Reynaud to sign an armistice. In so doing, they appeared to threaten the authority of civil government, and on 16 June Reynaud resigned. Pétain took over as premier and requested an armistice. Pétainism was born.

The Armistice was signed on 25 June. This divided France into two main zones. The zone occupied by the Germans was the larger of the two, including all the north and west of the country and extending down the Atlantic coastline to the Spanish border. It thus incorporated the most populated and prosperous areas of France. The unoccupied zone, which remained in French hands, stretched over central and southern France. At the same time, the Armistice left the French navy and colonies intact. The British, in turn, were worried that the navy might fall into German hands, and on 3 July British planes bombed the North African port of Mers-el-Kébir, where much of the French fleet was anchored. Meanwhile, a new French capital was established in the unoccupied zone at the little spa town of Vichy, where there were a sufficient number of hotels to house all the various ministries.

Although it had been Hitler who had dictated the terms of the Armistice, many French men and women were grateful to Pétain for having saved them from a harsher settlement. Certainly Pétain's desire for a cease-fire arose from his wish to avoid further bloodshed, and he was opposed to continuing the fight from North Africa. Yet it cannot be denied that he was an intensely ambitious man who had no liking for democracy, and who now sought to consolidate his personal control. This he achieved on 10 July when a majority of deputies, convinced that Pétain was the right man for the moment, suspended the Republican constitution and voted full powers to the Marshal.

So ended the Republic. In the months that followed, it became customary to blame defeat on the old democratic system. In February 1942 Vichy even put several former parliamentarians (including Daladier, Blum and Reynaud) on trial at Riom for having betrayed their country. But the trials had to be abandoned after the defendants skilfully turned the proceedings into an indictment of the Pétainist regime. Indeed, as we have seen, the defeat should be seen in military terms. In 1939 the Republic was no nearer to collapse than it had ever been.

Following the Liberation of France in 1944, Vichy became an embarrassment to its former supporters, and many argued that it was a passive government forced to accept Nazi directives. This was never the case. The Germans were largely unconcerned about what happened in the unoccupied zone, and allowed Vichy considerable autonomy in its internal affairs. Nor can it be maintained that Pétain was doing his best to shield France from German designs by secretly working for the liberation of his country. Instead, he welcomed the Occupation as an opportunity to promote the moral regeneration of the nation. In so doing, he enjoyed enormous personal popularity. There even developed a cult of the Marshal. This took several different forms: his portrait hung in all public buildings, and schoolchildren were taught the values of their elderly leader. In part, the strength of this cult may be explained as a quest for security.[18] In the wake of the German advance, over six million people took to the roads in what is known as the *exode*. Bewildered and frightened, they looked for a symbol of security, which they discovered in the figure of Pétain. Pétainism may also be seen as a triumph of Maurrassian values over the old Republic. Although the Marshal was never a member of the AF, he shared many of its beliefs, as did Vichy itself. Yet, most importantly, his cult symbolized a rejection of the Popular Front. It is highly significant that the most fervent Pétainists came from those elements of the peasantry and bourgeoisie who had no liking for the costly social measures of the Blum government.

A hatred of the Popular Front also characterized the policitians who made up the Pétain governments. But beyond that they were divided, with the ironic result that Vichy continued one tradition of the old Republic: a rapid turnover of cabinets. These ministries included Maurrassians, Catholics, former parliamentarians and even some figures from the Left. Perhaps the only time when Vichy possessed any semblance of unity was at the end of 1943, when it comprised several Fascists such as Philippe Henriot (Minister of Information and Propaganda), Marcel Déat (Minister of Labour), and Joseph Darnand (Secretary of State for the Maintenance of Order). Nonetheless, political divisions were deep-rooted, and it is difficult to label Vichy as 'Fascist'.

Together, this disparate collection of individuals attempted to promote a National Revolution based on the values of 'Work, Family, Country'. A key concern was education. A number of youth organizations were established to raise moral standards by providing young men of military age with a taste for hard work. Within schools, Vichy rooted out left-wing schoolteachers who were blamed for the defeat. At the same time Vichy restored former educational freedoms to the Catholic Church which, in the early months of the Occupation, was an ardent supporter of the regime. Yet there were limits to Vichy's clericalism, and in 1941 the government became less charitable to the Church. A further concern was the family. Building on Daladier's Family Code, Vichy made divorce more difficult and encouraged women to stay at home and raise families. Within the workplace the National Revolution attempted to rebuild the French economy along corporate lines. By organizing workers and employers into self-governing communities, Vichy hoped to end class conflict and the uncertainties of the liberal market. In practice, however, corporatism favoured producers at the expense of peasants and workers.

However, the most sordid aspect of the national Revolution was its racial policies. It is now clear that these measures were undertaken by Vichy itself, largely independent of German pressure. The French Right had a long history of anti-Semitism dating back to the Dreyfus Affair. As we have seen, the election of the Blum government hardened their prejudices. Subsequently, in 1940 Jews discovered themselves to be the object of official hostility. Legislation of 1940–1 deprived Jews of their French citizenship, prevented them from holding positions of public importance and confiscated their property. The intention of these laws was to rid France of 'unassimilable elements'; ultimately, however, Vichy contributed to the 'Final Solution'. Between 1942 and 1944 the regime handed over to the Germans some 80,000 Jews for deportation; of these, barely 3 per cent returned alive. Yet this was of little concern to Vichy, which regarded the Jews as a bargaining counter in its dealing with the Germans.

Negotiations with the Nazis remained a vital concern to Vichy throughout the Occupation. In October 1940 Pétain met Hitler at Montoire, where he declared that France had entered into a policy of collaboration with Germany. But little agreement existed as to what collaboration should entail. The Marshal hoped it would lessen the impact of the Armistice and allow him to pursue the goals of the National Revolution. Different concerns motivated Laval, who was foreign minister between July and December 1940. A former Socialist who had deserted to the Right, he was a long-standing advocate of Franco-German reconciliation, and believed that France could play a significant role in Hitler's new Europe. Yet his early forays into foreign affairs accomplished little in practice, and in December 1940 he was dismissed. He was eventually replaced by Admiral Darlan, who took charge of Vichy's foreign policy in February 1941. An ardent anglophobe, Darlan was a full-blown collaborationist who almost took France into the war on Germany's side. Yet, as always, the Germans refused his offers of assistance. In April 1942 Pétain was forced to recall Laval, this time as prime minister. Laval found the situation very different from that in 1940. By 1942 both the United States and the Soviet Union had entered the war, and a German victory looked less likely. In November 1942 Allied troops invaded North Africa and the Germans occupied all French territory. Even so, Laval continued making greater sacrifices to Hitler. Ultimately his policies led to the deportation of Jews, to the conscription of French workers for the Nazi war effort and to the subservience of the French economy to that of Germany. Still the Führer remained unresponsive. This was always the fatal flaw in Vichy's thinking. The regime never understood that it was

Hitler's intention to keep France in a weak position lest it attempt a war of *revanche*.

Similar problems beset those members of the far Right who chose to congregate at Paris rather than Vichy. This was a disparate group of individuals including Fascist intellectuals, journalists, and former members of the Left. Each had his own competing vision of how France should take its place in Hitler's Europe, but all welcomed the Occupation as an opportunity to further their own careers. At the same time there was a myriad of collaborationist groups. These included Déat's Rassemblement National Populaire, Doriot's PPF and the Légion des Volontaires Français contre Bolchévisme, which recruited Frenchmen to fight on the eastern front. Yet the most dynamic of these movements was the Milice Française. Founded in 1943 by Joseph Darnand, a distinguished war hero, the Milice was a paramilitary organization whose job it was to crush internal resistance. Darnand's services were welcomed by the Germans but, generally speaking, they were suspicious of collaborationist groups. Hitler feared that they might become popular movements which would rejuvenate French nationalism.[19] Thus the Nazis skilfully played off one faction against another. Vichy was also apprehensive about the collaborationists. Although Pétain shared many of their beliefs, he was frightened that they might form, with German backing, the nucleus of an alternative government. Accordingly, Vichy kept a close watch on their activities.

The history of the Resistance is also marked by diversity. The first resisters were an eclectic group of individuals united by nothing except their belief that France should continue the war. As has been shown, there were several factors which governed the emergence of resistance.[20] First, resisters had to overcome people's loyalty to Pétain. Although public opinion soon became disenchanted with Vichy, many retained their faith in Pétain until 1944. A further problem was the different nature of the two zones. The German presence in the north made it difficult for resisters to operate freely. Consequently, resistance was more marked in the south, at least until the total occupation of France in November 1942. The differences between town and countryside also had a bearing on resistance activities. To begin with, protest was concentrated in urban areas. This was because towns offered greater anonymity than the countryside. It was not until late 1942 that resisters, many escaping from Laval's obligatory work service, formed *maquis* groups in the hills. And, finally, it is significant that resistance was stronger in those regions, such as the Cévennes, which had a long tradition of protest against central authority, often from before the 1789 revolution.

Among the first resisters was General de Gaulle who, in June 1940, escaped to London to found the Free French. At the time, his position was remarkable, particularly when compared with Pétain. Unlike the Marshal, he had little experience of either politics or combat, and was best known for his unorthodox views on tank warfare. Even so, de Gaulle claimed to speak for France and questioned the legitimacy of the Vichy regime. Drawing on British help, the Free French built up a powerful base in the French colonies, and by the end of 1943 de Gaulle was widely acknowledged as the leader of the Resistance. Meanwhile, independent groups established themselves in metropolitan France. Among the most prominent in the northern zone were Organisation Civile et Militaire, Libération Nord and Ceux de la Résistance. Notable in the south were Libération, Témoignage Chrétien and Franc-Tireur. The only organization which had formal links with a political party and which operated over the two zones was the Communist-dominated Front National. Considerable controversy surrounds this movement. Several non-Communist historians argue that the PCF did not join the Resistance until the German invasion of Russia in June 1941. Before then the Communists had been held back by the terms of the Nazi–Soviet pact of 1939. Certainly the pact was an embarrassment to the party, which had been forced to adopt a neutral policy towards Germany. Even so, many Communists acted independently and engaged in resistance activities much earlier than June 1941. Thereafter the PCF played a formidable role in the Resistance, and took a leading part in the Liberation.

The lack of coordination between resistance organizations has often been criticized by historians. Yet it is difficult to see how they could have operated otherwise. Given the secretive nature of much of their work, resisters had to remain on their guard to prevent the infiltration of police informers. In any case, the Resistance did accomplish a large degree of unity. This was achieved by Jean Moulin, a former prefect of Chartres. In 1942, under de Gaulle's instructions, he established the Mouvements Unis de la Résistance, a loose federation which grouped together the non-Communist organizations. In May of the following year he persuaded the Communists to join the Conseil National de la Résistance, which was to plan for the Liberation. However, Moulin himself would never see the realization of its aim. In June 1943 he was betrayed to the Nazis and died at the hands of Klaus Barbie, the 'butcher of Lyon'.

Resistance groups engaged in several activities. These included industrial action, the production of clandestine newspapers, and the establishment of escape networks for Allied airmen shot down over France. Yet, as the Liberation drew nearer, military action became more significant. In the event, the D-Day landings of June 1944 ascribed little importance to the Resistance. This was because the Allied commanders had little knowledge of the strength of Resistance units and were unwilling to trust partisans with details of such a crucial operation. Nonetheless, the Resistance took an active part in the fighting and was instrumental in liberating large areas of Brittany and the south-west. More importantly, the Resistance had played a moral role. In its opposition to Nazism, it had demonstrated to the world that France had not relinquished the fight, and that it deserved a prominent role in the reconstruction of Europe.

In the wake of the Allied invasion, the Vichy government found itself under German guard and was held captive in the fortress of Sigmaringen. Eventually it was returned to France to stand trial. Several former ministers, including Laval and Pétain, were sentenced to death, although the marshal escaped execution on the grounds of age. Others fled abroad and lived in exile. The *épuration*, as it is known, has subsequently become one of the most sensitive episodes in French history. Former Vichyites claim that the Resistance summarily executed over 100,000 collaborators. A more accurate figure would be around 10,000. Indeed, France was excused the horrors of civil war. There was no wholesale purge of the civil administration and many former members of the regime returned to public life. Nor did the PCF, as de Gaulle later claimed, attempt to use the Liberation as a vehicle for revolution. It believed that there was no real alternative but to support the General, who ruled France for fourteen months after August 1944. Although de Gaulle was supposed to work in liaison with a consultative assembly, he enjoyed enormous personal authority and paid little heed to that body's opinions. Wanting to avoid the errors of the old Republic, he hoped that in future France would be governed by a political system which provided for a strong head of state and a weak legislature. This was not to be. The various political parties, in charge of drawing up a new constitution, were not united except in their desire to thwart the general's political ambition. In the event, the best they could do was to provide the Fourth Republic with a constitution remarkably similar to that of the Third.

The Third Republic survived for seventy years, longer than any other modern French regime. Its very longevity is a sign of its success. Certainly parliamentary democracy in France between 1918 and 1940 fared better than it did in Italy and Germany. As we have seen, the Republic was destroyed by the might of Hitler's armies and not by the failings of the Chamber of Deputies. How do we explain the Republic's success? To begin with, there is a great deal to be said for the view that France remained a calm country governed by overwrought politicians. Although in the 1920s France underwent significant economic change, it remained a nation dominated by small property owners who coveted social stability. Thus, unlike Germany, France never possessed a large number of *déclassés* who believed their only hope for the future lay in supporting political extremism. This is not to say that France escaped formidable ideological divisions. Even so, they were contained within the Republican system. Moreover, a faith in democracy remained strong and was only temporarily undermined by the defeat of 1940. To explain why, we need to reflect on the experiences of the nineteenth century. Since the 1789 revolution, France had experimented with a variety of regimes: Jacobinism, dictatorship and constitutional monarchy. Each of these had alienated a sizeable part of the political classes. Accordingly, a Republic came to be seen as the most suitable and least divisive form of government for France. This was underlined by the failure of the authoritarian regime of Vichy to win widespread public support. Since 1945 France has undergone further political upheaval, but has remained true to the Republican tradition. This tradition still supplies the form of government that divides French men and women the least.

NOTES

1 R. N. Gildea, *The Third Republic from 1870 to 1914* (London: Longman, 1988), p. 81.
2 M. Larkin, *France since the Popular Front: Government and People, 1936–1986* (Oxford: Clarendon Press, 1988), p. 36.
3 J. F. McMillan, *Dreyfus to de Gaulle: Politics and Society in France, 1898–1969* (London: Edward Arnold, 1985), p. 88.
4 Larkin, op. cit., p. 1.
5 D. Johnson and M. Johnson, *The Age of Illusion: Art and Politics in France, 1918–1940* (New York: Rizzoli, 1987), p. 9.
6 J. Jackson, *The Politics of Depression in France, 1932–1936* (Cambridge: Cambridge University Press, 1985), p. 23.
7 McMillan, op cit., p. 98.
8 Figures from A. Sauvy, *Histoire économique de la France entre les deux guerres, 1931–1939*, vol. 2 (Paris: Fayard, 1967), p. 554.

9 Jackson, op. cit., pp. 53–79.

10 M. Beloff, 'The sixth of February', in J. Joll (ed.), *The Decline of the Third Republic*, St Antony's Papers, no. 5 (London: Chatto & Windus, 1959), pp. 9–35.

11 P. Bernard and H. Dubief, *The Decline of the Third Republic, 1914–1938* (Cambridge: Cambridge University Press, 1988), p. 211.

12 Larkin, op. cit., pp. 48-9.

13 D. Johnson, 'Léon Blum and the Popular Front', *History*, 55(184) (1970), p. 201.

14 ibid.

15 J. Jackson, *The Popular Front in France Defending Democracy, 1934–38* (Cambridge: Cambridge University Press, 1988), p. 96.

16 McMillan, op. cit., pp. 112-13.

17 Larkin, op. cit., p. 62.

18 H. R. Kedward, 'Patriots and patriotism in Vichy France', *Transactions of the Royal Historical Society*, 5th ser., 32 (1982), pp. 175–92.

19 H. R. Kedward, *Occupied France: Collaboration and Resistance, 1940–1944* (Oxford: Basil Blackwell, 1985), p. 43.

20 These issues are discussed in H. R. Kedward, 'The French Resistance', supplement to *History Today*, 34 (1984 June issue); pp. not numbered.

FURTHER READING

An excellent introduction to the general history of twentieth-century France may be found in J. F. McMillan, *Dreyfus to de Gaulle: Politics and Society in France, 1898–1969* (London: Edward Arnold, 1985). Also helpful are M. Larkin, *France since the Popular Front: Government and People, 1936–1986* (Oxford: Clarendon Press, 1988), and T. Zeldin, *France 1848–1945*, 2 vols (Oxford: Oxford University Press, 1973-7). All of these studies contain their own bibliographies. For a general guide to French economic history see F. Caron, *An Economic History of Modern France* (New York: Columbia University Press, 1979).

An overview of the inter-war years is provided by P. Bernard and H. Dubief, *The Decline of the Third Republic, 1914–1938* (Cambridge: Cambridge University Press, 1988). On the 1920s, see J.-J. Becker and S. Bernstein, *Victoire et frustrations 1914–1929* (Paris: Editions du Seuil, 1990). Analysis of the 1930s is contained in S. Bernstein, *La France des années 30* (Paris: Armand Colin, 1989), and S. Hoffmann,

Decline or Renewal: France since the 1930s (New York: Viking, 1974). For the political impact of the Depression, see J. Jackson, *The Politics of Depression in France, 1932–1936* (Cambridge: Cambridge University Press, 1985). The same author has also written an excellent guide to the Popular Front: *The Popular Front in France Defending Democracy, 1934–1938* (Cambridge: Cambridge University Press, 1988). See also the collection of essays in M. Alexander and H. Graham (eds), *The French and Spanish Popular Fronts: Comparative Perspectives* (Cambridge: Cambridge University Press, 1989), and J. Joll (ed.), *The Decline of the Third Republic*, St Antony's Papers, no. 5 (London: Chatto & Windus, 1959). A good introduction to the Daladier ministry is J.-P. Azéma, *From Munich to the Liberation, 1938–1944* (Cambridge: Cambridge University Press, 1985).

French foreign policy in the inter-war years is considered by J. Néré, *French Foreign Policy, 1914–1945* (London: 1977), but the key study is J.-B. Duroselle, *La Décadence 1932–1939* (Paris: Imprimerie Nationale, 1979). On the origins of the war and the defeat of France, see A. Adamthwaite, *France and the Coming of the Second World War* (London: Cass, 1977); A. Horne, *To Lose a Battle: France 1940* (London: Macmillan, 1969); and J.-B. Duroselle, *L'Abîme, 1939–1945* (Paris: Imprimerie Nationale, 1982).

The best introduction to the Vichy regime remains R. O. Paxton, *The Vichy Regime: Old Guard and New Order, 1940–1944* (New York: Alfred A. Knopf, 1972). More succinct is H. R. Kedward, *Occupied France: Collaboration and Resistance, 1940–1944* (Oxford: Basil Blackwell, 1985). The world of collaboration is analysed by B. M. Gordon, *Collaborationism in France during the Second World War* (Ithaca: Cornell University Press, 1980), and P. Ory, *Les Collaborateurs 1940–1945* (Paris: Editions du Seuil, 1976). The Resistance is studied in H. R. Kedward, *Resistance in Vichy France* (Oxford: Oxford University Press, 1978). On the Liberation, see J. Simmonds and H. Footitt, *France 1943–1945* (Leicester: Leicester University Press, 1988).

Finally, two reference works are of use: D. Bell, D. Johnson, and P. Morris (eds), *A Biographical Guide to Modern French Political Leaders since 1870* (Hemel Hempstead: Harvester Wheatsheaf, 1990), and P. H. Hutton, *Historical Dictionary of the French Third Republic, 1870–1940*, 2 vols (London: Aldwych Press, 1986).

10 Hitler's war?
The origins of the Second World War in Europe

Philip Bell

The outbreak of the Great War and the coming of the Second World War in Europe present sharp contrasts. In 1914 the advent of war was rapid. A matter of eight days brought five great powers and two small ones into conflict. The coming of the Second World War was a long and uneven process, starting in 1939 and culminating in the German attack on the Soviet Union in June 1941. The events which are usually regarded in Great Britain as the start of the war (the German attack on Poland on 1 September 1939, and the British and French declarations of war on the 3rd) were clearly important, but marked only a stage in this process, producing a limited war involving four European states.

There are contrasts too in the historiography of these events. Historical writing on the origins of the Second World War in Europe has been less extensive and varied than that of 1914.[1] When the war began there was a general consensus outside Germany (and perhaps inside as well) that Hitler had caused and indeed planned the war. The historian G. P. Gooch, who had spent much of his professional life in unravelling the complexities of 1914, wrote in 1940 that the second conflict presented few difficulties: the guilt lay squarely on the shoulders of Hitler.[2] The judgement of the Nuremberg tribunal after the war confirmed this view. So did common sense. There was not the slightest doubt that between 1939 and 1941 Germany had repeatedly attacked other countries, and no hint that any other power had intended to attack Germany.[3]

It is true that things were never quite as simple as this. Even if the plain thesis of Hitler's guilt was accepted, there were, from an early date, disputes as to how far Hitler's responsibility should be shared by others. As early as 1948, for example, an American collection of documents on *Nazi–Soviet Relations* cast some of the blame for the outbreak of war in 1939 on Stalin as well as on Hitler.[4] Then in 1961 A. J. P. Taylor published his *Origins of the Second World War*, which still stands as a landmark in the historical debate for its direct attack on the straightforward 'Hitler thesis'. Since then discussion has developed along well-defined paths.

The events that require explanation may be stated quite briefly. During the 1920s it appeared that Europe was on the way to recovery from the effects of the 1914–18 war, and that some of the faults in the 1919 peace settlement were being remedied. Notably, the Treaty of Locarno (1925) brought stability to western Europe, and drew Germany back into the comity of European states. Similarly, the Dawes Plan (1924) took some of the difficulties out of the reparations question. Between 1925 and 1929 Germany prospered, reparations were paid, and Europe seemed set for better times. Then the great economic depression, which began in 1929, destroyed these hopes of economic and political stability, and set all the powers off on the road to self-sufficiency and economic nationalism. It also produced a rise in political extremism, and, above all, brought Hitler to power in Germany in January 1933.

Thereafter, events moved with accelerating speed. For a time Hitler consolidated his position at home and took stock of the situation in Europe. Then in March 1935 Germany openly proclaimed its rearmament, in defiance of the disarmament clauses of the Treaty of Versailles. In October 1935 Italy invaded Abyssinia. The League of Nations, led by Britain and France, imposed economic sanctions which were enough to hurt the Italians but not to stop them. Abyssinia was not saved, and Italy was driven towards an alliance with Germany. In March 1936 the Germans occupied and began to fortify the Rhineland, previously demilitarized under both the Versailles and Locarno treaties. This deprived France of one of the key elements of its security. In March 1938 Germany annexed Austria. In the summer of 1938 there was a great crisis over Czechoslovakia, ending at the Munich conference (29 September), where the Sudeten areas of that country were handed over to Germany with the active assistance of Britain and France. In March 1939 the remains of Czechoslovakia were broken up, and mostly came under German control. Meanwhile, from July 1936 to March 1939 the Spanish Civil War was being waged, attracting armed intervention from Germany, Italy and the Soviet Union, and threatening to spread into a wider European conflict. No sooner was the Spanish war over than, in April 1939, Italy kept the Mediterranean in commotion by occupying Albania. For some three years Europe lived with a sense of imminent conflict.

Then, on 1 September 1939, Germany attacked Poland. Britain and France declared war on Germany on 3 September. On 17 September the Soviet Union too invaded Poland, which succumbed rapidly to the joint onslaught. After a pause which we call the 'phoney war', German aggression was resumed. In rapid succession the Germans invaded Denmark and Norway (April 1940), and then the Netherlands, Belgium and France (May). In June Italy entered the war, and in October 1940 Mussolini attacked Greece. Germany invaded Yugoslavia and Greece in April 1941; finally, in June 1941, the German assault on the Soviet Union brought the long movement towards total European war to its climax.

This chain of events stretching from 1935 to 1941 has given rise to a number of interpretations. One broad question which has been in dispute is whether the Second World War was really a continuation of the First, and the final stage of a Thirty Years' War; or whether it was something separate, emerging essentially from the rise of Hitler. The other questions which have arisen about the origins of the war all pose similar problems of continuity or discontinuity. Was it Hitler's war, brought about by the aims and actions of one man; or was it another German war, in which Hitler was merely the new representative of long-standing forces and ambitions? Was it essentially an ideological conflict, or a war of a more familiar kind about material interests and the domination of Europe? Was it a planned, premeditated war; or did it come about by improvisation, opportunism, or even by accident? Was it an inevitable war; or was it, in Churchill's famous phrase, 'The Unnecessary War'?[5]

There are many questions. Yet there is also a good deal of agreement on two fundamental propositions. First, the war arose primarily from a German drive for expansion which was bound at some stage to be resisted. Second, other powers accepted that expansion up to a point where it could only be opposed by means of a major war. Much debate has therefore concentrated on the problems which lie behind these propositions: what were the causes of German expansionism? why did other powers first accept the growth of German power and then decide to oppose it? and was there an easily available alternative policy, as implied in the phrase 'unnecessary war'? Let us examine these three issues.

German expansionism clearly lies at the root of the matter, and it is crucial to reach some judgement on its causes. This raises the whole question of the place and significance of Hitler and Nazism in German, and indeed, in European history. There has been a strong tendency, especially in West Germany in the period immediately after the war, to see Hitler and the whole Nazi period as an aberration, completely outside the main course of German history. The historian Golo Mann published in 1958 a history of Germany in the nineteenth and twentieth centuries, in which he argued that Nazism was not really a chapter in German history.[6] Hitler came virtually from nowhere and imposed his authority on the German people – the Nazis behaved in their own country like foreign conquerors. Mann, like Gerhard Ritter before him, used in referring to Hitler the word 'demon'. There could be no more forcible way of asserting Hitler's absolute singularity and isolation. It followed from this that Hitler's foreign policy and conquests were also unique, and were the products of his own particular ideology and psychological make-up.

Against this there has been a strong school of thought placing Hitler firmly within the framework of German history. Alan Bullock concluded his massive biography of Hitler with the claim that Nazism was rooted in German history and that Hitler represented the logical conclusion of nationalism, militarism, the worship of force, and the exaltation of the state. Hitler, in fact, concentrated in himself the most sinister forces in German history[7], though he also in some ways embodied a malaise which was European as well as German. Fritz Fischer, in some pregnant passages in his book on *Germany's Aims in the First World War*, asserted the continuity between Germany's objectives in the two world wars.[8] Many similarities indeed leap to the eye. In 1914 Bethmann-Hollweg outlined a plan for *Mitteleuropa* under German control; in 1940 Hitler achieved it. In 1918, in preparing the terms to be imposed on Russia in the Treaty of Brest-Litovsk, Ludendorff aimed to detach the Ukraine and use its resources for German benefit, and also to plant a German colony in the Crimea. Hitler, too, aimed to conquer the Ukraine and exploit its resources, and he did actually plant a settlement (though only a short-lived one) in the Crimea. There were also close and direct links between Hitler's ideas of race and *Lebensraum* (living-space), and those propagated earlier by the Pan-German League.[9]

There can be no doubt that Hitler absorbed the ideas which were current in Pan-German and nationalist circles, or that he took up the broad aims advocated by Ludendorff and others during the war of 1914–18. What Hitler added was a speed, boldness and intensity of purpose not seen before; and also a new and ferocious commitment to ideas about race. Anti-Semitism existed in Germany (as elsewhere) before Nazism came to power; so did the concept of a racial struggle between Teuton and Slav. But previous German policies had not been set on the annihilation of the Jews, or the reduction of the Slavs to something like serfdom. The elements of continuity were strong, but

Hitler added his own contribution – for which the word 'demonic' does not come amiss.

How did Hitler conduct his foreign policy? The strongest case for seeing him as essentially an improviser, snapping up opportunities provided for him by others, was made in A. J. P. Taylor's *Origins of the Second World War*, where the author argued, for example, that in the Czechoslovakian crisis it was repeatedly Chamberlain who took the initiative – all Hitler had to do was react. In this interpretation, the war against Poland assumed the character almost of an accident, arising because Hitler made an error of timing by launching on 29 August 1939 a diplomatic manoeuvre which he should have begun on the 28th.[10]

Against this stands the concept of Hitler as a man with a programme. After the *Anschluss* with Austria in March 1938, Churchill told the House of Commons: 'Europe is confronted with a programme of aggression, nicely calculated and timed, unfolding stage by stage.'[11] Much later, the American historian William Shirer, who had worked as a journalist in Berlin during the Nazi period, wrote a massive best seller, *The Rise and Fall of the Third Reich*, in which he claimed that Hitler had devised a blueprint for aggression – a detailed plan, equivalent to the working drawings for building an aeroplane.[12]

Neither of these contradictory propositions has been found generally acceptable in its plain form. To claim that Hitler was nothing but an opportunist carries no conviction; but Nazi actions were much less carefully planned and timed than Churchill or Shirer made out. It is clear that in 1938 the timing and method of the *Anschluss* was forced on Hitler by circumstances, even though the ultimate absorption of Austria was one of his fixed ideas. Alan Bullock, who was in no doubt that Hitler had long-term aims, still found that in August 1939 he was contemplating three possibilities: another Munich, war with Poland alone, and war with the Western powers as well. What has emerged is a sort of compromise: a view of Hitler as a man with a systematic framework of thought and an outline scheme of foreign policy, into which the exigencies and opportunities of the time could be fitted. The West German historians Andreas Hillgruber and Klaus Hildebrand have argued that Hitler had an outline policy which can be defined in various stages: to restore Germany as a European power; to secure living-space in the east; to achieve racial objectives against both the Jews and the Slavs; and finally to organize a new Europe in order to wage a war against the United States for world supremacy.[13] It is far from clear that this last stage was ever formulated distinctly, and Hitler's views on the United States remain obscure.[14] Nonetheless, much of this interpretation arises from what Hitler in fact accomplished as well as from what he said and wrote, and a strong case has been built up for seeing Hitler as an improviser within a broadly outlined set of objectives. Those objectives would certainly involve war.

These explanations concentrate on Hitler's political objectives and ambitions. There is a different approach, which puts the emphasis on economic aims as the motive for German expansion. In simple terms, the argument is this. The recovery of the domestic German economy in the mid-1930s, together with large-scale and rapid rearmament, produced a heavy demand for imports of raw materials, fuel and food. Germany had neither the foreign exchange nor the exports to pay for these imports, and the result was a chronic balance of payments problem which was causing particular difficulties at the end of the 1930s. One way of coping with this problem was to conclude a series of 'clearing' agreements, which placed trade with some neighbouring countries largely on a barter basis; but by 1936 and 1937 these devices had exhausted their usefulness. Another method was force, using war as a means of resolving the balance of payments problem, or, put more crudely, war for gain.[15] At the so-called Hossbach conference in November 1937, Hitler explained the danger of a food crisis if Germany could not pay for its imports, and asserted that the acquisition of Austria and Czechoslovakia would stave off this threat. This was in fact a dubious proposition, because neither country was a major food producer; but food was not the only or even the major issue.

The problem, and its resolution, may be best illustrated by examining German imports of two vital commodities: oil and iron ore. In 1939, despite an ambitious programme for producing synthetic oil, Germany was still largely dependent upon oil imports. Its only significant source of oil not subject to naval blockade or the control of another great power was Romania; and in late 1938 and 1939 the Germans set themselves to secure a large proportion of Romanian oil exports. As long as the only means used for this purpose were economic, the Germans made little headway against British competition; but when Germany conquered large parts of Europe the position was transformed. In March 1940 Britain purchased 130,000 tons of oil from Romania, Germany 45,000 tons. In August, the British figure was a mere 6,000 tons, the Germany 187,000 tons.[16] It was not necessary for Germany to invade Romania to produce this reversal, but it was none the less the result of the use of force. In the case of iron ore, Germany's major source of imports was Sweden. Again, while the instruments used were economic and financial, Britain could compete with Germany on roughly equal terms, and was able to restrict Swedish exports to Germany; but when Germany invaded Norway in April–May 1940, cutting Sweden off from the outside world, the position changed. In July 1940 the Swedes had to sign a trade agreement on terms favourable to Germany. In both these cases, the indirect consequences of the use of force worked to Germany's economic advantage. At the same time, German conquests brought, as a direct result, the capture of the iron ore resources of Lorraine, and of stocks of many materials, including large quantities of oil. The Germans also controlled a vast reservoir of manpower, and by August 1940 about a million foreigners were working in Germany. Problems of foreign exchange were resolved by compelling occupied countries to accept a highly favourable rate of exchange against the mark. At least in the short run, war paid Germany well.

This economic impulse for expansion can be presented as being detached from the personality and policies of Hitler. It is true that the response of other states to the economic circumstances of the 1930s was to try for self-sufficiency, either by organizing their empires (as Britain and France did) or by aggression (as practised by Japan in the Far East). On the other hand, it would have been possible to ease the German balance of payments problem by slowing down the pace of rearmament, putting more resources into exports, and moving the country back towards a system of multilateral trade. Schacht, the economics minister and head of the Reichsbank, suggested such a policy in 1936; but Hitler would accept no relaxation of the armaments programmes, which he insisted must be pressed forward with the utmost speed. There was in fact a vicious circle, in which a policy of expansion required heavy armaments, and the armaments programmes brought economic difficulties, to which one solution was further expansion. That vicious circle was created by Hitler's policies.

In all these discussions, we find three basic lines of approach to the problems posed by German expansionism. One presents Hitler as virtually alone and unique; an aberration, or even a demon. This applies whether he is regarded as a planner or an opportunist in his methods. The second sees Hitler and the Nazi period as essentially a part of the continuity of German history, and the expansion which led to the Second World War as simply an extension of the war aims of 1914–18. The third sees German expansion as a response to the economic problems of the late 1930s, though here too Hitler's personal role cannot be avoided.

It is impossible to discuss these issues without raising moral questions, or encountering the powerful emotions which are still aroused by the deeds of Hitler and the Nazis. To present Hitler as a unique phenomenon may be seen as absolving all others (and notably all other Germans) from any responsibility for his actions – in this context, for the outbreak of war. This is naturally welcome to some observers, especially in Germany, but unwelcome to others. To place Hitler within some wider context in the continuity of German history is often seen as diminishing his personal responsibility, or even excusing his actions. Historical discussion of the forces behind German expansion touches many nerves which are still left raw after the events of the Second World War, and we are still far from any attempt at detached history.

Are we equally far from being able to strike a balance between these various explanations of German expansionism? It must surely be accepted that Hitler took up much that was already to be found in German history. It is a perfectly conceivable hypothesis that, without Hitler and the Nazis, some sort of military government in Germany might have attempted a repetition of the Great War. But this remains a matter of speculation, and in any case does not go far enough. Hitler represented something more than the elements of continuity. He was *sui generis*, adding a degree of intensity, fanaticism and sheer speed of action which had not been present before. As for the economic arguments, there can be no doubt that Hitler regarded himself as the master of economic forces, not their servant; and the economic motivation for expansion must be seen as supplementing, not displacing, the drive supplied by ideology. In the dispute over planning and improvisation, the extreme theses of unbridled opportunism and the detailed blueprint should both be discarded. Hitler had an objective, which was the domination of Europe and the conquest of the Soviet Union (world domination is a much more dubious proposition), but his route towards it contained a number of hesitations, improvisations and surprises. The manner and timing of the annexation of Austria in March 1938 were improvised. In September 1938 Hitler hesitated and drew back from launching an attack on Czechoslovakia at the very last minute, when some army units were already on their way to the frontier; and it is still not clear to us why he held back. In August– September 1939, on the other hand, he was firmly determined on war against Poland, but was taken aback to find Britain and France declaring war upon him. In June 1940 the extraordinary speed of the German victory over France took even Hitler by surprise, and there was certainly no blueprint ready for the invasion of Britain, or for the reorganization of Europe. But through all these uncertainties the drive and pace of German expansion continued unchecked, propelled by a powerful mixture of ideological and economic imperatives.

It is time to turn to our second main question. Why was the growth of German power and territory for so long accepted by other powers, so that ultimately it could only be opposed by means of a great war? In other words, why was the policy which we call 'appeasement' pursued by those states which might have been expected to resist the advance of Germany?

Any examination of this question must start with British policy, though it must not end there. Condemnation of 'appeasement' formed for a long time an essential ingredient in the view of the Second World War as 'the unnecessary war'. The phrase was Churchill's, and the theme of Churchill's first volume of memoirs on the Second World War has dominated popular British views on the subject for over forty years, extending by a kind of osmosis to many who have never read the book. The theme of that volume, *The Gathering Storm*, was: 'How the English-speaking peoples, through their unwisdom, carelessness and good nature, allowed the wicked to rearm.'[17] The essence of Churchill's argument was that Britain had tried to buy peace with Germany (and to a lesser extent with Italy) by a policy of one-sided concessions, which was both dishonourable and disastrous. It was dishonourable because it led to the betrayal of small states (Austria, and above all, Czechoslovakia); it was disastrous because it led in the long run to war in appalling conditions, when German power had grown almost too great to be resisted.

In recent years this Churchillian view of the policy of 'appeasement' has been subject to close and critical re-examination. This is partly because a mass of new evidence has become available, with the opening of government and private archives. There has also been a change in perspective with the passage of time and the advent of a new generation of historians. What has this reconsideration achieved for our understanding of 'appeasement'?

First and foremost, the constraints within which British policy operated, long visible in outline, have been revealed in convincing detail. In strategic matters, the long-standing general impression of British military weakness and unpreparedness for war has been filled out. The Cabinet papers showed how, in 1937, the Chiefs of Staff had conducted a gloomy review of the enemies threatening the British empire; Germany, Italy and Japan. British armed strength was inadequate to fight all three, and the Chiefs of Staff recommended that, until rearmament was well advanced, it should be the main task of foreign policy to diminish the number of Britain's enemies. Any review of the policy of 'appeasement' must take this stern and sober advice into account. We might indeed wonder why it was not more carefully followed, because

Britain did indeed eventually find itself at war with those three enemies, with calamitous results.

Rearmament was in fact pursued, though only slowly, from 1934 onwards; but that raised questions as to what sort of rearmament, and for what purpose? There was a difficult debate on the issue of limited liability versus a continental commitment as the basis for British strategic policy. 'Limited liability' meant engaging only small land forces in a European war, and putting the major effort into naval and air warfare, and into economic support for allies on the Continent. A continental commitment meant fighting a war like that of 1914–18, with casualties like those recorded on war memorials up and down the land. Neville Chamberlain told the Cabinet on 5 May 1937, just before he became Prime Minister, that he did not believe that the government could, ought, or indeed would be allowed by the country to fight a continental war on the same lines as the last war.[18] It was a short step to the conclusion that it would be best if war could be avoided if at all possible.

Economic and financial constraints operated in the same direction. Again, the examination of government records has filled in the detail of a position already known in outline. Large-scale and rapid rearmament would involve a heavy bill for imports (notably of raw materials and machine tools) while removing resources from the export industries which were needed to pay that bill. To create an army of continental size would demand manpower and equipment which could only come from elsewhere. Even to concentrate primarily upon the air force – which was in fact the policy from 1935 to 1938 – involved severe problems of skilled manpower, the availability of machine tools, and the design and testing of new types of aircraft. Such problems had disturbing political dimensions, because industrialists opposed the imposition of anything like a command economy (which the government did not want anyway), and the restrictive practices of trade unions obstructed change in the skilled trades. At the back of all government calculations on these questions lay the assumption that economic strength was itself the 'fourth arm of defence'. A future war would, in all probability, have to be sustained and financed without the benefit of loans from the United States which had been so crucial in the previous conflict. It would therefore be rash to commit great resources to a rearmament effort which could not be long maintained. Rapid rearmament was thus a policy involving grave problems, and it is easy to see why the government tried to avoid it for as long as possible. Once again, to avoid war seemed the best solution.

When these detailed strategic and economic considerations are added to the other well-known motives for 'appeasement' – public revulsion against war, an underestimation of the danger posed by Nazi Germany, and fear of communism, which war was likely to promote and against which Germany was a bulwark – the strength of the policy's roots becomes plain. Appeasement was not simply the work of one man, Neville Chamberlain. It arose from a calculation of British interests, as well as from sentiment; and an alternative policy based on rapid rearmament posed serious difficulties.

Let us turn to France, the country which (even more than Britain) should have opposed the advance of German power, but did not do so. French interests and security were directly threatened by the German occupation of the Rhineland in March 1936. Czechoslovakia was an ally of France, and it was French influence in central and eastern Europe which collapsed during the Czechoslovakian crisis of 1938. France was certainly the country with the greatest stake in the status quo established in 1919, and, yet between 1933 and 1939 France did nothing to sustain that status quo. The reasons for this inaction are plain enough, and have only been elaborated upon by recent research. The war of 1914–18 had been a catastrophe for France. The loss of 1,300,000 French dead in the course of the war, together with a dramatic fall in the number of births (an estimated deficit of 1,400,000 against normal totals), produced two depressing gaps in the population. France could not afford losses on such a scale again.

From this situation there followed strategic and political consequences. French strategic thinking in the period after the Great War was dominated by a defensive mentality – a mode of thought embodied in the concrete of the Maginot Line, constructed from 1929 onwards. Despite some genuflections towards ideas of attack and manoeuvre in the army manuals, the whole structure of the army was arranged for defence. Swift offensive action was virtually beyond its capacities. In political terms, the growth of German power after 1933 confronted France with an impossible dilemma. To resist that growth meant war, and France could not afford another victory like that of 1918, never mind defeat. But if it did not resist, the best that could be hoped for was that France would be eaten last, after Germany had devoured other states in Europe. Neither prospect was attractive. It is not surprising that French policy was sometimes reduced to almost complete passivity.

This passivity also arose from the state of French internal politics. It was no novelty for France to be divided; but the divisions of the 1930s were particularly conspicuous and noisy. There were groups on the Right which, if mostly not Fascist, were certainly Fascist-like.

Ideological sympathies even made parts of the French Right hesitant in their opposition to Germany, a development which would have been unthinkable before 1914. On the Left, the French Communist Party received a great boost from adopting the policy of the Popular Front, and polled 1.5 million votes in the election of 1936. The Party was thoroughly Stalinist, and acted visibly on the orders of Moscow, so that it had all the appearance of being a foreign army encamped on French soil. The extremes of Right and Left were bitterly opposed both to one another and to the parliamentary system of the French Third Republic, which operated with increasing difficulty during the 1930s. Between 1932 and 1935 there was a total of eleven changes of government, as one cabinet after another failed to grapple with the problems posed by economic depression. In 1936 the Popular Front (Socialists, Radicals and Communists) came to power, in theory giving France the chance of a new direction, but in practice making little headway. In foreign policy, the Socialists were trapped between their hatred of Nazism and Fascism and a strong residual pacifist instinct. Léon Blum, the premier of the Popular Front government, was a Frenchman, a Socialist and a Jew; but it was not until autumn 1938 that he became firmly convinced that all the three identities for which he stood were gravely menaced by the rise of Nazi Germany, which would have to be resisted by force if need be. Until then, the old enchantments of disarmament and the League of Nations had exercised a potent and paralysing spell over Blum, as they continued to do over some of his colleagues.

These weaknesses and divisions within France were not fatal. Jean-Louis Crémieux-Brilhac has demonstrated the striking difference in August and September 1939 between the nervousness and doubts of the politicians in Paris and the firmness of French opinion as a whole. At that point, Daladier (despite much that has been said to the contrary) gave a firm lead in favour of war, and the French people followed.[19] The disease of the 1930s was not terminal, but while it ran its course it was extremely debilitating. So, for all these reasons – psychological, strategic and political – France stood by in the 1930s and watched the growth of German power.

Thus the two powers with a stake in the European status quo watched it being dismantled until the point came when they could abstain no longer and had to make a stand. For Britain, 'appeasement' never meant peace at any price. For France, temporary paralysis did not mean that the German advance would be permitted to go on for ever. In an examination of the origins of the Second World War, the point is that the two powers accepted, and even assisted, that advance up to a point where it could only be resisted at the cost of a major war. The corollary of this, within the general thesis of the 'unnecessary war', has always been that there was another line of policy readily available. The case has repeatedly been put that there were lost opportunities to stop the German advance, either without war, or by means of an earlier and less costly war. In this hypothetical scenario, three occasions stand out: the Rhineland in March 1936, Czechoslovakia in September 1938, and the negotiations for a French–British–Soviet alliance in the summer of 1939.

Of these three occasions, the Rhineland is the favourite. The argument, reduced to its simplest form, is that when German forces moved into the previously demilitarized zone in the Rhineland, a 'police action' involving minimal use of force would have sufficed to expel the Germans and probably to bring down Hitler, whose prestige would not have survived failure. We cannot tell whether this would have been the case or not; the attempt was not made, and the question remains hypothetical. But it is highly unlikely that the Germans were bluffing and would simply have withdrawn without a fight at the mere sight of French uniforms. The forces involved in the occupation were not large, but neither were they trivial: they numbered about 10,000 soldiers and nearly 23,000 armed police, who were incorporated into the army on 8 March. The German army as a whole consisted of thirty infantry and three armoured divisions, though these were not yet fully trained or equipped since the rapid expansion begun in March 1935. There was a difference of opinion between Hitler and the principal generals involved, Blomberg and Fritsch, over the course to be adopted in the event of a French riposte; but the likelihood is that the German troops would have withdrawn to the line of the Rhine, where they would have stood and fought. The French High Command for its part had no intention of moving into the Rhineland, which General Gamelin had written off in advance of the event; and it proceeded to exaggerate the size of the German forces involved by treating some 235,000 auxiliaries as though they were regular troops. But in one sense the French General Staff was right: what they confronted in the event of action was not a military promenade, but a serious campaign.

Was it a lost opportunity? Yes and no. Yes, in that the German army was only partly formed and trained, and when it fought (as it surely would have done) it could probably be defeated. No, because a *simple* opportunity was not present at all. The French had neither the plans nor the type of forces for a powerful and rapid assault, and only an extremely bold and determined government would have been capable

of improvising one. What actually existed was a caretaker government, conscious that there were only two months to go before a
general election. Insofar as there was an opportunity at all, it was not
to carry out some police action, but to fight a serious campaign on
German territory, and then (if victorious) to maintain forces there for
an indefinite period. One can only wonder how much public support
there would have been for such a policy in the Britain and France of
1936.[20]

No one has claimed that Czechoslovakia in 1938 offered the chance
to stop Germany without war, but only that it would have been better
for the French and British to fight in September 1938 than in September 1939. This raises all sorts of hypothetical questions: whether
and for how long Czechoslovakia could have held out; whether the
French army could have mounted an effective attack in the west; and
whether the Soviet Union would have joined in. There can be no firm
answers, though there has been much interesting speculation.[21] The
war would surely have been a serious one, though doubtless not so
grave as that which actually came about. As a 'lost opportunity', the
unfought war of 1938 seems a dubious prospect.

The case of the French–British–Soviet negotiations during the
summer of 1939 is different. Here the hypothesis is that if a firm
military alliance between these three powers had been achieved, Germany, being presented with the threat of overwhelming force, would
have been deterred from any further aggression.

It is probably still the generally accepted view in Great Britain that
the British government sacrificed this opportunity to avoid war by a
mixture of dilatoriness, incompetence and anti-communist prejudice.
In all of these accusations there is much truth. The British conduct of
the negotiations was indeed both slow and inept. They began by
rejecting (on 8 May) the idea of a three-power treaty in favour of
separate unilateral guarantees to different countries, but then
accepted the concept of a treaty on 24 May. They then tried to insist on
concluding a political agreement first, after which a military convention could be negotiated at leisure. The Soviet Union demanded that
the two agreements should be signed and should come into force
simultaneously; eventually, on 23 July, the British agreed to this
concept in principle. But they did not nominate their delegation for
military talks for another eleven days. The British and French teams
travelled to Moscow by ship and train rather than by air; and neither
set of military negotiators was armed with authority to conclude an
agreement. The French, it is true, wanted to push the negotiations on
at a greater speed. They nominated their military delegation for the

talks in Moscow ten days ahead of the British, and gave instructions that a military agreement should be concluded in a minimum of time. Nonetheless, it was understandable that Litvinov, the Soviet foreign minister when the negotiations began, should think that the British government was undertaking them more as a concession to its own public opinion than with any serious intentions of pushing them through. The Soviet ambassador in Paris reported to his government in mid-July that three months of negotiations had shown that neither of the Western powers really wanted an agreement.

The methods were wrong, and, despite French attempts to instil some sense of urgency, the political will was lacking. The British, in particular, were unconvinced of the value of a Soviet alliance. The Soviet armed forces had been wrecked by the purges; the states of eastern Europe, terrified of the Russians, were likely to be driven into the arms of Germany; and insofar as moral considerations entered British thinking, Stalin was regarded as being at least as evil and dictatorial a ruler as Hitler – which was true.

But this is not the whole story. In a shrewd, and too little-known, analysis of the negotiations, the former French diplomat Jean Laloy argued that the only hope for the negotiations would have been for the British and French to tackle outright the question of the mutual distrust of the two sides and the issue of Soviet territorial claims in eastern Europe.[22] It is not easy to see how distrust could have been dealt with – trust is a difficult coin to mint – but territory is another matter. It was quite clear in the course of the negotiations that one thing the Soviet Union wanted was a sphere of influence in eastern Europe stretching from Finland in the north to Romania in the south. They also probably wanted to press territorial claims on Poland which had been outstanding since the Treaty of Riga in 1921, which had been very unfavourable to the Soviet Union. For the British and French to meet such demands would have called for bold and ruthless diplomacy. Would the British public have supported such a move? And did the two governments have the power to act in such a way? It was notable that, at the end of August, the French did not have sufficient influence in Warsaw to persuade the Polish government to accept the entry of the Red Army into Polish territory in advance of the outbreak of war. Colonel Beck maintained, with much reason, that if the Russians entered Poland they would never go away; and there the French had to leave it.

The other aim which the Soviet government pursued in 1939 appears to have been to keep out of a major European war. They were, after all, already engaged in serious fighting with the Japanese in the Far

East. What could the British and French offer on this score? An alliance with them *might* deter Germany from going to war, but if it did not, the Soviet Union would be involved in conflict at once. From all Stalin's actions it is apparent that this was far from being his intention. From Stalin's point of view, therefore, the Germans were in a position to offer him a better bargain. Instead of a substantial risk of being involved in war, they could guarantee certain neutrality. In terms of territory and spheres of influence, they were willing to make definite proposals, and to yield at once to Stalin's request for more – for the whole of Latvia rather than a part, as Ribbentrop at first proposed. Moreover, once the bargain had been agreed upon, the Germans were willing and able to deliver the goods. The British and French could deliver nothing.

The upshot is surely that even if the British and French had played their hand with the combined diplomatic skills of a Talleyrand and a Bismarck, it is highly unlikely that they would have succeeded, because the hand was weak. Stalin took the better offer. In doing so he joined the ranks of the appeasers in that he accepted the growth of German power and territory in the hope of buying peace, or at any rate, a respite. Stalin's name is not usually bracketed with that of Chamberlain, but at the time of the Nazi–Soviet Pact that is where it should be.

In all the circumstances, this final and much vaunted 'lost opportunity' to deter Hitler from going to war looks like a broken reed. The speculation which continues to surround it contains a large element of wishful thinking – though it is natural enough that we should wish that events could have turned out otherwise in 1939.

With the passage of time the case for 'appeasement' has strengthened, as historians have examined the constraints under which British and French governments operated. In the long run, of course, the policy of 'appeasement' stands under the final condemnation – it did not work; but we can increasingly see why it was tried. Equally, the 'lost opportunities' now look less than convincing. But the stronger the case for 'appeasement', the more insistent becomes the final question: why was the policy changed, and German expansion resisted, after so long a period of yielding?

It was Poland which brought the powers to the point of decision. For the first time Hitler encountered a government and people who could not be bullied or shaken by a war of nerves. Earlier, Nazi tactics had been as successful as Nazi strategy. Schuschnigg had been harried and harassed, and Austria had been taken over virtually as a result of threats over the telephone. Benes and Czechoslovakia had yielded to pressure, as much from their so-called friends as from their enemies. In March 1939 Hacha had allowed himself to be summoned to Berlin and browbeaten in the middle of the night. No such treatment would be accepted by the Poles. There may well have been some flexibility in their approach to the precise status of Danzig, but on issues involving their independence or territorial integrity, the Poles were immovable, and astonishingly confident in their capacity to defend themselves.

Hitler was right in thinking that Poland was not like Czechoslovakia, and that this time there would be fighting. German policy in the summer of 1939 moved, with only one temporary pause, towards war with Poland. This in turn brought Britain and France to the sticking-point. On 31 March 1939 the British government guaranteed the independence (though not the territorial integrity) of Poland, in which they were joined by France. In the event, they stood by that guarantee. They did so only after some delay. Poland was attacked on 1 September, and Britain and France did not declare war until the 3rd; even then, they did nothing practical to help the Poles by military or aerial operations. Nonetheless, they went to war, and stayed at war even when Poland was overwhelmed. There has been much discussion of the intentions and motives behind these British and French actions.

One interpretation has been that the British and French governments did not change their fundamental policy at all, and that even the guarantee to Poland was appeasement in another guise. An extreme form of this argument may be found in Gilbert and Gott's *The Appeasers*, which maintains that appeasement continued to be Chamberlain's true policy right through the 'phoney war', up to his resignation as Prime Minister in May 1940. A more cautious and careful statement of the case may be found in a recent work by Anna Cienciala, in which she concludes that the policy behind the guarantee to Poland was a continuation of appeasement, because it was intended to lead to negotiations in which Hitler would get what he wanted and peace be saved. It failed, not through any Anglo–French determination, but because the Poles would not be bullied and Hitler would not wait.[23] British and French actions were thus decided by circumstances over which they had no control, and by the pressure of parliamentary and public opinion in Britain, which pushed Chamberlain in a direction that he did not want to take.

Another line of explanation is that the British government, led by Chamberlain, acted on a combination of traditional thinking (or perhaps instinct) about the balance of power and on personal distrust of Hitler. Very simply, Germany could not be allowed to dominate

Europe by force, and it had become clear (somewhat belatedly, it might be thought) that there could be no secure peace in Europe while Hitler was in control of Germany. The main evidence for this view lies in the change that came over British thinking and actions as early as February 1939. The previous assumption of the British government had been that Hitler's aims were limited. This changed, and it began to be assumed that the next German move against another state would signify that their aim was the dominaton of Europe. There was no hesitation in deciding that such an attempt must be resisted, by force if necessary. On 1 February the Cabinet agreed that Britain must go to war if Germany invaded either the Netherlands and Switzerland, which were thought to be the countries most under threat at the time. On the same day the Cabinet decided to open detailed staff talks with France, and on the 6th Chamberlain stated in the House of Commons that 'any threat to the vital interests of France … must evoke the immediate co-operation of Great Britain.' Later that month the Cabinet accepted a Chiefs of Staff paper arguing that British security was bound up with that of France, and that Britain would have to accept, in the event of war, a large, continental-style army – in other words, the end of limited liability.

As regards Hitler, Chamberlain felt the repudiation of the Munich agreement as a personal blow – in Churchill's words, 'he did not like being cheated'. Chamberlain told the Cabinet on 18 March, 'No reliance could be placed on any of the assurances given by the Nazi leaders.' It is notable that after the war had begun Chamberlain insisted that there could be no peace with Hitler. Cadogan, the permanent head of the Foreign Office, wrote in his diary that his war aim was to 'Get rid of Hitler.'[24] This corresponded to a growing feeling among the British people that something must be done to stop Hitler. This was, perhaps, an oversimplification and over-personalizing of the issues, but it was a belief which was both widely and deeply held.

It is true that British policy continued to follow a double line. There was always some hope that a negotiated solution to the German–Polish problem could be found. In July 1939 there were secret conversations in London between Wohlthat, an official of the German economics ministry, and Chamberlain's confidant Sir Horace Wilson. In the final crisis, the self-appointed Swedish intermediary Dahlerus was welcomed in London. But there was no serious sign that the fundamental British determination altered: if necessary they would fight. They were not even shaken by the diplomatic bombshell of the Nazi–Soviet Pact.

In this revulsion of both feeling and policy, Britain took the lead. But it is clear that in France, too, opinion changed and hardened. In

July 1939 a public opinion poll produced a 76 per cent 'Yes' reply to the question, 'If Germany attempts to seize Danzig, do you think we should prevent it, if necessary by force?' In prefects' reports on opinion at the time of the German attack on Poland, there was a frequently noted remark that one could not go on being mobilized every three months. In other words, the constant crises would have to be stopped. Compared with the situation in September 1938, the pacifist movement was silent – there was no equivalent to the vast petition against war organized at the time of Munich. Bonnet searched desperately for a way out of war, but Daladier was determined on it, and his will prevailed. As the current saying went, 'Il faut en finir'.[25]

This second explanation is simpler than the first. It also fits the main facts better, for the facts which have to be explained are not only those of September 1939, but those of the months and years ahead. The great European war was not about Danzig, nor even about Poland, but about the fate of the continent.

The principal origins of the war thus emerge with considerable clarity. There was a powerful German drive for expansion, arising partly from ambitions present well before 1914, partly from Nazi ideology, and partly from economic motives – all shaped by Hitler's powerful personality. This drive was continuous, and did not halt even in 1940 when Germany was in control of the whole of central and western Europe. It was not checked from outside at an early stage, because of the constraints and inhibitions which guided the policies of Britain and France and caused them for a long time to try to reach an accommodation with Germany by methods of concession and negotiation. But this never meant peace at any price, so that a conflict was certain at some time. Germany's opponents had opportunities to fight an earlier war and to deter Germany by means of an alliance, but did not take them. However, these opportunities were neither as simple nor as painless as they have been made to appear, and it is easy to see why they were passed over. For Britain and France to be convinced that they would have to fight another European war, the necessity had to be overwhelming. It was only the persistence of German expansion which created that necessity.

NOTES

1 The writer's views on the historiography of the subject are set out in P. M. H. Bell, *The Origins of the Second World in Europe* (London, 1986), chs 1–4.

2 G. P. Gooch, 'The coming of the war', *Contemporary Review*, July 1940, p. 9.

3 The case that Stalin was preparing to attack Germany in the summer of 1941 has been set out in E. Topitsch, *Stalin's War: A Radical New Theory of the Origins of the Second World War* (London, 1985), and in V. Suvorov, 'Who was planning to attack whom in June 1941: Hitler or Stalin?' *Journal of the Royal United Services Institute*, June 1985. So far, it carries little conviction.

4 US Department of State, *Nazi–Soviet Relations, 1939–41: Documents from the Archives of the German Foreign Office* (Washington, DC, 1948).

5 Winston S. Churchill, *The Second World War*, vol. 1: *The Gathering Storm* (London, 1948), p. viii. Churchill used the phrase in a message to Roosevelt, and went on to add, 'There never was a war more easy to stop!'

6 G. Mann, *A History of Germany since 1789* (London, 1968); German original published in Frankfurt am Main in 1958.

7 A. Bullock, *Hitler: A Study in Tyranny* (Harmondsworth: Pelican, 1962), pp. 805–8.

8 F. Fischer, *Germany's Aims in the First World War* (London, 1967); see esp. the preface.

9 See the discussions in W. D. Smith, *The Ideological Origins of Nazi Imperialism* (Oxford, 1986); G. Stoakes, *Hitler and the Quest for World Dominion: Nazi Ideology and Foreign Policy in the 1920s* (Leamington Spa, 1986).

10 A. J. P. Taylor, *The Origins of the Second World War* (London, 1961); see esp. p. 278.

11 Hansard, *House of Commons Debates*, 5th ser., vol. 333, col. 95 (10 Mar. 1938).

12 W. L. Shirer, *The Rise and Fall of the Third Reich* (London, 1960).

13 See E. Jaeckel, *Hitler's Weltanschauung: A Blueprint for Power* (Middletown, Conn., 1972); K. Hildebrand, *The Foreign Policy of the Third Reich* (London, 1973), which includes an exposition of Hillgruber's views.

14 See Stoakes, op. cit., pp. 221, 234–6, arguing that Hitler did not contemplate actual world conquest or a military invasion of the US, but rather the replacement of Britain as the pre-eminent world power. Cf. M. Hauner, 'Did Hitler want a world dominion?', *Journal of Contemporary History*, 13 (1978).

15 See D. E. Kaiser, *Economic Diplomacy and the Origins of the Second World War* (Princeton, 1980).

16 P. Marguerat, *Le IIIme Reich et le petrole roumain, 1938–40* (Geneva, 1977), pp. 192–3, 200.

17 Churchill, op. cit., vol. 1, p. v, 'Moral of the work'.

18 Quoted in P. J. Dennis, *Decision by Default: Peacetime Conscription and British Defence, 1919–1939* (London, 1972), p. 98.

19 J.-L. Crémieux-Brilhac, *Les Français de l'an 40*, 2 vols (Paris, 1990), vol. 1, pp. 55-134.

20 For the Rhineland, see J. T. Emmerson, *The Rhineland Crisis, 7 March 1936* (London, 1977); for further details on the military position, J. Defrasnes, 'L'événement du 7 mars 1936', in *Les Relations franco-allemandes, 1933–1939* (Paris, 1976), esp. pp. 251, 254–5.

21 See, e.g., W. Murray, 'Munich 1938: the military confrontation', *Journal of Strategic Studies*, 2(3) (Dec. 1979).

22 J. Laloy, 'Remarques sur les négociations anglo-franco-soviétiques de 1939', in Comité d'Histoire de la 2 Guerre Mondiale, *Les Relations franco-britanniques de 1935 à 1939* (Paris, 1975), pp. 403–13, esp. pp. 412–13.

23 M. Gilbert and R. Gott, *The Appeasers* (London, 1963); A. Cienciala, 'Poland in British and French policy in 1939: determination to fight or avoid war?', *Polish Review*, 34 (1989).

24 See Bell, op. cit., pp. 247–8, 253; D. Dilks (ed.), *The Diaries of Sir Alexander Cadogan, 1938–1945* (London, 1971), p. 221 (entry for 7 Oct. 1939).

25 Crémieux-Brilhac, op. cit., vol. 1, pp. 55–68.

FURTHER READING

Recent general discussions of the origins of the war may be found in P. M. H. Bell, *The Origins of the Second World War in Europe* (London, 1986), and in a wide-ranging collection of essays (including a valuable historiographical review) edited by R. Boyce and E. M. Robertson: *Paths to War: New Essays on the Origins of the Second World War* (London, 1989). A. J. P. Taylor, *The Origins of the Second World War* (London, 1961; reprinted with new preface, 1963), remains highly readable and a key element in the historical discussion; see the essays in G. Martel (ed.), *The Origins of the Second World War Reconsidered: The A. J. P. Taylor Debate After Twenty-five Years* (London, 1986).

On the crises of the 1930s, see G. W. Baer, *Test Case: Italy, Ethiopia and the League of Nations* (Stanford, 1977); J. T. Emmerson, *The Rhineland Crisis, 7 March 1936* (London, 1977); T. Taylor, *Munich: The Price of Peace* (London, 1979); H. Thomas, *The Spanish Civil War*, 3rd edn (London, 1977). An up-to-date review of the war crisis, at once detailed and reflective, is provided by D. Cameron Watt, *How War Came: The Immediate Origins of the Second World War, 1938–1939* (London, 1989); the much shorter treatment in C. Thorne, *The Approach of War, 1938–1939*, (London, 1967), remains useful.

On individual countries and their policies, see the following. **France**: A. P. Adamthwaite, *France and the Coming of the Second World War, 1936–1939* (London, 1977). **Germany**: among many books, see the short analysis in W. Carr, *Arms, Autarky and Aggression: A Study in German Foreign Policy, 1933–1939* (London, 1972); and the detailed exposition in G. L. Weinberg, *The Foreign Policy of Hitler's Germany*, vol. 1: *Diplomatic Revolution in Europe, 1933-1936*; vol. 2: *Starting World War II* (London, 1970 and 1980). On questions of interpretation, see A. Hillgruber, *Germany and the Two World Wars* (London, 1981); and the perceptive discussion in I. Kershaw, *The Nazi Dictatorship: Problems and Perspectives of Interpretation* (London, 1985). **Great Britain**: K. Middlemas, *Diplomacy of Illusion: The British Government and Germany, 1937–39*; W. R. Rock, *British Appeasement in the 1930s* (London, 1977). **Italy**: H. MacGregor Knox, *Mussolini Unleashed: Politics and Strategy in Fascist Italy's Last War* (Cambridge, 1982); D. Mack Smith, *Mussolini* (London, 1981). **Poland**: A. M. Cienciala, *Poland and the Western Powers, 1938–1939* (London, 1968); A. Prazmowska, *Britain, Poland and the Eastern Front, 1939* (Cambridge, 1987). **Soviet Union**: A. B. Ulam, *Expansion and Co-Existence: The History of Soviet Foreign Policy, 1917–1967* (London, 1968); J. Haslam, *The Soviet Union and the Struggle for Collective Security in Europe, 1933–1939* (London, 1984). **United States**: R. W. Dallek, *Franklin D. Roosevelt and American Foreign Policy, 1932–1945* (Oxford, 1979).

On economic affairs, C. P. Kindleberger, *The World in Depression 1929–1939* (London, 1973), remains an excellent general guide; D. E. Kaiser, *Economic Diplomacy and the Origins of the Second World War*, is indispensable. On strategic issues see D. Cameron Watt, *Too Serious a Business: European Armed Forces and the Approach to the Second World War* (London, 1975); W. Murray, *The Change in the European Balance of Power, 1938–1939* (Princeton, 1984).

11   Europe in the Second World War

Philip Bell

The First World War was essentially a European War which spilled over into other continents, and in which non-Europeans (notably the United States and Japan) intervened. The Second World War was very different. Its first phase was indeed European – *The Last European War*, as John Lukacs called it.[1] This lasted from September 1939 to December 1941, when the Japanese attack on Pearl Harbor brought the United States into the war, drawing two separate conflicts in Europe and East Asia into a genuinely world-wide war. The second phase began in 1942, when, despite German victories, the initiative passed to the Allied side, and continued in a period of Allied victories, though also of stubborn German resistance which prolonged the war until May 1945. The conflict ended with Europe in ruins, and with the armies of the United States and the Soviet Union (the first certainly, and the second arguably, a non-European power) meeting in the heart of the continent.

These phases define the broad strategic pattern of the war. Each phase comprises what were in effect a number of separate conflicts, most of which even now present problems of understanding and interpretation. In general, the second phase has probably attracted more attention in British historical writing, partly because it is more agreeable to contemplate victory than defeat, and partly because the events of 1942–5 have been ransacked in search of the origins of the 'Cold War'. This chapter, by contrast, puts its emphasis on the first phase of the war, which was in many ways of crucial importance. It will also look as much at questions as at answers; it is surprising how little we know, even now, about some aspects of the Second World War.

The First Phase, 1939–41

The first distinct war within this phase was that which took place in Poland from 1 September to early October 1939, which deserves to be remembered as more than a mere prologue to later events. It was the first example of German *Blitzkrieg* methods – fast-moving attacks delivered by a small but effective tank force, supported by overwhelming air power. It also provided the fascinating spectacle of active cooperation between Germany and the Soviet Union; and precise details of how that collaboration worked have yet to be elucidated. Partition between Germany and the USSR wiped Poland off the map, and began the process of massacre and deportation which was to afflict the Polish people for years to come. These were the first signs of what total war was to mean. The Polish government showed its recognition of the sort of war which was being waged by leaving the country and continuing the struggle, first from France and later from Britain. New Polish forces were raised, and fought through the whole of the war. Just as importantly, underground resistance to both the German and the Soviet occupation began at once.[2]

The Polish compaign has also raised one of the many speculative questions of the Second World War: what would have happened if the French had launched a serious offensive in the west while the Germans had only a thin screen of forces there? The reasons why they did not do so lay in the slowness of French mobilization, the defensive nature of their strategic thinking, and above all in the conviction that the war was bound to be a long one, in which a prolonged defensive period accompanied by economic pressure would precede any offensive action. In France and Britain there was a widespread hope that an economic blockade might in itself suffice to defeat Germany, and the war would be won without the blood-letting of 1914–18.

These illusions were shattered by the next stage of the war: the victorious German campaigns in Norway, the Low Countries and France in April–June 1940. These successes, and above all the defeat of France in six weeks, remain astonishing and, to a large degree, baffling. On the military aspect of the fall of France, historical examination has done much to shed light. It is now (or at any rate ought to be) common knowledge that the Germans had fewer tanks than the Allies in the battle of France, and that in terms of quality the French tanks could at least hold their own. The issue was not so much one of materials as of how it was used. It was once widely believed that French morale had rotted almost to the point of collapse before the German blow fell; but recent work, based on the French army's postal censorship reports, reveals a picture of much greater steadiness and determination than was previously thought to exist. It remains difficult to strike the balance as to how far this was a campaign won by the Germans, who used their armour brilliantly, or lost by the French, who appear to have committed every mistake that can be conceived of by the historian of war.[3] Moreover, do we yet comprehend the links between the military defeat of the French army and the political collapse of the Third Republic, which abdicated its authority to the new regime set up by Marshal Pétain? The weaknesses of the Third Republic were obvious enough: short-lived governments, a stagnant economy, political and social divisions. Yet it is surely an open question whether the Republic was fundamentally in a worse state in 1939–40 than in 1914–18, when it endured with success the terrible ordeal of the Great War. The trouble was that in 1940 the speed and intensity of the German attack struck precisely at the weak points of the regime, and offered no time for recovery. The crisis demanded tough decisions, speedily carried out and bearing the stamp of complete moral authority. Reynaud's government could not provide them. The premier was conscious that he held only a doubtful majority in the Chamber; his cabinet was divided; and in the flight from Paris it met irregularly and lost all administrative grip. Moral authority and executive capacity both disappeared, and military defeat turned into political collapse.[4]

The consequences of the fall of France were far-reaching – it was the war's first great turning-point. The widespread assumptions that the war would follow the pattern of the previous conflict were overthrown. There would be no western front against Germany for a long time to come. Outside Europe the effects spread far and wide. The United States was suddenly stricken with fear for the control of the Atlantic. The Soviet Union congratulated Hitler on his victories, but moved to consolidate its power in eastern Europe by annexing the Baltic states and Bessarabia. Far away in the Pacific, Japan saw an opportunity for expansion which might never recur. Within a mere six weeks Germany had achieved more than it ever managed during the whole of the 1914–18 war. Germany controlled the whole of western Europe, and sent shock waves round the world.

The fall of France was decisive in shaping the war. The survival of Britain decided that the war would continue. This was not something to be taken for granted. All over Europe, in the summer of 1940, there was a strong and natural tendency for governments to adjust to the new situation and come to terms with German predominance. Soon after Churchill became premier the British War Cabinet briefly but agonizingly considered (on 26, 27 and 28 May) the possibility of making an approach to Mussolini, which would inevitably lead to talks with Germany. They rejected the idea, and under Churchill's leadership they prepared to continue the war even if France fell, as was soon to happen. The British then faced the threat of invasion, and the struggle for air supremacy which we call the Battle of Britain. The margin of victory in that battle was narrow, but it was enough. The *Luftwaffe* was unable to gain the superiority to cover a seaborne invasion, or to deliver a knock-out blow by itself.[5] This was crucial. If Hitler had beaten Britain in 1940, the course of the war would have been completely changed and Germany would surely have won. As it was, Britain survived as the rallying-point for others, and as the base for future offensives. Meanwhile, the British continued to fight a separate campaign in the Mediterranean and North Africa, and to maintain control of the Middle East, its oil resources, and the Suez Canal.

With Britain undefeated, Hitler had then to decide on his next step. Various options were briefly considered or attempted: a grand coalition, stretching from Madrid to Tokyo by way of Moscow, which would overawe the British into surrender; an attack on Gibraltar, to close the Mediterranean; a Middle East campaign. But from as early as September 1940 the favourite was an attack on the Soviet Union. This assault actually began on 22 June 1941. The immediate success of Operation Barbarossa was enormous. The Soviet air force was caught on the ground. The Red Army was cut to pieces by the German armoured forces, leaving vast numbers surrounded; the Germans took an estimated three million prisoners by the end of September. The German army captured Kiev, besieged Leningrad, and by December was barely twenty miles from Moscow. This tremendous conflict, involving millions of men along a front some two thousand miles long, was to prove the decisive struggle within the Second World War, and its greatest killing-ground. The events of 1941 have left three great problems which historians have yet to resolve: why did Hitler launch the invasion? why was Stalin caught so utterly by surprise? and how narrow was the margin between victory and defeat at the end of 1941?

First, why did Hitler do it? From much debate, the elements of an answer emerge clearly enough; it is in the balance between them that the problem lies. Ideological explanations hold one of the commanding heights. Hitler had a deep-set cast of mind, visible from the earliest time when we can catch glimpses of his thought, in which living-space in the east, a racial war with the Slavs, and an ideological struggle with Bolshevism were all involved. There is another interpretation which concentrates on economic ambitions and calculations: the German desire to have Soviet oil, foodstuffs and minerals directly under their own control, instead of having to be dependent on the fulfilment of economic agreements. Third, there was a set of disputes over influence in eastern Europe which grew more acrimonious between Molotov's visit to Berlin in November 1940 and March 1941. The countries involved were Finland, Romania and Bulgaria; and the friction was quite severe enough to show that the Nazi–Soviet agreements of 1939 were in danger of breaking down. Fourth, Hitler himself insisted that one of his major reasons for attacking the Soviet Union was that it was the surest way to defeat the British, who were clinging to the hope of ultimate help from Russia. How to strike the balance, and decide on the weight to be attributed to these different explanations, continues to elude historians. The strategic argument about Britain seems implausible; the British, after all, were looking across the Atlantic for succour, not towards the frosty ramparts of the Kremlin. Yet we cannot dismiss the possibility that Hitler *believed* it to be true. The economic arguments were very finely balanced: a successful invasion would secure long-term control of Soviet resources, but the certain short-term effect would be to shut them off, and meanwhile the flow of supplies under the economic agreements was moving smoothly. If neither of these considerations was decisive, we are driven towards ideological and racial fixations, with the immediate disputes in eastern Europe helping to decide the timing. This appears the most likely explanation, though no clear-cut resolution of the problem is yet possible.[6]

The second question – why Stalin was taken so utterly by surprise – remains one of the great puzzles of the war. Of the extent of the surprise there is no doubt, but the circumstances remain baffling. The massing of some 190 German and Romanian divisions could scarcely go unobserved; but when Soviet generals reported it they were told to take it easy – the Boss knew all about it. Stalin certainly had every opportunity to know. British and American warnings of an imminent German attack reached him, though they may well have been discounted as coming from tainted sources. More importantly, he had ample information from his own intelligence sources, including a sound description of the German order of battle and the correct date for the attack. Yet all this was disregarded by a man whom we would normally regard as the epitome of caution and realism. Why? We do not know; though there will presumably be something to be learned from Soviet archives if or when they become available. So far, the most plausible explanation is that Stalin believed that the German military concentration was the prelude, not to an attack, but to a demand for Soviet concessions. In these circumstances, he seems to have been putting his trust in appeasement, by fulfilling all his economic commitments to Germany and expelling from Moscow the diplomatic representatives of states conquered by the Germans. If this was Stalin's belief, it represents a miscalculation of monumental proportions. The puzzle remains. A gap of interpretation yawns between the Nazi–Soviet Pact of August 1939 – which made excellent sense, if the object was to keep the USSR out of war for as long as possible and to gain time and territory in the meantime – and the surprise of June 1941, which threw away all the advantage gained.[7]

How near did the Germans come to victory in 1941? Indeed, what constituted victory? Would the capture of Moscow have been enough? If the crucial questions were in the sphere of morale and will, as is often the case, the margin may have been narrower than is often recognized. The key moment was the panic in Moscow between 15 and 19 October, when in Erickson's words 'Moscow's nerve snapped', and when Lukacs estimates that 'the vast majority of the people of Moscow expected the Germans to arrive at any moment'. This episode has gone largely unregarded; yet it was probably the nearest the Soviet state came to collapsing under the German assault.[8] But the collapse did not take place; the Red Army held on. The restoration of morale was signalled by holding the customary parade in Red Square on 7 November, in Stalin's presence; by December 1941 the German attack on Moscow had been held. The Germans had failed to win the war in Russia within the year. Time was to prove that this meant they could not win it at all. It was another turning-point.

Talk of turning-points is of course speculative, and there is room for discussion as to whether Germany had real opportunities to achieve conclusive victory in 1940–1.[9] Yet is is surely the case that in this first phase of the Second World War there were four turning-points. Two decided the shape of the war: the fall of France and the German attack on the Soviet Union. The other two decided its outcome: the successive German failures to defeat Britain and the Soviet Union. If Britain had fallen in 1940, it seems certain that Hitler would have controlled Europe. If there had been no eastern front after 1941, it is almost inconceivable that the British and Americans could ever have launched a successful invasion of western Europe. In these various ways, the first phase of the war was crucial.

THE SECOND PHASE 1942–5

At first sight, the year 1942 did not appear to herald the final phase of the war and the tide of Allied victory. At the beginning of the year the Japanese humiliated a British army at Singapore. In the summer the Germans advanced to the bend of the Volga at Stalingrad, and swept south into the Caucasus. In North Africa they came within sixty miles of Alexandria. But behind the scenes the balance of strength shifted against Germany. In 1942 the aircraft production of the United States, the Soviet Union, Great Britain and the Commonwealth was about 105,000; that of Germany 15,400. German tank production in 1942 was 9,400; the United States produced 25,000; the Soviet Union nearly 24,700.[10] Churchill wrote later in his memoirs that after the United States entered the war, everything that followed was 'merely the proper application of overwhelming force'.[11] We may marvel at the word 'merely', and object that the mere possession of overwhelming material force does not in itself decide great conflicts; but the conclusion must surely stand. By the end of 1942 overwhelming force was becoming available to the Allies, and it began to be applied at Stalingrad, at Alamein, and in the Anglo-American invasion of French North Africa. The tide had turned.

'Closing the ring' on Germany (another of Churchill's phrases) involved the prosecution of three further wars: on the eastern front in 1942–5; in North Africa and Italy over the same period; and in France and north-western Europe in 1944–5.

The fighting on the eastern front deserves the greatest emphasis. Like the western front in 1914–18, it saw the defeat of the main body of the German army; and for the same reason, it was immensely costly in casualties. As late as 1944, it has been estimated, the Red Army was losing five or six dead for every German killed. But the task was accomplished. Stalingrad in February 1943 saw the first surrender of a German army in the course of the war, with results which were psychological as much as physical. The legend of German invincibility was broken. From the battle of Kursk in July 1943, when the Red Army won the greatest armoured battle of the war, the sequence of Soviet victories was virtually unbroken. That summer, the Russians recovered Kharkov, Smolensk and Kiev. In January 1944 they lifted the siege of Leningrad after nineteen months. Between June and September 1944 the German dead on the eastern front numbered a known 215,000, with another 627,000 missing; and yet the name of Operation Bagration, which inflicted these dreadful casualties, is little known in the English-speaking world. At the turn of the year 1944–5 the Red Army was fighting its way into Budapest; in April it reached Vienna; and in May 1945 the Russians fought their way into Berlin. By January 1945 it has been estimated that along the whole eastern front, from Hungary to the Baltic, the Russians could muster 5,000,000 men and 50,000 guns, against 1,800,000 Germans with only 4,000 guns. On the night before Barbarossa was launched, Hitler had said that he felt he was 'pushing open the door to a dark room never seen before, without knowing what lay behind the door'. What lay behind it was this terrible war, on an unprecedented scale, which finally destroyed the German army.[12]

During the same period the ring was being closed round Germany in the Mediterranean and western Europe. In November 1942 Anglo-American forces landed in French North Africa. By May 1942 they had met the British Eighth Army advancing from Egypt, and received the surrender of 275,000 German and Italian troops in Tunisia. There followed the invasion of Sicily in July 1943, and the long-drawn-out battle for Italy. This was a frustrating campaign for the Allies, who fought their way up the peninsula through difficult terrain and two severe winters. It saw moments of triumph, notably the capture of Rome in June 1944, and ended with the surrender of the German armies in northern Italy in May 1945. But it has left several persistent questions, ranging from the issues of strategy and morality involved in the fighting for the ancient monastery at Cassino, to the fundamental problem of whether the whole campaign was well conceived. Did it fulfil its purpose of pinning German forces down in Italy, and so easing the path of the main western invasion; or did it delay that operation unnecessarily, and use up resources which could have been better employed elsewhere?[13]

This takes us to the war in western Europe, which began with the British, American and Canadian landings in Normandy on 6 June 1944 and ended with the Allied armies in central Germany and on the shore of the Baltic – but not in Berlin. The planning and execution of these operations have left behind them another crop of disputed questions. The most far-reaching, leading to all kinds of speculations, is whether the cross-Channel invasion could have been successfully mounted at an earlier date.

The first great strategic decision reached by the Americans even before the United States was engaged in the war, was that in the event of their involvement the USA would concentrate its efforts primarily against Germany rather than against Japan. This was the vital decision on 'Germany First', which was precious to the British, who were afraid of seeing American efforts turned towards the Pacific. But it left Churchill with a delicate problem. In the nicely-chosen phrase of John Keegan, Churchill wanted 'Germany First – but not quite yet.'[14] He bore in his heart and mind the experiences of the western front in the previous war, which he was determined not to repeat. He was therefore determined that the cross-Channel attack should be postponed until it could be launched with a very great superiority of force, and with the near-certainty that the Allies could build up their armies more rapidly by sea than the Germans could by land. The British thus pursued a strategy of dispersing German forces through the Mediterranean campaign, and through the postponement of a landing in France. The Americans, on the other hand, favoured concentration on what they saw as a decisive point – northern France; and the earliest possible cross-Channel invasion. This strategic argument dragged on for most of 1942 and 1943. In 1942 the British at first agreed to a small-scale attack on the Cotentin peninsula (Operation Sledgehammer), but later retracted and got the plan called off. They then pressed successfully for campaigns in French North Africa, Sicily and Italy, which absorbed so many resources in men, ships and landing-craft that the cross-Channel attack was put off from 1943 to 1944. Finally, at the three-power conference at Teheran (at the end of November 1943), the Americans and Russians combined to forbid any further postponement.

The arguments are finely balanced and must remain hypothetical. On the one hand, it is just conceivably possible that if the Mediterranean operations had been closed down earlier, an invasion of France could have been successfully mounted in 1943, with far-reaching consequences in Europe. Could the Anglo-American armies have met the Russians somewhere on the Oder, or even the Vistula? On the other hand, the battle of the Atlantic, vital for the build-up of forces and supplies for the invasion, was not won by the Allies until the middle of 1943. It is highly likely that a cross-Channel attack would have been impossible in 1943, or, if attempted, would have ended in a failure which could not have been redeemed. Even in 1944 the battle was hard-fought, and the race to build up forces was a close-run thing. The strategic case for postponement to 1944 seems strong; but once it was accepted the political consequences were unavoidable. Soviet supremacy in eastern Europe was not mainly brought about by Roosevelt's ineptitude or illness at the Yalta conference, but by the relative positions of the Soviet and Anglo-American armies; and they were decided by the date of the Normandy invasion.[15]

Other stratetic-cum-political questions have continued to arouse controversy. One was the issue of whether to attempt the invasion of Germany on a narrow front in the north, which would have enabled the British to strike for Berlin, or on a broad front, which would have eased the problems of supply and enabled more forces to be brought into action. A northern attack was tried in the Nijmegen–Arnhem airborne operations in September 1944. It failed, and afterwards General Eisenhower, the Allied Supreme Commander, insisted on the broad-front approach. In April 1945 there was another chance for the western forces to try for Berlin. The American Ninth Army crossed the Elbe at great speed, and its advanced units were only fifty miles from the German capital; but Eisenhower regarded Berlin as a political, not a military target, and halted the attack. Berlin was left for the Russians.[16]

While these various and largely separate wars were being fought, two others went on continuously. The first of these – the war at sea – affected all the rest. The heart of it, which we call the battle of the Atlantic, was the least spectacular of all campaigns, fought in innumerable small-scale engagements amid long periods of slog and boredom. Many of the decisive developments came behind the scenes, in the application of radar technology or in the obscure worlds of intelligence and code-breaking. The indicators of success and failure were the statistics of merchant ships and German U-boats sunk and launched. Results could be measured by the apparently inhuman plotting of lines on graphs; yet the human element in the conflict is nowhere clearer than in this long struggle. For Britain, and for the whole western war effort, the results were crucial. Success for the U-boats would have meant the strangulation of British imports, and perhaps even starvation and surrender. Success for the Allies meant keeping the British going, and the steady build-up of the armies which invaded France in 1944. It is a war which, despite much that has been written, still awaits its master historian.[17]

Another war was fought in the air. Air power affected every aspect of the conflict, and an attempt to use it as a decisive weapon in its own right was made in the Anglo-American strategic air offensive against Germany. The objective was either to strike a decisive blow against the German economy (for example, by knocking out a vital industrial target like a production centre of ball-bearings or oil), or to sap the morale of the German people by repeated area bombing. Neither objective was achieved. German war production went up steadily until the end of 1944, despite an increasing weight of bombs dropped; while morale, though undoubtedly affected at times, speedily recovered when attacks moved elsewhere. Bombing undoubtedly gained some successes. The so-called 'interdiction' campaign, to cut German communications with the invasion area in Normandy in June 1944, was highly effective; so too, in late 1944 and early 1945, was the attack on oil production and refining. But the bomber offensive never produced the results for which the advocates of air power had hoped; and it has provoked a sharp and difficult debate on its morality and on the degree of its effectiveness.[18]

A striking aspect of the Second World War in Europe was the role of clandestine and irregular forces. 'Resistance' was a term virtually invented during the war, to describe the movements which arose throughout German-occupied Europe. The activities of resistance groups extended across a spectrum from the production of clandestine newspapers, through sabotage, intelligence-gathering, and the running of escape routes, to guerrilla warfare and open uprisings. It usually proved disastrous to challenge the German army in open combat. The Warsaw Rising (August–September 1944) was the most dramatic attempt, and proved a sad though heroic failure. Even in Yugoslavia, where Tito's partisans achieved some successes, no decisive result was secured. The main effects of resistance lay in the moral and political consequences for the countries concerned, whose peoples could claim to have contributed to their own liberation.[19]

All the time, at least two other forms of warfare were being waged behind the scenes. One was the war of intelligence, espionage and code-breaking, in which the British success in breaking the German 'Enigma' cipher system is now well known. The value of this in the conduct of particular operations has now been closely examined by Ralph Bennett; but the problem of assessing the relative importance of each belligerent's intelligence successes remains to be resolved.[20] The other form of war without bullets was psychological warfare: the constant attempt to sustain the morale of one's own population while subverting that of one's enemies by means of propaganda. All the belligerent states maintained ministries of propaganda or information; all used the widest possible range of means available in films, radio, press and leaflets; all delighted in the ingenuity of their methods, especially in subversion and black propaganda. None seems to have achieved the scale of results which were hoped for. No regime was undermined by propaganda alone – defeat was far more effective – but the consolidating effect of propaganda working with the grain of existing opinion was considerable, and there is evidence of the distinct effect of particular campaigns. The war of words retains its fascination, especially for those who live by words and images.[21]

THE POLITICS OF THE WAR

The military aspects of the war in Europe were extremely complex. About a dozen different aspects of the conflict have been reviewed above. All affected one another, and all were linked to the politics of the war. Yet the political issues involved were, by contrast, simple. They turn on two broad questions. What sort of Europe did Hitler set out to create? and what was the nature of the alliance which defeated him, and so left its own imprint upon the continent?

What would Hitler's Europe have looked like, if it had lasted? How far was there a political and economic plan to go with the tremendous military successes of 1940 and 1941? The political shape of Europe, as it was outlined between 1940 and 1942, was a sketch-map for German domination. At the centre lay Greater Germany, made up of the Germany of January 1938 plus Austria, the Sudetenland, western and northern Poland, Alsace-Lorraine, Eupen, and Malmedy. Within this solid block of German territory, German-speaking peoples from outside (notably from the former Baltic States and the South Tirol) were gathered. In the course of time it is likely that others would have been added from Transylvania, and even from the German Republic on the Volga. Outside Greater Germany lay some territories under direct military rule: occupied France, Belgium, and large parts of eastern Europe captured from the Soviet Union. The Government-General of Warsaw had a particular status, with a German governor ruling over territory used as a dumping-ground for Jews and other peoples to be purged from the new Europe. Bohemia-Moravia was called a 'protectorate'; though Slav in character, it was destined for Germanization. Norway and the Netherlands were granted some privileges in self-administration, with the possibility that their peoples might be treated as Germanic; indeed, the Dutch were treated as potential colonizers of eastern Europe. Denmark was occupied, but retained its own government. Vichy France, also under its own government, was not occupied until November 1942. Finland, Romania, Hungary and Bulgaria were very junior allies. Italy was in theory an equal ally, and in 1940 set out to wage a 'parallel war' by asserting its control over the Mediterranean, as Germany did over Europe north of the Alps. But this theoretical division of spheres of influence rapidly broke down. German forces had to be sent to rescue the Italians when the Italians were in difficulty in Greece and North Africa; and by 1942 Italy had become a subordinate rather than an ally of Germany.

Economically, Europe was organized for short-term exploitation by Germany. Prices and exchange rates were fixed so as to meet German needs. Other countries were to accept specialization of functions so as to serve the German economy by providing agricultural produce, raw materials and fuel, while Germany concentrated on industrial production. Romania, for example, was to concentrate on the production of cereals and oil. Its exports came to be directed almost entirely towards Germany – nearly 99 per cent in 1943, as against 63 per cent in 1940. In France, occupation costs were set at 20 million marks per day – well above the actual cost of the operation – and the surplus was used to make purchases from the whole of France on conditions set by the Germans. Denmark (an occupied country), Finland (an ally) and Sweden (a neutral, but surrounded by German-held territory) all accepted trade agreements on German terms before the end of 1940. Denmark provided foodstuffs, Finland nickel and timber, and Sweden iron ore. The whole of occupied Europe, and German's allies too, were used to provide workers either at cheap rates or as forced labour. In the comparatively short period of German predominance, there emerged no fully coherent economic policy. The immediate needs of the war sometimes worked against longer-term objectives; and in Poland and the Ukraine, occupation policy had the effect of reducing agricultural production even though German economic interest certainly lay in increasing it. What might have happened if western Europe had remained under German economic control, and eastern Europe had been systematically Germanized and colonized, we cannot tell.[22]

What is certain is that the purpose of the 'new Europe' was German predominance. There was a good deal of talk in German propaganda, especially after the opening of the war against Russia, about a new Europe; and there was at least some genuine response to the idea among non-Germans, as well as a widespread and natural desire to run to the aid of the victor. In retrospect, the amount of collaboration with Germany during the years of victory in 1940–2 has almost certainly been underrated, and for a long time it was not a popular subject for study. But whatever collaborators thought or hoped, the 'New Order' in Europe was to be German even more than Nazi; certainly the foreign Nazi parties, even in the Netherlands or Norway, received short shrift in their dealings with the Germans.[23]

It is often said, correctly, that there was no 'blueprint' for the New Order; but the outline of what Hitler intended is clear enough. In the short run, the new Europe was organized for two purposes which were achieved to a remarkable degree: to wage war and to exterminate the Jews. The extent of the German war effort has already been noted; but it bears repeating that Germany fought for nearly four years against an overwhelming coalition, and succumbed only after a most tenacious resistance. The holocaust of European Jewry accompanied this long struggle, and demands separate attention.

It was not Hitler's initial intention to murder all the Jews in Europe. Nazi policy passed through phases of harassment and discrimination against Jews within Germany, and then to the concept of their forced emigration, perhaps to the United States, but more likely to Madagascar – a scheme which was seriously discussed by German government departments in the latter part of 1940. In 1940 and 1941 the Jewish population in the areas under German control was transported into ghettoes, mainly in Poland, where in 1941 the Warsaw ghetto contained over 400,000 Jews. At the time of the invasion of the Soviet Union it became German policy to massacre Jews in occupied Soviet territory; and in January 1942, at a conference at Wannsee under the chairmanship of Heydrich, bureaucratic requirements for the policy of total extermination were agreed. A Jewish historian has written, with an almost unnerving calm, that 'a spirit of administrative efficiency informed the proceedings at Wannsee, for the annihilation of the Jews had now moved beyond ideology.'[24] The means of mass extermination by gassing was now available, and had been tried out. Camps were constructed for the purpose, Europe was combed for the victims, and trains ran regularly to transport them. Large numbers of SS guards were employed in the running of the camps and the perpetration of the massacres, even when Germany was in dire need of military manpower. There is no decree bearing Hitler's signature to confirm his authorship of these deeds, but in the structure of Nazi Germany it is impossible to conceive that they could have been pursued without his active support. Given the history of his thought and speeches, there can be no doubt that his impulse lay behind the whole dread procedure.

These events still confront historians of the Second World War, and every student of that history, with the grimmest reflections. The death toll was enormous. John Grenville has written, 'Mass murder was so huge in extent that historians cannot tell for certain even to the *nearest million* how many people perished.' The generally accepted figure is about six million.[25] Insistent questions still confront us. How much did the German people know of these events? What was the role of institutions and individuals in rounding up, or on the other hand sheltering, Jews? What lay behind the public silence of the Vatican? We now know that the Allied governments had evidence about the 'final solution' in 1942; could they have done something to get Jews out of occupied Europe, or to save those in the camps?[26] We cannot be the judges of the generation which had to struggle with these issues in the flesh; but we must surely reflect upon these questions.

A further point remains. John Lukacs has written, 'It is now universally thought that Nazism was much more criminal than Communism. Now this argument, taken for granted by the liberal mind, will stand *only* because of the Jewish issue.'[27] The lot of the German people under Hitler was better than that of the Soviet population under Stalin. The record of mass slaughter under the two regimes probably puts a heavier toll down to Stalin's Russia. It was the massacre of the Jews that separated the two. Is this enough to draw a clear line between Hitler's Europe and the Grand Alliance, or must a moral ambiguity cloud our view of both sides?

It is time to turn to the politics of the Grand Alliance. Our main concern is with Europe, and therefore with Britain – the United States is a non-European power, the Soviet Union half-and-half. It will help us to look separately at Anglo-American and at Anglo-Soviet relations, before examining the triangular partnership.

Anglo-American relations played a crucial part in the British experience of the Second World War, and have occupied a large place in historical writing about it. The alliance, and above all the personal friendship between Churchill and Roosevelt, created the continuing idea of a 'special relationship' between the two countries. The questions of how well the alliance worked, and how close the friendship was, have therefore more than simply a historical significance. In his weighty and influential war memoirs, Churchill presented a roseate view of Anglo-American relations, playing down or omitting much of the friction which arose, and painting a romantic picture of his friendship with Roosevelt; Christmas at the White House in 1941 is an unforgettable scene.[28] For many years this interpretation held the field, and there remains a solid foundation for it. The Churchill–Roosevelt correspondence, and their seven meetings (plus two jointly with Stalin) in three and a half years, illustrate a form of cooperation rarely seen among allies.[29] The two men and their staffs hammered out, despite many difficulties, a common strategy, which was put into effect by the Combined Chiefs of Staff and the integrated Allied commands, which had no precedent in the history of war. On the economic side, the arrangements to coordinate shipping, and purchases in other countries, were remarkable in their efficiency. None of this can or should be gainsaid.

But eventually a reaction set in against this roseate view, which went too far in claiming an identity of interest between the two countries. Beyond the immediate and crucial interest of beating the Germans, this was not the case. A great deal of friction arose from American resentment against the British empire, and the tariff system embodied in Imperial Preference. The American government used the leverage of lend-lease to undermine that system. They used their immense advantages in civil air traffic to take over air services previously run by Imperial Airways. Their oil companies pushed into Saudi Arabia, competing with British firms in controlling the oil supplies of the Middle East. Equally, and for similar reasons, there was much Anglo-American dispute over the future status of France. Britain wanted to restore France as a major European and imperial power; the United States did not. More immediately serious than any of this was the rift that developed from 1943 onwards between Churchill and Roosevelt in their dealings with Stalin. In mid-1943 Roosevelt tried to arrange a meeting alone with Stalin, and deceived Churchill as to what he was doing. At the Teheran Conference later in the year, the President ostentatiously courted Stalin and was cool to Churchill, seeking to demonstrate that the Americans and British were not 'ganging up' against the Russians. From the American point of view, this was perfectly reasonable. By the end of the war the Soviet Union was going to be a stronger power than Britain, playing a greater role in world affairs, and it was a shrewd move to come to terms with the rising star. But it was a course which did serious damage to the Churchill–Roosevelt relationship, and imposed a strain upon the alliance.

Anglo-Soviet relations between 1941 and 1945 presented a very different aspect from those between Britain and the United States. The tone of the correspondence between Churchill and Stalin was often harsh and acrimonious. No strategic cooperation of any depth or closeness was achieved, and little information was exchanged. In the background lay over twenty years of ideological hostility and deep-rooted suspicion. The upshot was an alliance which was plagued by strategic and political difficulties, and yet was held together by a strange combination of grim necessity and what now appears to be superficial optimism. The whole subject is still far from being properly understood.[30]

Strategically, the western allies and the Soviet Union fought separate wars. This was mainly the result of geography, which made direct cooperation almost impossible. In September 1941 Stalin made an astonishing appeal for the deployment of large British forces in the Caucasus, only to be reminded by Churchill of the logistic obstacles in the way of such an operation. The supply routes to Russia, whether by way of the Arctic, through Iran, or across the Pacific to Vladivostok, were long and difficult. From 1941 onwards Stalin repeatedly demanded the opening of a 'second front' (meaning a cross-Channel invasion) in the west to divert German forces from Russia. This the British government resolutely refused to do until it judged the time was right, thus causing much friction. The British felt that they were being pushed towards a hazardous operation by a Soviet government which did not understand amphibious warfare. The Russians felt that they were being condemned to sustain the whole land war alone, and doubtless also suspected that the British government was happy to see them bleed provided they did not collapse. This dispute was in effect never resolved, because when the Normandy landings eventually took place in June 1944 the Red Army had largely won its war, and was driving the Germans out of Soviet territory.

The political difficulties besetting the alliance were serious, but by no means so grave as might have been thought at the time, or as they have been made to appear since. The overriding question was that of the western frontiers of the Soviet Union, along with the associated issue of a Soviet sphere of influence outside those frontiers. The Soviet government always insisted, even with the German army at the gates of Moscow, that at the end of the war it would accept nothing less than the frontiers of June 1941, which included the former Baltic states of Estonia, Latvia and Lithuania, the former Romanian province of Bessarabia, and (most serious of all from the British point of view) the eastern half of pre-war Poland. Again, Stalin repeatedly insisted that Poland (whatever territorial shape it was to assume) must have a government 'friendly' to the Soviet Union. Yet Poland was Britain's ally. In 1939 Britain had guaranteed Polish independence; and Polish forces had never ceased to fight alongside the British with the greatest courage – as they did in the Battle of Britain, in Italy and in Normandy. There were thus the makings of a serious dispute between the Soviet Union and Britain on the twin questions of the Polish–Soviet frontier and Polish independence – for there was no doubt that a Polish government friendly to the Soviet Union meant in practice one under Soviet control.

In the event, though these problems produced some serious disputes, the British moved steadily towards acceptance of the Soviet demands. By the time of the Teheran Conference at the end of 1943, they had accepted the so-called Curzon Line (which was not far from the Molotov–Ribbentrop Line) as the basis for the Polish–Soviet frontier. At the Yalta Conference in February 1945, both Churchill and Roosevelt agreed that the Soviet-nominated Lublin government should form the basis of a new government of Poland – though with an assurance of free elections to be held as soon as possible. Between these meetings, Churchill met Stalin at Moscow in October 1944 and concluded an agreement by which he accepted that Russia was to have predominant influence in Romania and Bulgaria, and similarly Britain in Greece. In short, Churchill accepted a substantial Soviet sphere of influence in eastern Europe, provided that it did not extend into the Mediterranean. It was at this time Churchill's view, contrary to what is often thought, that considerable Soviet territorial expansion and the growth of Soviet influence must be accepted – after all, what choice was there? In the last months of the war he sought to limit Soviet influence in *central* Europe, but in *eastern* Europe he accepted it. It was also a constant British view that the Soviet Union was bound to play a major part in any post-war settlement, and that a stable peace depended on Soviet cooperation with the western Allies. This was the theme stressed by both Churchill and Roosevelt when they returned to their respective countries after the Yalta Conference.

For these reasons, the political difficulties in Anglo-Soviet relations were kept in check during the war. The same was true of the moral questions which lurked not far beneath the surface of the alliance. The British government was aware as early as 1940 of the policies of deportation – often leading to deaths in vast numbers – being pursued by the Soviet Union in eastern Poland and in the Baltic states. When the mass graves of Polish officers at Katyn were revealed by the Germans in April 1943, Churchill and the responsible Foreign Office officials knew to a near-certainty that the officers had been murdered by the Russians. In the summer of 1944 the suspicion was strong that the Red Army had deliberately halted outside Warsaw, and that the Russians had refused to allow American aircraft to use their airfields for supply flights, in order to ensure the massacre of the Polish Home Army in the Warsaw Rising. Yet none of this deterred the British government from its policy of maintaining the Soviet alliance, without which Germany would not be defeated and hopes for a post-war settlement would vanish into dust. In war, morality must often take second place to expediency. When Churchill returned from Moscow in October 1944 – barely three weeks after the agony of Warsaw – he seems seriously to have believed that during his visit he had got on terms with Stalin, and had achieved a genuine personal understanding which would produce valuable results in the future.

The Grand Alliance was a three-sided relationship. In the perspective produced by the 'Cold War', it became easy to think of that alliance as consisting of the Americans and British over against the Soviet Union; but this was a false picture of events at the time. The truth was of a meshing of interests and a criss-cross of disputes; not a clear divide, but a sort of cat's cradle of tangled threads. Roosevelt sought to work closely with Stalin, and so did Churchill. Each was prepared to do so, on occasion, against the other. Churchill, for example, knew full well that his 'spheres of influence' diplomacy in Moscow in October 1944 would be unwelcome to Roosevelt. The British were in dispute with Russia about the Second Front; but equally they were in conflict with the Americans on the same issue. The Americans and Russians both wanted an early invasion, the British wanted to put it off. The alliance was made up of disparate and difficult partners, but it worked as well as alliances usually do, and achieved its aim. Germany was defeated, which, even with over-whelming material and numerical superiority, was no easy task.

Germany was defeated; and after nearly six years the Second World War in Europe came to an end. What were its consequences for the continent? The casualties were heavy, and more numerous even than in the war of 1914–18. Among the defeated, the German dead amounted to about 5,000,000, the Italian to about 330,000. The figures for Soviet war dead present problems; the conventional figure is 20 million, but the statistics are uncertain and it is not easy to distinguish war dead from other casualties. Another figure is about 14 million, half of them civilians, which is terrible enough. Similarly for Poland, the losses are difficult to enumerate, but there were probably about 6 million dead, almost one-fifth of the pre-war population. Great Britain escaped lightly, with just over 300,000 dead including 60,000 civilians. France suffered some 600,000 dead, of whom only 200,000 were soldiers.[31] The material damage was enormous. Parts of the Soviet Union were fought over four times, and cities lay ruined. Warsaw was about three-quarters destroyed, its population killed or removed. Many German cities were bombed to rubble, and the country had been fought over as it was not in 1918. The economic cost of the war was incalculable. It was unevenly spread, but in general the whole conti-nent had paid the price. Industrial production was low, and in some places non-existent. Transport – except for the armies – was often at a standstill. Agricultural production in Europe could not feed the peoples of Europe, and in some parts there had been famine – the fate of the northern half of the Netherlands in the winter of 1944–5 is a grim example.

This catastrophic situation was made worse by a movement of peoples such as had not been seen in European history for fifteen hundred years. This process had begun in the early phases of the war, when Germanic peoples were moved into the Reich from outside, and other Germans were moved into Poland. At the same time the Soviets deported vast numbers from Poland and the Baltic states, as well as shifting Germans from the Volga and Tartars from the Crimea. But it was at the end of the war that the greatest movement came about, with the advance of the Red Army into central Europe. First there was a flight of Germans from east Prussia and occupied Poland; then there was the systematic expulsion of Germans from areas where they had lived for generations, but which were now to become part of Poland or the Soviet Union. Somewhere between 12 and 14 million were driven out westwards. East of the Oder–Neisse line, and in the reconstituted Czechoslovakia, there remained only tiny German populations. The problem of German minorities had been 'solved' with a brutal finality, and the ethnographic map of Europe had been drastically redrawn.

This ruined continent was about to be divided between East and West. In the East, the Soviet Union was to impose a new empire. In the West, the former imperial powers (France, the Netherlands, Belgium, and even Britain) were so reduced in resources and worn down in will-power that they could not long sustain their overseas empires.

The First World War was supposed to be the war to end war. The Second World War seemed likely to be the war which had ended Europe. Yet in a strange way there were signs of resilience. In France, the birth rate had actually gone up during the years of the war. All across Europe, resistance movements emerging into the open set out, not merely to reconstruct their countries, but somehow to make them anew. They did not succeed; but it remains astonishing that they hoped for so much and achieved at least something. Not the least of the puzzles remaining from the Second World War is what actually happened to the peoples of Europe while it was going on, and what enabled them to rebuild their continent from the ruins of 1945. Europe, despite the devastation, proved to be still alive.

NOTES

1 J. Lukacs, *The Last European War, September 1939–December 1941* (London, 1976). This chapter owes much to this deeply pondered and illuminating book. May its title prove a true prophecy!

2 J. Garlinski, *Poland in the Second World War* (London, 1985), pp. 26–60.

3 On the question of tanks and other war material, the key article is R. H. S. Stolfi, 'Equipment for victory in France in 1940', *History*, vol. 55 (Feb. 1970). See also the valuable up-to-date discussion and review of the literature in M. Alexander, 'The fall of France, 1940', *Journal of Strategic Studies*, 13 (Mar. 1990). On the question of mistakes, see E. A. Cohen and J. Gooch, *Military Misfortunes: The Anatomy of Failure in War* (New York, 1990).

4 We await books on Daladier by E. du Réau (Université du Maine, Le Mans, France), and on Reynaud by J. Jackson (University College, Swansea).

5 A valuable recent summary of the Battle of Britain may be found in J. Keegan, *The Second World War* (London, 1989), pp. 91–102.

6 See the recent summing-up by B. Wegner, 'The road to defeat: the German campaigns in Russia 1941–43', *Journal of Strategic Studies*, 13(1) (Mar. 1990), esp. pp. 106–8; and the excellent review of the whole issue in R. Cecil, *Hitler's Decision to Invade Russia, 1941* (London, 1975).

7 For an early dissident Soviet discussion of the problem, see V. Petrov, *June 22 1941: Soviet Historians and the German Invasion* (Columbia, SC, 1968); J. Erickson, *The Road to Stalingrad* (London, 1985), pp. 118–42.

8 See the vivid accounts of this largely neglected episode in Lukacs, op. cit., pp. 151, 389; Erickson, op. cit., pp. 305–8.

9 Wegner, op. cit., pp. 122–3. For the question of whether or not there were opportunities for a German victory, see A. J. Levine, 'Was World War II a near-run thing?', *Journal of Strategic Studies*, 8(1) (Mar. 1985).

10 P. Kennedy, *The Rise and Fall of the Great Powers* (London: Fontana, 1989), p. 455; H. Michel, *La Seconde Guerre mondiale*, vol. 2, *La Victoire des allies, 1943–1945* (Paris, 1969), pp. 48, 70, 163.

11 Winston S. Churchill, *The Second World War*, vol. 3: *The Grand Alliance* (London, 1950), p. 539.

12 For a detailed account of the war on the eastern front, 1943–5, see J. Erickson, *The Road to Berlin* (London, 1983); for relative casualties in 1944, Kennedy, op. cit., p. 449; for Operation Bagration, Keegan, op. cit., pp. 479–82, 503; for opposing forces in Jan. 1945, Michel, op. cit. p. 315. Hitler's remark is quoted in J. Fest, *Hitler* (Harmondsworth: Pelican, 1977), p. 961.

13 Accounts of the Italian campaign may be found in W. G. F. Jackson, *The Battle for Italy* (London, 1967), and J. Strawson, *The Italian Campaign* (London, 1987).

14 Keegan, op. cit., p. 312.

15 A case for launching an invasion in 1943 has been argued in W. Scott Dunn, jun., *Second Front Now, 1943* (University of Alabama Press, 1980). Churchill made his own powerful case for delay in his war memoirs. For the landings and the battle of Normandy, see C. d'Este, *Decision in Normandy* (London, 1983).

16 There is a vivid account of these events in C. Ryan, *The Last Battle* (London, 1966).

17 S. W. Roskill, *The War at Sea, 1939–1945*, 3 vols (London, 1954–61), is among the best of the British official histories, but is now

somewhat dated. A moving account of a particular episode is M. Middlebrook, *Convoy: The Battle for Convoys SC122 and HX229* (Harmondsworth: Penguin, 1978). A valuable study of the German navy, with a good deal on the U-boat campaigns, is C. S. Thomas, *The German Navy in the Nazi Era* (London, 1990). A recent article by M. Milner, 'The battle of the Atlantic', *Journal of Strategic Studies*, 13(1) (Jan. 1990), concludes that putting the Atlantic battle in its full context 'remains as a challenge to historians' (p. 64).

18 J. Terraine, *The Right of the Line* (London, 1985), is a history of the RAF during the Second World War, including much discussion of the bomber offensive. Cf. N. Frankland, *Bomber Offensive* (London, 1970); M. Hastings, *Bomber Command* (London, 1987).

19 M. R. D. Foot, *Resistance: An Analysis of European Resistance to Nazism, 1940–1945* (London, 1976), is a masterly survey.

20 R. Bennett, *Ultra in the West* (London, 1979), and *Ultra and Mediterranean Strategy, 1941–1945* (London, 1989).

21 For a general history of propaganda, see P. M. Taylor, *Munitions of the Mind: War Propaganda from the Ancient World to the Nuclear Age* (Wellingborough, 1990). For the Second World War specifically, see M. Balfour, *Propaganda in War, 1939–1945* (London, 1979); I. McLaine, *Ministry of Morale: Home Front Morale and the Ministry of Information in World War II* (London, 1979); P. M. H. Bell, *John Bull and the Bear: British Public Opinion, Foreign Policy and the Soviet Union, 1941–1945* (London, 1990).

22 Lukacs, op. cit., pp. 345–57; the best account of the economic organization of Europe under German control is in A. S. Milward, *War, Economy and Society, 1939–1945* (London, 1977).

23 For the best-known of all European collaborators, see P. M. Hayes, *Quisling: The Career and Political Ideas of Vidkun Quisling, 1887–1945* (Newton Abbot, 1971); for reactions to the idea of a 'new Europe', Lukacs, op. cit., pp. 487–500.

24 L. Dawidowicz, *The War against the Jews, 1933–1945* (Harmondsworth: Pelican, 1977), p. 179.

25 J. A. S. Grenville, *A World History of the Twentieth Century* (London: Fontana, 1980), pp. 515–16. Grenville puts the figure at between 5 and 6 million; Dawidowicz, p. 480, at 5,933,900.

26 On Allied knowledge of what was happening, see W. Laqueur, *The Terrible Secret* (London, 1980); M. Gilbert, *Auschwitz and the Allies* (London, 1981).

27 Lukacs, op. cit., p. 452.

28 Churchill, op. cit., vol. 3, pp. 587–8, 593–4.
29 W. F. Kimball (ed.), *Churchill and Roosevelt: The Complete Correspondence*, 3 vols (Princeton, 1984), is a prime source for the whole working of the alliance, and Kimball's introduction is an illuminating discussion of Anglo-American relations, as well as of the personal friendship.
30 See M. Kitchen, *British Policy towards the Soviet Union during the Second World War* (London, 1986); J. Beaumont, *Comrades in Arms: British Aid to Russia, 1941–1945*; Bell, op. cit.
31 See the rather different sets of figures in Michel, op. cit., vol. 2, pp. 432–3, and Keegan, op. cit., pp. 590–1. For a formidable catalogue of ruin, see D. Cameron Watt, *How War Came: The Immediate Origins of the Second World War, 1938–1939* (London, 1989), pp. 3–8.

FURTHER READING

Excellent general accounts of the war (including the Pacific theatre) may be found in J. Keegan, *The Second World War* (London, 1989), and P. Calvocoressi, G. Wint and J. Pritchard, *Total War*, revised edn (London, 1989). On the early stages of the war, up to Dec. 1941, J. Lukacs, *The Last European War, September 1939–December 1941* (London, 1976), is an unusual and perceptive book.

The military defeat of France in 1940 is still best dealt with, in English, by A. Horne, *To Lose a Battle* (London, 1969), and G. Chapman, *Why France Collapsed* (London, 1968). The vast campaigns on the Russian front are dealt with on the Soviet side by J. Erickson, *The Road to Stalingrad* (London, 1975), and *The Road to Berlin* (London, 1983); the German side may be followed in A. Seaton, *The German Army 1939–1945* (London, 1982), and O. Bartov, *The Eastern Front, 1941–1945: German Troops and the Barbarisation of Warfare* (London, 1985). The Mediterranean campaigns are best approached by way of M. Howard, *The Mediterranean Strategy in the Second World War* (London, 1968) – succinct and lucid. Particular episodes are dealt with in K. Sainsbury, *The North African Landings, 1942* (London, 1976), and J. Strawson, *The Italian Campaign* (London, 1987); the impact of Ultra is analysed in R. Bennett, *Ultra and Mediterranean Strategy, 1941–1945* (London, 1989). The Normandy campaign of 1944 is covered by W. G. F. Jackson, *'Overlord': Normandy 1944* (London, 1978), which examines the origins and planning of the operation, and C. d'Este, *Decision in Normandy* (London, 1983), which analyses the fighting. R. Bennett, *Ultra in the West* (London, 1979), is a detailed discussion of the effect of Ultra on the campaign in France, taking the story through to 1945.

The war at sea is well described from the British point of view (before Ultra) in the official history by S. W. Roskill, *The War at Sea 1939–1945*, 3 vols (London, 1954-61). J. Terraine, *Business in Great Waters: The U-Boat Wars, 1916–1945* (London, 1989), takes into account British, Canadian, American and German standpoints. C. S. Thomas, *The German Navy in the Nazi Era*, is a fascinating account of its subject, both before and during the war. On the war in the air, J. Terraine, *The Right of the Line: The Royal Air Force in the European War, 1939–1945*, is large-scale and vivid; M. Cooper, *The German Air Force* (London, 1981), deals with its subject more briefly. A special issue of the *Journal of Strategic Studies*, vol. 13, no. 1, Mar. 1990, entitled *Decisive Campaigns of the Second World War*, provides up-to-date reviews of our knowledge of the 1940 campaign in France, the battle of the Atlantic, North Africa (1940–3), the Russian campaigns (1941–3), the Italian campaigns, and the Allied air offensive against Germany.

Books on the political leaders during the war must, from a British point of view, start with Churchill. Winston S. Churchill, *The Second World War*, 6 vols (London, 1948–54) remains illuminating and immensely influential; M. Gilbert, *Finest Hour* (London, 1983) and *Road to Victory* (London, 1986), are the two wartime volumes of his massive biography of Churchill. A. Bullock has recently reflected in great detail on two leaders, in *Hitler and Stalin: Parallel Lives* (London, 1991), which includes much material on the Second World War. F. W. D. Deakin, *The Brutal Friendship: Mussolini, Hitler and the Fall of Italian Fascism* (London, 1962), deals with the Rome-Berlin Axis and relations between Mussolini and Hitler. On the Grand Alliance, H. Feis, *Churchill, Roosevelt, Stalin: The War they Waged and the Peace they Sought* (Princeton, 1957), and W. H. McNeill, *America, Britain and Russia: Their Co-operation and Conflict, 1941–1946* (London, 1953), remain remarkably useful; their source material is of course dated, but they have the great advantage of being primarily concerned with the war, and not with 'Cold War' interpretations. R. Edmonds, *The Big Three* (New York, 1991), is an up-to-date discussion. W. F. Kimball (ed.), *Churchill and Roosevelt: The Complete Correspondence*, 3 vols (Princeton, 1984), is a marvellous piece of editing and is full of illuminating detail. M. Kitchen, *British Policy towards the Soviet Union during the Second World War* (London, 1986), and V. Mastny, *Russia's Road to the Cold War: Diplomacy, Warfare and Communism, 1941–46* (New York, 1979), deal with the Soviet side of the Grand

Alliance from different points of view. Economic aspects of the war are dealt with by A. S. Milward in *War, Economy and Society, 1939–1945* (London, 1977), and *The German Economy at War* (London, 1965). C. Barnett, *The Audit of War: The Illusion and Reality of Britain as a Great Nation* (London, 1986), is a critical analysis of British economic performance during the war.

On German-controlled Europe, N. Rich, *Hitler's War Aims: The Establishment of the New Order* (New York, 1974), remains the fullest general account. On the Holocaust, M. Gilbert, *The Holocaust: The Jewish Tragedy* (London, 1986), and L. Dawidowicz, *The War Against the Jews* (London, 1977), provide starting-points.

12 Mind at the end of its tether: political ideology and cultural confusion, 1914–45

Michael Biddiss

In 1920 the novelist and scientific popularizer, H. G. Wells, published his best-selling *Outline of History*. This survey of mankind from the earliest times to the twentieth century concluded with a chapter that looked forward, envisaging 'The Possible Unification of the World into One Community of Knowledge and Will'. Twenty-five years later the dying Wells produced a final essay that was meant to update his history. He gave it the gloomy title *Mind at the End of its Tether*, and in it he surveyed 'a jaded world devoid of recuperative power'.[1] Both the earlier optimism and the later pessimism were exaggerated. Yet each tells us something important about the ideological and cultural experience of Europe during the epoch of the two world wars.

The conflict which ended in 1918 was, in a crucial sense, quite different from that which had started four years before. At that earlier and more innocent epoch Crown Prince Wilhelm of Germany had expressed his anticipation of a bracing, even 'jolly', combat. Such enthusiasm, popularly shared in 1914, reflected images of swiftly decisive struggle moulded by the Bismarckian era. During 1915, however, Europeans started to realize that they had become bogged down – often quite literally – in the mire of a Great War. This was a conflict characterized not by rapid mobility but by slow attrition, nowhere more so than amidst the desolate landscape of the Western Front whose trenches, craters, and barbed wire dominate even now our collective 'memory' of the whole catastrophe. They convey, in short, the world of Wilfred Owen, not of Rupert Brooke. By the time that the guns fell silent – at the eleventh hour of the eleventh day of the eleventh month of 1918 – perhaps eight million people had been directly killed through battle, while rather more than three times that number had been left disabled. If greater precision eludes us here, it is all the more tragic to note that this would not be the last time during Europe's history down to 1945 when estimates of killing and maiming, on the later occasion inflicted by Stalinist and Hitlerian persecution as well as by renewed warfare, must contain margins of error and be scaled to 'the odd million' or so. The extent of destruction between 1914 and 1918 also helps to suggest how far the First World War reflected the conditions of that emergent mass society which sociologists like Le Bon and Tarde (see p. 95) had been analysing ever more keenly since the 1890s. An increasingly conscripted soldiery had been subjected to indiscriminate and impersonal carnage, to the point where it suddenly appeared quite fitting to recognize that even heroes were nameless, and to pay post-war homage in London or Paris at the tomb of an Unknown Warrior. Equally, the lines between combatant and civilian had been more than ever blurred. Systematic bombardment and blockade had ignored distinctions of age, sex or class; and, once attrition was the priority, it had also become imperative to mobilize through such means as mass propaganda, every kind of human as well as material resource.

Those who survived what Henry James called 'this abyss of blood and darkness'[2] were witnesses to the way in which the wonders of industrial advance had suffered gigantic conversion from productive to destructive purposes. What price, now, the idea of progress – especially towards the Wellsian vision of 'one world'? The question needed to be all the more sharply pursued precisely because a war of such length and scope came to assume, during the course of its fighting, far deeper ideological significance than Europe's leaders had anticipated at its outset. The victorious western powers directing the processes of 'peacemaking' at Paris in 1919 might take comfort from the fall of the more autocratic Hohenzollerns, Habsburgs and Romanovs. However, the tough task of securing the future of the domains previously ruled by the first two dynasties was made worse by the fact that the battered empire of the third had eventually fallen into the hands of the Bolsheviks. Lenin certainly had ideas about progress, but not ones which tallied with the liberal-democratic aspirations being variously revived by the leaders of France, Britain and the USA.

It was the 'Fourteen Points', first stated in January 1918 by President Woodrow Wilson, which set the tone for the post-war treaties. There he offered the formula of 'national self-determination' as a force for freedom and peaceful felicity. But how well would this work, granted especially the unstable character of the power vacuum created in central and eastern Europe by a war that surprisingly ended with *all three* of the region's great powers – Germany, Austria-Hungary, and Russia – being, in one sense or another, defeated? It is arguable that, on such matters, Wilson simply demonstrated a Mazzinian innocence without the excuse of living in the Mazzinian age, when the linkage of nationalism and liberalism had seemed so natural; and that he was naïve to suppose that the nationalism which had so troubled Europe before 1914 would now, quite suddenly, find its fulfilment not in war but in peace. Clearer still is the fact that Wilson implemented self-determination inconsistently, and failed to rally either the US Congress or his allies properly to its cause. The French had no intention of allowing to Germany a principle of national choice which left themselves vulnerable; and the British soon saw the perils of a universalistic commitment that might rebound against them almost anywhere from Ireland to India. The resulting 'patchwork Wilsonism'[3] with its gaps between the professions of principle and the realities of implementation, helped to undermine confidence in the legitimacy of the settlement – and, even more generally still, in the liberal-democratic values which it claimed to uphold. The tragedy of the Versailles Treaty in particular was not that it annoyed men like Hitler (for nothing more reasonable would have satisfied them), but that it alienated many more moderate Germans and, even more remarkably, failed ultimately to retain the respect of so many within the victor nations themselves.

Some liberal critics spoke early: for example, J. M. Keynes, who resigned from the British team at Paris so as to issue *The Economic Consequences of the Peace* (1919), an international best seller highlighting the counter-productivity of massive reparation demands. From the mid-1920s at any rate, there were certainly signs of a positively creative revisionism that served to promote material recovery and to lessen diplomatic tensions. Amidst the atmosphere of the Locarno and Kellogg–Briand Pacts, and of the Dawes and Young Plans, there were hopes of refurbishing the liberal idea 'that politics is the art of the peaceful settlement of diverging interests, and that its method is democratic decision by the majority, ensuring protection for the minority and the right of opposition'.[4] But the Great Depression of the early 1930s, triggered by the Wall Street Crash of October 1929, transformed the whole scene. For the second time within a generation, vast forces appeared to be escaping from human control, even from all rational understanding. The catastrophe of 1914 had been readily blamed on autocratic emperors. Now these were no longer available as scapegoats for the unprecedented scale of an economic collapse that threatened to shatter every familiar orthodoxy about the essentially self-balancing mechanisms of liberal capitalism. Keynes was, again, particularly notable among those liberals who, often not far removed from such democratic socialists as Léon Blum, accepted the need to redefine the relationship between the values of individualism and the pressures for a greater governmental role in economic planning. *The General Theory of Employment, Interest, and Money* (1936) eventually crystallized Keynes's own 'struggle of escape from habitual modes of thought and expression'.[5] Meanwhile, however, it was not only the dole queues that grew. So too, through much of Europe, did the allure of more radical substitutes for the seemingly discredited principles of liberalism in politics and economics alike. It was, as Karl Bracher says, 'a fateful coincidence of overestimation and underestimation of democracy that gripped political thought between the wars and made people look around for false alternatives'.[6]

The Bolshevik revolution provided the first of two principal sources of new inspiration, managing to do so even despite the evident harshness of the Soviet experiment. Lenin and his colleagues bore no blame for the horrors of the Great War, and offered a comprehensive humanitarian ideal that also promised to restore substance to the notion of 'progress'. Until the Bolsheviks' triumph, the main thrust of Marxism had appeared as a critical and negative one, reflecting a force potentially subversive of all established governments. But in 1917 it lost its political virginity. Within one of Europe's greatest states, the communist creed now supplied the ideological basis for a ruling cadre. How well would it survive this translation from the sphere of theory to that of power and practice, especially in regard to a less industrially oriented society than Marx had envisaged for such a pioneering revolutionary role? Any answer was sure to be marked with the distinctive stamp of the Bolsheviks – that emphasis on organization élitism described in an earlier chapter (see p. 158). On the very eve of their takeover this was one of the points that Lenin himself was most firmly reiterating in *The State and Revolution*. His text made plain that, so long as any traces of the old class system still survived, it was largely idle to talk about greater democratic freedoms. After the October revolution his Bolshevik party machine maintained a certain distance from the proletariat in whose name, but beyond whose control, it operated. Such autonomy eased its embarkation upon a task whose theoretical status was disputable – that of using political power as the instrument of radical transformation in Russia's supposedly substructural economic conditions. It was soon clear, especially after such events as the suppression of the Kronstadt rising in February 1921, that the Bolsheviks remained utterly ruthless in the pursuit of their objectives. They would tolerate no rival political organization, socialist or otherwise, nor any significant separation between party and government. Even the much vaunted federal constitution of the new USSR could hardly obscure the realities of their imperial-dictatorial centralization.

Both within and beyond the Soviet Union a major issue was that of revolution's likely spread. While the Paris peacemakers had feared this prospect, the Russian communists with their newly-founded Third International were conversely confident about its imminent realization. However, once the Marxist risings of 1919 in Berlin, Bavaria and Budapest had failed to take permanent root, the Bolsheviks needed to improvise responses to an unexpectedly protracted period of revolutionary isolation. This whole topic became central to ideological conflicts within the Soviet leadership after the death of Lenin in January 1924. Joseph Stalin, who emerged as his successor, wanted to give priority to the consolidation of 'socialism in one country'. Leon Trotsky argued, conversely, that this was a recipe for bureaucratic stagnation, and that the USSR should adopt instead a strategy of 'permanent revolution' involving ceaseless activism on an international scale. In 1929 Stalin had his rival deported. By then he had already launched the first of his Five-Year Plans. This embodied a programme of massive industrialization, coupled with schemes of agricultural collectivization. The dynamism of the former made more immediate propaganda impact than the follies of the latter. Thus it was hardly surprising that, at the very epoch when most of Europe was entering the Great Depression of the capitalist system, the USSR's version of idealistic 'progress' looked all the more alluring to many otherwise dispirited foreign observers.

The persistence of such appeal well into the 1930s is perhaps harder to explain. The full scale of Stalin's tyranny was as far as possible concealed by a huge apparatus of secrecy and censorship, while the more patent sufferings were skilfully depicted as the unavoidable price for revolutionary survival amidst the hostile climate fostered by capitalist states. By 1934 the Soviet Communist Party Congress could be told that, within the USSR at any rate, there were no enemies left. However, this assessment did not deter Stalin from unleashing a reign of internal terror that climaxed around 1936–8. Millions suffered arbitrary arrest, followed by condemnation to labour camp or to death or – in effect – both. These purges, preceding the worst of the Nazis' own barbarities, even swept through the Party itself, 'liquidating' all who (like Trotsky or Nikolai Bukharin) might conceivably rival Stalin in their ideological authority. The 1930s were also the decade during which Soviet communist discourse accelerated its descent into the crudest and most dogmatic versions of dialectical materialism. The survival of any more self-critical Marxist tradition thus became dependent during the inter-war period on thinkers operating beyond Russia: for instance, the Hungarian György Lukács (up to 1930, the time of his abject 'recantation' in Moscow), the Italian Antonio Gramsci, and in Weimar Germany such figures of 'the Frankfurt School' as Max Horkheimer, Walter Benjamin and Theodor Adorno.

The leaders of that Frankfurt circle were forced into exile by the Nazis in 1933, and Gramsci (imprisoned since 1926) died in one of Mussolini's gaols four years later. All were leftist victims of a new Fascist style of dictatorship which provided, now roughly from the Right, the second major threat to the politics of moderation. In fact, the elements of novelty in the movements led by Mussolini and Hitler confused not only liberals but many communists and democratic socialists too. Those on the Left who viewed Fascism principally as a symptom of decay within the capitalist system were often tempted to let it pursue its destruction of liberal-democratic values. Orthodox Stalinists were certainly among those who initially (as well as again in the period of the Nazi–Soviet Pact, 1939–41) underestimated the scope of the threat against their own movement, to the extent that until the mid-1930s the Kremlin delayed allowing communist parties abroad to participate in forming broad-based 'popular fronts' against the rising Fascist peril. At such points, historical analysis based simply on a polar opposition between Stalin's 'extreme Left' and the 'extreme Right' of Mussolini and Hitler hardly suffices. For we must note also some measure of similarity between the broadly 'totalitarian' aspirations common to all three of their regimes. Each dictator used the machinery both of propaganda and of violence to mobilize mass support behind a leader who expressed hostility to every form of effective representative democracy and to any conception of politics as an arena for consensual compromise. All of them sought to impose through the power of the single-party state a standardized mode of life and thought, where every meaningful distinction between the public and private realms would be annihilated and every prompting of individual conscience nullified. Moreover, the various ideologies which justified these aims, and offered a reinvigorated sense of purpose and progress, themselves became closed intellectual systems. Thus each of the totalitarian creeds was built on assumptions of absolute and unquestionable certainty, about the past struggles and future destinies of the particular class, or race, or nation-state championed, respectively, by Stalin, Hitler and Mussolini.

During the 1920s it was the 'Duce' who set the tone for a general style of Fascist politics, which non-Italians too could loosely adapt to their own various national purposes. Imitative movements of a minority nature developed in parts of western Europe, while in such countries as Spain, Hungary, and Romania there was a tendency for Fascist techniques of political mobilization to be absorbed within stronger forces of traditional authoritarianism. Most significantly of all, by the 1930s contemporaries were readily viewing Nazism as Germany's particular manifestation of a wider 'European' Fascism. Everywhere greatest support came from those whose anxieties about status were most acute, especially the hitherto uncoordinated ranks of peasants and smaller bourgeoisie threatened by organized labour. But industrial workers too were not entirely immune to the Fascist spell: Mussolini had begun as a socialist, and Hitler's movement had that same term in its very title. Essentially, Fascism sought to go beyond the familiar rhetoric of 'Left' and 'Right', so as to realize a vision transcending both socialism and capitalism as hitherto understood. It aspired to make irrelevant the habitual confrontation between conservative and revolutionary, by offering them a new and higher form of shared community. However, such union was also conceived in a spirit of national or racial exclusiveness that set it apart from the humanely universalistic ideals espoused not just by liberalism, but by socialism and communism too. The violent cult of élitist domination within Fascism never embodied that note of apology – those allusions to mere temporary expediency – intermittently observable even in Stalinism. Moreover, though fundamentally contemptuous about the claims of intellect, Mussolini and Hitler proved readier than most of their opponents to grasp the principles of mass psychology and propaganda, and to appreciate the power of ideas once harnessed to mass emotion. Fascism gained a measure of support from intellectual circles precisely because it drew so aptly from the wells of irrationalism enlarged before the Great War. In this sense, the aggressive modernity of its élite-inspired myths helped to encourage within its believers an epic and redemptive state of mind.

Mussolini's classic statement of his movement's meaning was an article on 'The Doctrine of Fascism', drafted with help from the philosopher Giovanni Gentile and embedded in the *Enciclopedia Italiana* of 1932. Here the Duce argued that only the State itself – organized in 'corporatist' terms and operating with the discipline symbolized by the *fasces*, or lictors' rods – had the potential to become a true spiritual reality. It must embrace, synthesize and trascend all other social phenomena; it should therefore respect individuals only insofar as these identified themselves with its own higher purposes. As Mussolini went on:

If liberty is to be the attribute of the real man, and not of the abstract puppet envisaged by individualistic liberalism, Fascism is for liberty. And the only liberty which can be a real thing, the liberty of the State and of the individual within the State. Therefore, for the fascist, everything is in the State, and nothing human or spiritual exists, much less has value, outside the State. In this sense Fascism is totalitarian, and the Fascist State, the synthesis and unity of all values, interprets, develops, and gives strength to the whole life of the people.[7]

Whereas in the Italian case ideology tended to be extracted from prior action, Hitler's policies were directed towards the implementation of a no less anti-individualistic world-view that was largely complete in outline from a much earlier stage. This centred not on state glorification as such, but rather upon that concept of race which had already loomed large in the political thinking of the pre-1914 era (see pp. 91–2). Within the Nazi interpretation of history this played the same pivotal role as class did for the Marxists. As the 'Führer' explained in *Mein Kampf* (1925–6):

All the human culture, all the results of art, science, and technology that we see before us today, are almost exclusively the creative product of the Aryan. This very fact admits of the not unfounded inference that he alone was the founder of all higher humanity, therefore representing the prototype of all that we understand by the word 'man'.[8]

From this it was easy to argue, conversely, that non-Aryans were something less than fully human, and that struggle between the higher and lower stocks must constitute the principal determinant of human development.

Even in that early book Hitler was outlining a continental 'new order', more consistent than Woodrow Wilson's and potentially even more inhumane than Stalin's. By 1945 Europe's Jews had become the principal – though far from exclusive – victims of this Nazi ideology focused on racial hierarchy. Debate continues about whether full-scale genocide was, even from the outset, the fate which the Führer was determined to inflict upon them. What can hardly be disputed, though, is the logic behind the eventual physical annihilation of those Jewish communities once they had been identified as an 'anti-race', as a lethal biological threat to Aryan mastery. Every brand of racism, in generating rigid typologies to which its enemies must conform, strips its victims of any claim upon personal individuality. But during the early

1940s, at Auschwitz and the other Nazi extermination camps, the process was pushed to a still more horrific stage – from depersonalization to dehumanization. Here types became, at best, merely animal. In that form they might be dispatched all the more readily to the abattoirs of Hitler, Himmler and the SS.

Those mass murders were not the work of 'savages' in the sense that Europeans had usually given to the word. They were perpetrated from the heartlands of civilization, as commonly understood, and by members of the nation that was most directly endowed with the legacies of Bach and Beethoven, Goethe and Schiller. Amidst all the turmoil of the first half of the twentieth century, Germany's Third Reich was certainly unique in the pitch that its barbarities attained. Even while inflicting his own vast terror, Stalin had never forsworn certain ultimately humane aspirations; and not even he had brought theory and practice so perfectly into murderous alignment as did Hitler. It is easy to see why, when the horrors of the Holocaust became fully revealed around 1945, there occurred such general outcry against Germany. Yet that should not be allowed to erase the bravery of those Germans who did resist Hitler. Equally, it must not obscure those senses in which Nazism had merely intensified a mood of anti-Semitic and other brutality already well-developed across Europe at large. Here is the way in which Alan Bullock wisely concluded the earliest major scholarly biography of the Führer:

> The condition and state of mind which he exploited, the *malaise* of which he was the symptom, were not confined to one country, although they were more strongly marked in Germany than anywhere else. Hitler's idiom was German, but the thoughts and emotions to which he gave expression have a more universal currency.[9]

Let us remember that, both in Hitler's 'satellite' countries and in many of the regions more directly subjugated, the Nazis conducted their anti-Jewish and other atrocities with help fron indigenous cohorts, whose lust for violent action often far exceeded any promptings of compulsion. Nor should we forget the indirect collaboration of those – Germans and non-Germans alike – who, despite their growing suspicions especially about genocide, endeavoured merely to keep their own eyes, ears and mouths closed.

If the experience of a generation that had stumbled from Ypres to Auschwitz was hardly reconcilable with simple faith in political or social improvement, it was similarly obvious by 1945 that any assumptions about the steady 'advance' of intellectual and creative achievement must be severely questioned. Had it really been wise to evolve over the centuries forms of discourse stressing the distance, rather than the proximity, between 'barbarism' and much of what, for example, the Germans sought to conceptualize as *Kultur* or the French as *civilisation*? In essence, had Europe's long march of 'progress' turned out to be merely the sort of grand circular manoeuvre mapped so dramatically by Oswald Spengler's effort at global history, *The Decline of the West* (1918–22)?

Back in August 1914, intellectuals and artists had certainly been no less susceptible than others to the jingoistic intoxication of the moment. Some, such as the Italian futurists, or the German novelist Ernst Jünger (author of a semi-autobiographical 'diary', *The Storm of Steel*, published in 1920), continued, even to the end of hostilities, their celebration of the bracing experience of conflict. However, especially as the lengthening battles began to take an exceptionally heavy toll upon the most talented cadres of a whole generation that was just emerging into maturity, this heroic romanticization was rivalled by a more sombre tendency. Its tone of anguished lamentation was increasingly heard in the work of the major British war poets, not least that of Wilfred Owen before his own death in the very last days of the fighting. From France there came Romain Rolland's *Above the Battle-field* (1915), a Nobel Prize-winning essay advocating international pacifist solidarity amongst intellectuals, and the novel *Under Fire* (1916), in which Henri Barbusse detailed the grim realities of survival and non-survival in the trenches. The theme of revulsion at mindless slaughter was similarly pursued after the war by the German novelist Erich Maria Remarque, whose *All Quiet on the Western Front* (also soon adapted for the cinema) met with swift international celebrity when published in 1929. The course by which, ten years later, Europe was turned once more into a battlefield owed something to each of these broad mentalities; the enthusiasts who were bent upon preserving struggle as a whole way of life would never have got as far as they did during the 1930s without the appeasing propensities of others who were prepared to pay almost any price in order to escape the horrors of renewed warfare.

The conflict of 1914–18 seared the consciousness of Europeans, to the extent that thereafter the idiom of 'pre-war' and 'post-war' became swiftly current as a means of expressing their sense of having crossed some huge watershed. But, in many matters of concern to intellectual history, the phasing of such shift was actually more complex. As chapter 4 sought to show, even before 1914 a sense of cultural disorientation was already gaining ground, and a major revolution against established patterns of thought and expression had begun. So, here, the First World War is less important as an igniter than as an accelerator to the motor of change. The battles did more than works of imaginative talent by themselves ever could to accentuate disillusionment with a civilization that appeared to have failed, and to enhance not only the urgency but also the popular acceptability of the case for radical rethinking in many spheres. With some particular reference to modernism in literature and the arts, Malcolm Bradbury observes that 'what had once seemed to be rarified and outrageous experiments not took on a different character; they now looked like necessary means for grasping the fevered and accelerated spirit of the postwar world'.[10] Thus much of the intellectual and cultural history of the 1920s and 1930s deals with ideas that were projected from the turn of the century and were then refracted, first through the experience of the Great War and then subsequently through the turmoil of economic collapse and totalitarian dictatorship as well.

The full significance of that process, driving eventually towards a great politicization of cultural endeavour, can only be grasped if we also remember the senses in which this conclusion ran counter to much of the original modernist impulse. Part of the legacy from the pre-1914 epoch was a questioning as to whether the creative activity which went on *amidst* public events should also be directed *towards* them. In short, how essential were social engagement and remedial prescription? Within modernism there were many elements of abstraction and introspection, including a distancing from positivistic realism and an inclination towards 'art for art's sake', which served to support initially negative answers.

One striking response of this kind stemmed from two poets, the Romanian Tristan Tzara and the German Hugo Ball. During 1916 they formed at neutral Zurich a circle of artists and writers who then became notorious in Paris, and Berlin too, during the immediate post-war period. They took the label 'Dada' – a nonsense word reflecting, but hardly redeeming, a nonsense world. The group aimed to shock, whether by reproducing the Mona Lisa with beard and obscene caption, or by staging 'events' (including brawls, and exhibitions at lavatories) that were offered as acts of artistic creativity in themselves. Much of this same spirit carried over into a movement led by the French poet André Breton. Influenced by the symbolists and by Freud, he explored conditions of incomplete consciousness with a view to converting the superficially contradictory states of dream and reality into a sort of higher absolute, or 'surreality'. Breton's first manifesto of 1924 defined this surrealism as follows:

Pure psychic automatism, through which it is proposed to express verbally, in writing or in any other manner, the real functioning of thought. Dictated by thought, in the absence of any control exercised by reason, outside of any aesthetic or moral consideration.[11]

René Magritte, a Belgian, was outstanding among the painters who soon gave these promptings visual shape. Like the rest of surrealism in its opening phases, his nightmarish incongruities seemed just as remote from constructive social concern as the otherwise very different experiments with the vertical and horizontal lines of non-representational 'pure form' geometry that were also being conducted during the 1920s by the Dutch artist, Piet Mondrian.

This was not, however, an epoch during which it was easy to sustain for long any position of intellectual or artistic disengagement from public issues. The pressures towards politicization obviously proved strongest within the areas that fell directly beneath the control of the new totalitarian dictators. Under Stalin and Hitler especially, the fanatical political party became central to the operation of the repressive state. Every channel of propaganda was mobilized in support of ideological orthodoxy, and the new media of the cinema and radio broadcasting were exploited to especially striking effect. The dictatorships also politicized the rapidly developing spheres of mass sport and leisure, as well as every level of the formal education system. Through their very nature, totalitarian governments sought to make truly independent thought itself unthinkable, and to render equally incomprehensible the case for individuality of literary or other creative output. Thus by the mid-1930s virtually any habit of behaviour or expression on the part of those subject to such rule – whether they adopted this in a spirit of dissent, of enthusiastic commitment, or even just of conformist acquiescence – was likely to carry a political meaning.

From its earliest days the Soviet regime insisted that culture, like everything else, should serve the purposes of communist advance. Yet it is notable that, initially, this view did manage to preserve some potential for experimentation with those avant-garde forms which had developed, even in the West, as part of the modernist critique of bourgeois civilization. The Bolsheviks urged Kandinsky into a temporary return to Russia so that he might supervise picture purchasing for the state museums, and on May Day 1918 they bedecked Moscow with the abstract images of Kasimir Malevich and other 'suprematists'. Creative innovation was also outstandingly characteristic of early Soviet film-making, inspired by directors such as Vsevolod Pudovkin and Sergei Eisenstein. Here was a genre technological in its basis, industrial in its organization, and popular in its appeal – not least, a medium as uncluttered as the regime itself by any associations with the previous hegemony of autocratic or bourgeois values. When Eisenstein completed *Battleship Potemkin* in 1925, it was still possible to argue for some congruence between political revolution and cultural experimentation. However, as Stalin consolidated his authority thereafter, the remaining scope for literary and artistic independence rapidly vanished. The regime increasingly demanded conformity of production in terms of 'socialist realism', a revamped naturalism concerned with easily accessible descriptions of proletarian muscles, hard hammers, sharp sickles, and Fascist fiends. This was the new orthodoxy that even such an accomplished author as Maxim Gorky chose to serve by going back to Russia at the end of the 1920s and chairing a Union of Soviet Writers that soon made issues of literary judgement and party discipline inseparable from each other. Novelists were encouraged to glorify the technological achievements of the Five-Year Plans, yet were prohibited from recording the tragedies ensuing from Stalin's terroristic methods of implementation. A similar blight fell upon theatre, film, and the visual arts. Even music could not escape: when *Pravda* condemned modernistic 'chaos' and demanded works in a more popularly accessible idiom, the USSR's two leading composers of the later 1930s and 1940s, Dmitri Schostakovich and Sergei Prokofiev, found it only prudent to comply.

On the Fascist side, Mussolini never attained a comparable degree of effective control. It is true that, from early on, those who proposed to earn their living from intellectual or artistic activities within the new corporate state were obliged to join the appropriate *sindicati*. Yet it was only after 1935, with the formation of the Ministry of Press and Propaganda (from 1937, the Ministry of Popular Culture), that such controls began to mesh with a more sustained campaign directed towards great standardization of content and technique. By then the Duce was already feeling the pressures to ape Hitler, rather than to continue acting with more dignity as the Führer's mentor in developing dictatorial techniques. The leading jackboot was now, so to speak, on the other foot. Quite simply, the Nazis had been just as rapid and ruthless in matters of intellectual purging as in the other spheres where they were similarly pursuing *Gleichschaltung*. That policy – essentially one of crushing everything down into flat uniformity – brought a swift end to the creative excitement characteristic of Germany during the Weimar period, when political and aesthetic innovation had seemed to run hand in hand, and Berlin had become a city second only to Paris as a cultural focal point for Europeans of many nationalities.

After 1933 many exiles from the Third Reich endeavoured to salvage something of worth elsewhere. Inside Germany, however, only the hollow-heroic and the sickly-sentimental survived as weapons with which to combat the perceived menace of *Kulturbolschewismus*. A subversive assault was launched even against language itself, by a regime which made the discourse of 'Nazi-Deutsch' ('final solution', 'protective custody', and much else besides) instrumental not in clarifying, but in obscuring thought and action alike. Literature and painting, music and film, were all dragooned into celebrating the sacredness of Aryan blood and soil, the imminent triumphs of the master race. Hitler's cultural propagandists thrust modernism aside – for example, condemning Van Gogh, Munch, and Picasso as the epitomization of 'degenerate art' – and returned to forms of pedantic naturalism in order to project their doctrines of strength and joy. In the last resort, paintings of Nazi-Aryan muscle and of Soviet-proletarian muscle manifested all too many similarities; and in both the German and the Russian cases they stood a good chance of being used to decorate new public buildings notable only for the tasteless monumentality of their own architecture.

It was natural that, granted their almost limitless ambitions, the two principal totalitarian dictatorships should also aim to extend their control across other intellectual domains. From the outset the Bolshevik regime had conferred an unhealthily monopolistic status upon Marxist approaches to knowledge. Under Stalin even these were further narrowed, into one particularly arid version of dialectical materialism. Thus the method which Lenin had commended for every context now became the only one tolerated within each, whether involving the study of philosophy or history, linguistics or genetics. In Nazi Germany it was anti-Semitism and the rest of racist biology that similarly spread and tainted every area of scholarship, often producing a powerfully alluring mysticism semi-disguised by the mantle of scientific pretension. Here the debauchment of intellect penetrated even the superficially apolitical world of theoretical physics, with what eventually proved to be very counter-productive effect. Condemnation of 'Jewish physics' would have been indefensible at any time; but in an era when Jews deserved their prominence amongst the best in the field such attacks were also, in a precise sense, self-defeating. Whatever the status of the alternative 'Aryan physics' may have been, a regime so disdainful of scientists like Einstein did not, even for that reason alone, deserve to survive. Moreover, survival was indeed at stake. The racial persecutions by the Nazis helped spur a flight of talent from those universities – most notably Göttingen and Berlin – which

during the 1920s had rivalled Cambridge on the leading edge of research into the structure and potency of the atom. By the time the
military relevance of all this was becoming plainer, many of those
exiles were working alongside scientists in countries hostile to Hitler.
As for Nazi Germany, it was fitting that a regime so contemptuous of
true scholarly values should have debilitated those same centres of
research which might otherwise have helped to produce – amidst an
alliance between science, technology and ruthless military planning – a
uniquely powerful instrument for the very domination which the
Führer craved.

Whether it was from Left or Right that the dictators exploited the
confused aftermath of war or economic collapse, they embodied increasingly forceful styles of government, which by the later 1930s,
were concentrating minds upon public issues even in the countries
lying still beyond the direct ambit of authoritarian control. This height-
ening of political consciousness could only be speeded by an influx of
fugitives from tyranny. Retreat (mainly but not entirely by Jews) from
actual or imminent Nazi rule reached a particularly large scale, and
included a significant proportion of talented artists, scientists and
thinkers. Overall, the rising quantity of those persecuted, whether or
not they sought refuge, helped to stimulate greater social engagement
amongst those European intellectuals who still enjoyed freer conditions for expression. Even within the ranks of the latter there were
some who did indeed willingly succumb to the spell of Fascism. A
rather larger number saw it as a threat which needed to be countered
by adopting or strengthening allegiance to a Marxism more humanely
inspired; these tended to treat whatever there might be of substance in
tales of Stalinist terror as matters of temporary aberration or passing
necessity. But among others, probably most numerous of all, a distate
for Fascism and Communism alike prompted renewed awareness of
the continuum between individual political liberties and the freedom
of creativity and intellect at large. Even for them, what the Great
Depression had encouraged the divisions of ideology underlined: a
realization that, at this epoch, any intellectual or artistic activity which
simply spurned social commitment must be accounted mere frivolity.

In such a climate, it was not surprising to find the Churches under
some particularly heavy pressure to give guidance. But who were
they to identify as the real enemies of 'Christian civilization'? The
anti-clerical and secularizing force of liberalism was undoubtedly a
long-standing foe. However, the atheistic values now being projected
from the Kremlin were even more plainly menacing. So great, indeed,
was the communist threat that Hitler's anti-Bolshevism won him an

otherwise inexplicable degree of ecclesiastical sympathy, within Protestant and Catholic circles alike. There were brave voices of dissent, such as Martin Niemöller and Dietrich Bonhoeffer of the Protestant 'Confessing Church'; and some signs of protest from the Catholic hierarchy too, especially over Hitler's 'mercy killing' of 'defectives' around 1939–40. In the main, however, the Reich and the churches at large found themselves playing for time, with neither side eager to enter prematurely into a situation of total and open hostility. These compromises, manufactured by religious leaders for the sake of institutional damage limitation, were bought at almost incalculable moral cost to Christianity as such. According to James Joll, 'The Churches in general did not, and perhaps could not, rise above the prejudices of most of their members, who had welcomed or accepted the rise of National Socialism, just as other Germans had done and for the same reasons.'[12] In Italy, moreover, the Vatican strove harder to accommodate Mussolini's regime than it had ever done to support any government within the whole 'liberal' era since the 1860s. Similarly, General Franco's victory over 'Red' republicanism in the Spanish Civil War of 1936–9 – earned with vital help from the Führer and the Duce – was a triumph that the Catholic Church took for its own.

As for secular philosophy, this was scarcely in a better condition to offer unconfused wisdom about the political and moral dilemmas of the epoch. Its more analytic practitioners, much influenced by the so-called Vienna Circle, had difficulty in reversing their preference for concentrating upon the kind of logical and linguistic concerns that seemed strictly technical within their discipline, rather than upon ones that reached out from academic philosophy towards broader public issues. Conversely, the less analytic styles of thinking which cultivated more intuitive understanding (for example, phenomenology and existentialism) did encourage such wider prescriptions – but with such frequency as to produce only a welter of contradictory imperatives that denied any consensus about the principles actually deserving of commitment. And when Freud – through *The Future of an Illusion* (1927) and *Civilization and its Discontents* (1930) – outlined the vision of social life which must complement the psychoanalytic image of man himself, the apocalyptic tone in which he presented the current scene of civilizational crisis was far more impressive than any of the pseudo-scientific remedies he purveyed.

Where, finally, did imaginative literature – so central to the European cultural tradition throughout half a millennium – become most significantly engaged by the ideological conflicts which increasingly absorbed this particular generation? It must first be noted that, during the earlier 1920s especially, some of the most stimulating work did remain politically detached, or at least politically ambiguous. The poetry of Rainer Maria Rilke in German, and of Paul Valéry in French continued Mallarmé's symbolist disdain for worldly involvement. After the American-born T. S. Eliot had published *The Waste Land* from Britain in 1922, he felt obliged to hint at its private meanings, as a way of restraining those who acclaimed it too simply as an essentially public statement about the aridity of contemporary civilization. The Sicilian playwright Luigi Pirandello also won sudden post-war renown through dramas suggesting that no single reading of reality could ever be deemed authoritative. As for the novel, Proust's progress through the cycle started by *Swann's Way* (see p. 99) certainly confirmed his technical virtuosity, but also his lack of enthusiasm for registering political messages. The year in which he died, 1922, was not only that of *The Waste Land*, but also the one in which James Joyce issued from Paris his own principal contribution to the modernist upheaval. The huge text of *Ulysses*, once notorious for its sexual explicitness, encompassed just a single day of pre-war Dublin life. It was narrated through forms of prose-poetry which blended naturalistic detail with symbolist inspiration, and carried the art of interior monologue to new heights. Thus did the Irish author represent those 'streams of consciousness' which thereafter surged so strongly through many other European novels too. With *Finnegans Wake* (1939) his assault on literary convention stretched even to the radical fracturing and luxuriant re-creation of language itself. Joyce was plainly involved in a revolution, but a cultural not a political one. Nor could straightforward ideological intent be attributed to the paradoxical tales written in German by Franz Kafka, who died in 1924. Only later would hindsight allow readers to marvel at how, while living originally under Habsburg rule, this Czech Jew had succeeded in prefiguring so much of the totalitarian world of nightmare necessity. As time passed, such works as *Metamorphosis, The Trial* and *The Castle* (published in 1915, 1925 and 1926 respectively) looked ever more chilling in their newly-assumed relevance. Soon – in reality, and not in anguished imagination – millions did become identified as vermin, distinctions between guilt and innocence did get wilfully confused, and vast bureaucratic labyrinths were indeed constructed at dictatorial whim.

Even in countries still free from these terrors, the pressures towards the politicization of literature rapidly increased from the later 1920s onward. Most of what resulted was anti-Fascist in tone. But this is not to say that the minority who offered sympathy, or indeed fuller support, to the radical Right were derisory either in number or quality.

For example, among writers in English, Eliot came to share (albeit more briefly and less frenziedly than his brilliant but half-deranged poetical associate, Ezra Pound) some of D. H. Lawrence's enthusiasm for Italian Fascism as an agent for the regeneration of a civilization that was tending to become not only rightly disillusioned with liberalism, but also wrongly enchanted by the socialist or communist visions. In France, Henri de Montherlant and Charles Maurras were similarly notable for encouraging much the same kind of authoritarian solution to the problem of protecting culture from mass debasement. There, the Vichy regime of the early 1940s soon confirmed the hollowness of any aspiration to use broadly Fascist values for the purposes of reconciling creative spontaneity with the requirements of order in art and politics alike.

Among those who counter-mobilized against Fascism, none asserted the social responsibility of literature more stridently than Bertolt Brecht. Through such pieces as *The Threepenny Opera* (1928), with its laboured parallels between capitalism and criminality, this German Marxist playwright began to create a new form of epic theatre. Didactic slogans and interpolated commentaries were soon 'distancing' Brecht's audience from any habitual empathy with the characters portrayed. Here drama was 'real', not to the extent that it managed some illusory imitation of the world outside, but only according to the measure of its success at creating within the theatre an occasion for intensified social and ideological awareness. For another major German literary figure, who similarly exiled himself from Nazi rule, the road towards a far less radical brand of politicization was much more tortuous. An earlier chapter mentioned (see p. 97) how Thomas Mann, in his pre-1914 stories, had expressed anxiety about the tendency for creative activity to be contaminated by excessive concern with social issues. The post-war years saw his emphasis shifting, albeit painfully. The sanatorium of *The Magic Mountain* (1924) supplied the setting for a great – if ultimately inconclusive – debate about the choices confronting a civilization behind whose own tubercular bloom there ravaged forces of inner decay. In 1930 Mann published *Mario and the Magician*, a hostile commentary upon Mussolini's version of hypnotic Fascism. Then, through the quartet of *Joseph* novels (1933–43) about exile, as well as in *Doctor Faustus* (1947), with its allegorical treatment of the diseased spirit of modern Germany, he revealed still more of his conversion to the view that some reconciliation between creativity and democratic political commitment was inescapable. By thus gradually accepting that the season for what he had earlier defended as 'unpolitical man' was now over, he came to epitomize the most significant modulation in the cultural history of these decades.

Even before much of Europe again became a battlefield from 1939 onwards, the preceding three years of conflict in Spain had served to sharpen the responses of writers and others to the ideological confrontations of the era. Upon that country's own cultural life the Civil War inflicted deep wounds. The slaughter spurred Picasso into painting the masterpiece of *Guernica* (1937), but it was now as exiles that such distinguished figures as Picasso and the philosopher José Ortega y Gasset (especially notable for *The Revolt of the Masses*, 1930) would pursue their careers. Worse still, the young Republican poet and dramatist Federico García Lorca was only the most renowned of many talented Spaniards who died in action or, like himself, suffered political murder. Foreign writers also felt greatly involved, and many came to the battle zones as participants or observers. No novel inspired by the struggle was more widely read than the American Ernest Hemingway's *For Whom the Bell Tolls* (1940); and outsiders also wrote documentary accounts of lasting value, such as Arthur Koestler's *Spanish Testament* (1937) and George Orwell's *Homage to Catalonia* (1938). As the English poet Stephen Spender recalled, the Civil War offered every European an experience comparable to '1848' – an opportunity to stand and be counted. But, just like the European revolutions of that earlier epoch, the Spanish hostilities complicated some issues even while clarifying others. Not least, they underlined the ambiguities still remaining within the essentially triangular relationship between Fascism, Communism, and liberal or moderate socialist democracy. In countries where freedom to choose still survived, most support from intellectuals went to the Republic. Yet it was also amongst those on the Left that the Civil War did most to stimulate a revision of the naïve idealism which had hitherto suffused so much of their assessment of the great Soviet experiment. Here many became alert to the manner in which a popular Spanish movement had been cynically exploited for Stalinist ends. Of all novels, it was Koestler's *Darkness at Noon* (1940) – a vivid depiction of revolutionary hopes corrupted within Russia itself – which best conveyed an author's personal experience of this disillusionment with the communist faith.

Nonetheless, only five years after that book appeared, the advance of the Red Army into much of eastern and central Europe had greatly extended the area of Stalinist control. From the summer of 1941, when Hitler violated the Nazi-Soviet non-aggression agreement that he suddenly concluded back in August 1939, the USSR was linked to Britain (and soon to the USA as well) in military efforts to crush the

Fascist regimes. However, the relief from open warfare which followed the completion of that task was destined to be insecure; one kind of dictatorial threat had been removed only at the price of enlarging another. In 1945, even as Wells was brooding upon an exhausted world at the end of its tether, another British author – younger but similarly ailing – published a timely allegorical tract against the menace of Stalinism. Through *Animal Farm* George Orwell explored (as Koestler had done) the betrayal of revolutionary idealism, this time in a setting where pigs could suffer no more hideous fate than that of becoming indistinguishable from humans. More complex was the message of his last novel, *Nineteen Eighty-Four* (1949), which did not simply condemn totalitarianism but also warned against mass capitalist society's own capacity for drifting towards unthinking conformism. During those later 1940s the self-regenerative possibilities for liberal democracy, and its prospects across Europe at large, looked generally less favourable than they had done in the immediate, Wilsonian, aftermath to the battles of 1914–18. Now the conquest over Nazism, followed by the rapid onset of the 'Cold War' between the communist victors in the East and the capitalist ones in the West, had produced a new configuration of ideological tensions. But it had not reversed the tendency, clear from around 1930 at latest, for some brand of confrontation between ideologies to constitute the principal feature of Europe's political and intellectual condition. That was a situation which would indeed outlast the fall of Hitler by more than forty years – until, at the end of the 1980s, an internal collapse of the whole communist system of ruling and thinking brought the next major phase of European history to its own dramatic close.

NOTES

1 H. G. Wells, *Mind at the End of its Tether* (London: Heinemann, 1945), p. 30.

2 Quoted in M. Bradbury, *The Modern World: Ten Great Writers* (London: Secker & Warburg, 1988), p. 16.

3 H. Nicolson, *Peacemaking 1919*, reprint of revised edn of 1943 (London: Methuen, 1964), p. 70.

4 K. Bracher, *The Age of Ideologies: A History of Political Thought in the Twentieth Century* (London: Methuen, 1985), p. 166.

5 *The Collected Writings of John Maynard Keynes*, vol. 7 (London: Macmillan, 1973), p. xxiii.

6 Bracher, op. cit., p. 175.

7 In A. Lyttelton (ed.), *Italian Fascisms: From Pareto to Gentile* (London: Cape, 1973), p. 42.
8 A. Hitler, *Mein Kampf* (London: Hutchinson, 1961), p. 263.
9 A. Bullock, *Hitler: A Study in Tyranny*, revised edn (Harmondsworth: Penguin, 1962), p. 808.
10 Bradbury, op. cit., pp. 19–20.
11 In J. Pierre, *Surrealism* (London: Heron, 1970), p. 98.
12 J. Joll, *Europe since 1870: An International History* (Harmondsworth: Penguin, 1976), p. 341.

FURTHER READING

As with chapter 4, the principal recommendation must be to follow up the various 'primary sources' already mentioned in the text. Useful extracts from such material can be sampled in W. W. Wagar (ed.), *Science, Faith and Man: European Thought since 1914* (New York, 1968), and in the two documentary volumes edited by Arthur Marwick and Wendy Simpson for the Open University's Course A318, *War, Peace, and Social Change, 1900–1955* (Buckingham, 1990). As for secondary literature, much of the further reading suggested at the end of that same earlier chapter spreads into the 1914–45 period too, and such items are not listed again here.

General histories that do justice to the intellectual and cultural developments of the inter-war years include: R. J. Sontag, *A Broken World, 1919–39* (New York, 1971); J. Joll, *Europe since 1870: An International History* (Harmondsworth, 1976); and G. Barraclough, *An Introduction to Contemporary History* (Harmondsworth, 1964). Particularly helpful reference works are A. Bullock, O. Stallybrass, and S. Trombley (eds), *The Fontana Dictionary of Modern Thought*, 2nd edn (London, 1988); A. Bullock and R. Woodings (eds), *The Fontana Biographical Companion to Modern Thought* (London, 1983); and J. Wintle (ed.), *Makers of Modern Culture* (London, 1981).

Among the stimulating studies devoted to the impact of 1914–18 are P. Fussell, *The Great War and Modern Memory* (London, 1975); F. Field, *Three French Writers and the Great War* (Cambridge, 1975); and M. Eksteins, *Rites of Spring: The Great War and the Birth of the Modern Age* (London, 1989). Other good treatments of the European intellectual and artistic scene during the inter-war period include: P. Gay, *Weimar Culture: The Outsider as Insider* (Harmondsworth, 1974); W. Laqueur, *Weimar: A Cultural History, 1918–33* (London, 1974); G. Steiner, *In Bluebeard's Castle* (London, 1971); G. Brantlinger, *Bread and Circuses: Theories of Mass Culture as Social Decay*

(Ithaca, NY, 1983); and two works by H. Stuart Hughes, *The Obstructed Path: French Social Thought in the Years of Desperation, 1930–1960* (New York, 1966) and *The Sea Change: The Migration of Social Thought, 1930–1965* (New York, 1975).

A number of works about the conditions prevailing within the major dictatorships of the era have already been mentioned in the notes to chapters 7 and 8, and these are not further cited here. H. Arendt, *The Origins of Totalitarianism*, 2nd edn (London, 1958), remains a splendidly provocative point of departure for comparative discussion of the authoritarian systems. Useful source-books for ideas prevalent on the Right are A. Lyttelton (ed.), *Italian Fascisms: From Pareto to Gentile* (London, 1973), and G. Mosse (ed.), *Nazi Culture: Intellectual, Cultural, and Social Life in the Third Reich* (London, 1966). A. D. Beyerchen, *Scientists under Hitler: Politics and the Physics Community in the Third Reich* (London, 1977), demonstrates well just how far ideological colonization could spread. In the huge literature about the Nazi leader's own ideas and influence, J. P. Stern, *Hitler: The Führer and the People* (London, 1975), and I. Kershaw, *Hitler* (London, 1991), are especially worthy of study. Note also the 'parallel lives' presented in A. Bullock, *Hitler and Stalin: Parallel Lives* (London, 1991). Another area of comparison within the overall framework of totalitarian control is explored in R. Taylor, *Film Propaganda: Soviet Russia and Nazi Germany* (London, 1979). For the development of left-wing ideas within and beyond the USSR, see L. Kolakowski, *Main Currents in Marxism: Its Origins, Growth, and Dissolution*, vol. 3 (Oxford, 1978); and, for the problems of creative expression under conditions of dialectical materialism, B. Thomson, *The Premature Revolution: Russian Literature and Society, 1917–1946* (London, 1972). Notable amongst other works focusing on aspects of the Left are: R. H. S. Crossman (ed.), *The God that Failed: Six Studies in Communism* (London, 1950); D. Caute, *Communism and the French Intellectuals, 1914–1960* (London, 1964); and B. Crick, *George Orwell: A Life* (London, 1980). S. Ellwood, *The Spanish Civil War* (Oxford, 1991), provides a valuable recent introduction to the conflict of 1936–9.

Index

The following abbreviations are used: WW1 = World War One; WW2 = World War Two.